Manual of Dermatologic Therapeutics

With Essentials of Diagnosis

Third Edition

Kenneth A. Arndt, M.D.

Associate Professor of Dermatology,
Harvard Medical School; Dermatologist-in-
Chief, Department of Dermatology,
Beth Israel Hospital, Boston

Little, Brown and Company
Boston/Toronto

To Anne, David, and Jennifer

Contents

Preface

The textual material in this manual was originally prepared in a less detailed form for use by physicians, nurses, and other health care personnel at the Harvard Community Health Plan. The reception given such practical therapeutic guidelines by clinicians of various specialties, by medical students at the Harvard Medical School, and by house officers at several of the Harvard teaching hospitals encouraged me to write this more comprehensive work.

The first and second editions of the *Manual of Dermatologic Therapeutics* have been greeted enthusiastically. It is gratifying to realize that such an approach to rational therapeutics has become widely used in the United States, and to know that the information will find good use throughout the world through the Spanish, Portuguese, Italian, Indonesian, and Taiwanese editions.

The third edition has been significantly revised and rewritten, and much new material has been added. It continues to be surprising how so much changes in so short a time, especially in regard to the pathophysiology and approach to the treatment of cutaneous disease.

The *Manual* presents up-to-date information on the pathophysiology, diagnosis, and therapy of common cutaneous disorders. Dermatologic diagnostic procedures and surgical and photobiologic techniques are explained in both theoretical and practical terms. The pharmacology, structure, and optimal use of dermatologic and selected systemic medications are included along with current costs for both trade and generic drugs. Information in greater depth about some subjects may be found in several excellent comprehensive works.* Entities that require specialized therapy, such as malignant tumors of the skin, and conditions seen primarily in the hospital patient have been purposely omitted.

The first portion of the *Manual* is organized so that each entity is initially defined and its pathophysiologic features are discussed; each disease is then subdivided into subjective data (symptoms), objective data (clinical findings), assessment, and therapy sections, according to the problem-oriented record system in use in many institutions throughout the country. The rest of the text is concerned with procedures, techniques, treatment principles, and discussion of the pharmacodynamics and usage of specific medications employed in treating cutaneous disease.

I would like to express my appreciation to several colleagues across the country for their review of the material. Drs. Arthur Z. Eisen, John H. Epstein, David S. Feingold, Thomas B. Fitzpatrick, Irwin M. Freedberg, and Silas E. O'Quinn all offered constructive criticism on the first edition. Dr. Barbara A. Gilchrest reviewed the second edition. Dr. Jeffrey Bernhard carefully read the third edition and made numerous helpful suggestions about both syntax and content. He is also responsible for the first draft and much of the material in the sections on The Principles of Normal Skin Care and the Use of Systemic Steroids in Dermatology. Jeffrey P. Ross, B.S., R.Ph., offered valuable advice about current pharmaceutical pricing and pharmacy practices. My thanks go to the Schering Corporation, Kenilworth, New Jersey, 07033 for permission to reproduce some of the color illustrations.

*Such references include:
Demis, D. J., Dobson, R. L., and McGuire, J. (eds.). *Clinical Dermatology.* Hagerstown, Md.: Harper & Row, 1981.
Fitzpatrick, T. B., Eisen, A. Z., Wolff, K., Freedberg, I. M., and Austen, K. F. (eds.). *Dermatology in General Medicine* (2nd ed.). New York: McGraw-Hill, 1979.
Moschella, S. L., Pillsbury, D. M., and Hurley, H. J., Jr. (eds.). *Dermatology.* Philadelphia: Saunders, 1975.
Rook, A., Wilkinson, D. S., and Ebling, F. J. G. (eds.). *Textbook of Dermatology* (3rd ed.). Oxford: Blackwell, 1979.

Common dermatologic diseases: diagnosis and therapy

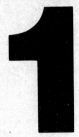

Acne

I. **Definition and pathophysiology.** Acne, a very common, self-limited, multifactorial disorder involving the sebaceous follicles, is usually first noted in the teenage years. Lesions may begin as early as age 8–10 at "sebarche" and are usually seen 2 years earlier in girls. Severe disease affects boys 10 times more frequently (up to 15% are involved), increases in prevalence steadily throughout adolescence, and then decreases in adulthood.

Severity of involvement can most often be correlated with the amount of sebum secreted; patients with severe acne will usually have large and active sebaceous glands with consequent prominent follicle openings ("pores") and oily skin ("seborrhea"). However, there is much variation and overlap in sebum secretion between unaffected control subjects and acne patients, and no evidence has yet been found that sebum in acne patients differs qualitatively from that of normal persons.

Androgens are the only stimulus to sebaceous gland development and secretion, but acne patients do not have higher plasma levels of androgens. At puberty, hormonal stimuli lead to increased growth and development of sebaceous follicles. In those who develop acne there is presumably a heightened responsiveness of these glands to androgenic stimulation. This heightened end-organ response of the sebaceous glands results in increased conversion of testosterone to dihydrotestosterone (DHT) and other 5 alpha-reduced metabolites; acne-bearing skin has been shown to produce up to 20 times more DHT than normal skin for corresponding areas.

The enlarged gland secretes sebum into a dilated follicle that contains a disproportionately large quantity of normal cutaneous bacteria. Sebum contains free and esterified fatty acids as well as unsaponifiable lipid components. It is the free fatty acid (FFA) fraction of sebum, produced in the sebaceous follicle by the action of enzymes associated with the anaerobic diphtheroid *Propionibacterium (Corynebacterium) acnes,* that acts as the primary irritating substance in inflammatory acne. In addition, *P. acnes* produces chemotactic factors that, together with those present in comedonal material, attract mononuclear cells. Patients with severe acne demonstrate cell-mediated immunity directed toward *P. acnes,* and other evidence for immune mechanisms includes the observation of complement component C3 in the walls of dermal blood vessels and the basement membrane zone of acne lesions. Attraction and killing of leukocytes by comedonal components, the resultant inflammatory cascade, and specific immunologic events probably all contribute to the final appearance of an inflammatory acne lesion.

Disordered shedding of the cells that line sebaceous follicles is another factor in the pathogenesis of acne lesions. Large numbers of desquamating horny cells tend to stick together, rather than flow to the surface with sebum. The resultant impacted lipid and keratin mass expands to fill the lumen and forms a solid plug in the dilated opening, becoming a closed comedo ("whitehead"). If this comedonal mass protrudes from the follicle, it is recognized as an open comedo ("blackhead"). Its dark color is due to oxidized lipid and to melanin within the mass of horny cells; this plug is **not** dirt. As follicle walls leak or rupture, sebum, with its irritant and chemoattractant factors, keratin, bacteria, and hair are released into the dermis and result in an inflammatory mass (papule, "pimple," pustule, nodule, cyst, and/or abscess). Most acne papules or pustules result from rupture of an intrafollicular microcomedo, rather than a visible one. Patients with large numbers of comedones usually have only small numbers of inflammatory lesions, whereas patients with severe cystic acne usually have few comedones. In adult life the cells lining the follicle presumably become less susceptible to comedogenic materials. The spontaneous disappearance of acne may also be related to a decreased dermal reactivity to irritant substances.

As many as a third of adult women are affected by a low-grade acneform eruption that may start de novo or merge imperceptibly with preexisting adolescent acne. The eruption may be induced by chronic exposure to comedogenic substances such as isopropyl myristate, cocoa butter, and fatty acids present in some creams and moisturizers, by androgenic stimuli from progestogens present in some oral contraceptives, by recent cessation of oral contraceptives ("postpill acne"), or from unknown causes.

Acne may lead to pitted or hypertrophic scarring. If left alone, most inflammatory acne tends to disappear slowly in the early twenties in men and somewhat later in women. Adequate therapy will in all cases decrease its severity and may entirely suppress this disease.

II. Subjective data

A. Patients' complaints may be related to inconspicuous lesions that nevertheless cause considerable social embarrassment. As with all medical and psychologic conditions, the patient's perception of the severity of the problem is an important guide to treatment, and judgmental decisions by the physician about the severity of objective disease must be evaluated in this context.

B. Inflammatory lesions of acne may itch as they erupt and may be very painful on pressure.

C. Pustules and cysts often rupture spontaneously and drain a purulent and/or bloody but odorless discharge.

III. Objective data (See color insert.)

A. Noninflammatory lesions. The initial lesion is the closed comedo, visible as a 1- –2-mm white dot (whitehead) most easily seen when the skin is stretched. If follicle contents extrude, a 2- –5-mm, dark-topped, open comedo (blackhead) results.

B. Inflammatory lesions. Erythematous papules, pustules, cysts, and abscesses may be seen. Patients with cystic acne also tend to show "double" or polyporous comedones, which result from prior inflammation during which epithelial tongues have caused fistulous links between neighboring sebaceous units. Acne lesions are seen primarily on the face, but the neck, chest, shoulders, and back may be involved. One or more anatomic areas may be involved in any given patient, and the pattern of involvement, once present, tends to remain constant.

C. The skin, scalp, and hair are frequently very oily.

IV. **Assessment.** Several points regarding etiology or therapy should be considered with each patient:

A. Are endocrine factors important in this patient?

1. Are menstrual periods regular? Is there any hirsutism? (Stein-Leventhal syndrome, Cushing's syndrome, and other endocrinopathies are frequently accompanied by acne.) Men and women with severe cystic acne, especially those who do not respond to conventional therapy, may have elevated plasma testosterone and/or dehydroepiandrosterone sulfate levels.

2. Is there a premenstrual flare-up? The sebaceous duct orifice is significantly smaller between days 15–20 of the menstrual cycle, leading to increments in duct obstruction and resistance to flow of sebum. Many of these women tend to do well on anovulatory drugs.

3. Is the patient on oral contraceptives, or has she stopped taking these pills within the past few months? When were the pills started? Which ones? During the first two or three cycles on oral contraceptives acne may flare up. Postpill acne may continue for as long as a year after birth control pills are stopped. Although anovulatory drugs may provide excellent therapy for acne, the various pills differ enormously in their effect on the sebaceous gland (see p. 11). Oral contraceptives that contain the androgenic and antiestrogenic progestogens norgestrel, norethindrone, and norethindrone acetate may actually provoke an acneform eruption. Ovral is cited particularly frequently in this regard.

B. What is the effect of seasonal changes? Has the patient recently been in a hot and humid environment? Is sunlight beneficial? Most patients find that summer sunlight will diminish the activity of their acne. However, very humid environments or heavy sweating will lead to keratin hydration, swelling, decrease in the size of the sebaceous follicle orifice, and partial or total duct obstruction. It is thus not always good advice to "get out into the sun," except in a dry climate. A small number of people overly exposed to sunlight will develop an acneform papular eruption related to abnormal follicular keratinization ("Mallorca," miliary, actinic acne).

C. Is the patient exposed to heavy oils, greases, or tars? These comedogenic agents will initiate lesions, as can some greasy substances used for hair care (pomade acne). Certain oily or greasy cosmetics and creams can also exacerbate acne.

D. Does the patient wear occlusive or tight clothing or have any habits that will initiate or aggravate the disease? Mechanical trauma (pressure, friction, rubbing, squeezing) as from clothing or athletic wear or from behavioral habits will also cause lesions. For example, an individual with the habit of cradling the chin in his or her hand may develop unilateral lesions at that site.

E. Has the patient been on any medications known to cause acne? The most prominent among these are corticosteroids, ACTH, androgens, Danazole, iodides, and bromides. Other possible stimuli include trimethadione, Dilantin, INH, lithium, halothane, vitamin B_{12} cobalt irradiation, and hyperalimentation therapy. Corticosteroids, both systemic and topical, are not directly comedogenic; they do appear to sensitize—to "prime"— the follicular epithelium to the comedogenic effects of sebum. Steroid acne starts as uniform red papules, which are then succeeded by closed comedones, and later by open comedones. Chronic steroid acne shows all three types of lesions.

F. How has the patient's acne been treated in the past? Have antibiotics been used? If so, what were the instructions, dosage, duration, and effect of these therapies? Was tetracycline inadvertently taken with meals instead of on an empty stomach? Was the dosage adequate? (See Antibiotics, p. 9.)

An unusual complication of chronic tetracycline administration is the development of a **gram-negative folliculitis.** Such patients will notice a sudden change in their acne, with the appearance of pustules or large inflammatory cysts that, on culture, usually grow *Proteus, Pseudomonas,* or *Klebsiella* species. Since acne cysts are sterile on routine bacteriologic culture, a sudden change in morphology warrants Gram's stain and culture of cyst/abscess contents. Gram-negative folliculitis usually responds to ampicillin, 1 gm/day, after which tetracycline can again be started.

G. Is there any effect from stress or emotional upsets on acne activity? An acutely stressful situation may cause acne to flare up suddenly (but "nerves" are **not** the cause of the disease).

H. The number and type of lesions should be roughly quantitated in order to assess further therapeutic responses.

V. Therapy

A. Mild involvement (few to many comedones)

1. **Bacteriostatics** are thought to improve acne by decreasing the formation of harmful by-products, but not necessarily the actual number, of *P. acnes* bacteria. These should be applied twice daily to the point of mild dryness and erythema but not discomfort. The gel-based benzoyl peroxide products are the agents of choice for the usual case.

   a. **Benzoyl peroxide** (see also p. 239) has a potent antimicrobial effect. It is hypothesized that this agent is decomposed by the cysteine present in skin, after which free radical oxygen is capable of oxidizing proteins in its vicinity. These proteins include the bacterial proteins of the sebaceous follicles, thus decreasing the number of *P. acnes* and consequently the amount of free fatty acids. Topical 5% benzoyl peroxide lowers FFA 50–60% after daily application for 14 days and decreases aerobic bacteria by 84% and anaerobic bacteria (primarily *P. acnes*) by 98%. Benzoyl peroxide will also reduce the size and number of comedones present and may inhibit sebum secretion. Contact sensitivity is observed in 1–3% of patients.

      (1) **Benzoyl peroxide products.** Clear aqueous gel (Desquam-X); clear alcohol gel (Benzagel, PanOxyl); clear acetone gel (Persa-gel); clear oil-based lotion (Benoxyl, Persadox).

b. **Topical antibiotics** (see also p. 240) may affect acne lesions by their antibacterial action or because of suppressive effects on the inflammatory response. Papular and pustular lesions respond best; the activity of comedonal or cystic acne may not be altered. There are no studies comparing the relative effectiveness of these drugs. It would appear that clindamycin and erythromycin are easiest to use and probably most helpful, tetracycline next, and then meclocycline. All topical antibiotics are applied twice daily.

(1) Clindamycin phosphate is available in 1% concentration in a hydroalcoholic vehicle as Cleocin T lotion (30 ml or 60 ml). Cleocin hydrochloride solutions can be compounded extemporaneously by dissolving the contents of Cleocin capsules into other vehicles such as Neutrogena Vehicle N (e.g., four 150-mg capsule contents in 50-ml vehicle = 1.2%; contents of 8 capsules = 2.4%). The drug has not been detected in the blood after topical use, but there have been two reports of pseudomembranous colitis after topical use of clindamycin hydrochloride. Patients with inflammatory bowel disease should avoid topical clindamycin use and all patients should be warned to discontinue therapy if intestinal symptoms occur.

(2) Erythromycin base applied topically is moderately effective and nonsensitizing. It is available as 1.5% solution (Staticin, 60 ml); and 2.0% solution (Ery Derm, 60 ml, and A/T/S, 60 ml).

(3) Tetracycline hydrochloride (Topicycline, 70 ml) may produce a temporary yellow discoloration of the skin that may be washed off 1 hr after application with no decrease in drug effectiveness. Skin with tetracycline on the surface will fluoresce when viewed under long-wave ultraviolet light (e.g., black lights in discos). The serum level after continuous 2id application is 0.1 mcg/ml or less.

(4) Meclocycline sulfosalicylate, an oxytetracycline derivative, is the only topical antibiotic manufactured in a nonalcoholic, nonlotion base. Meclan Cream (20-gm tubes) is less drying, but has an unpleasant smell and may be less effective than other topical antibiotics.

c. **Aluminum chloride hexahydrate** (Xerac A-C) is an effective antiperspirant that also has an antibacterial effect. It may be useful in cases of acne in which sweating is prominent or appears to be aggravating the disease but its effects have not been well studied.

d. Although the administration of systemic antibiotics will reduce comedo formation in experimental animal systems these drugs play no role in the therapy of the usual patient with comedonal acne.

2. **Exfoliants.** These agents, such as elemental sulfur, resorcinol, and abrasives, produce irritation and consequent peeling and exfoliation. Not all topical irritants have the property of decreasing the presence or formation of new comedones. Most are a source of additional injury to already inflamed skin. Also, they are ineffective at removing comedones that are too deeply rooted to be affected by surface measures. Tretinoin is the most effective comedolytic agent, followed by salicylic acid and benzoyl peroxide.

a. **Abradant cleansers.** Apply 1–2id. These products incorporate finely divided particles with cleansers and wetting agents. They are not indicated in most cases but may be used in the patient who appears to respond to them empirically.

   (1) **Products.** Polyethylene particle cleanser (Pernox scrub or lotion); aluminum oxide particle cleansers (Brasivol, fine, medium, rough); sodium tetraboxate decahydrate particle cleanser (Komex). These particles dissolve on use and thus their abrasiveness is limited.

b. **Topical exfoliants and irritants.** Clear gels or lotions (Acne Aid, Komed, Saligel, Transact; tinted creams (Acne Aid, Acnomel, Fostril, Sulforcin); tinted lotions (Acne Aid, Liquimat).

B. Mild or moderate involvement (few to many comedones, some papules and/or pustules)

1. Benzoyl peroxide gel, and/or

2. **Tretinoin** (trans-retinoic acid; vitamin A acid), the most effective comedolytic agent, used alone or in combination with benzoyl peroxide gels, may offer unique beneficial effects for those who can tolerate its use. The irritant effects of tretinoin sometimes limit its usefulness, but these can be minimized by the correct method of application. Tretinoin, which does not function as a vitamin in its therapeutic applications, increases epidermal cell turnover and decreases the cohesiveness ("stickiness") of horny cells, thus inhibiting the formation of comedones while helping existing comedones to become loosened and expelled. Tretinoin not only changes follicular keratinization, but decreases the number of normal cell layers of the stratum corneum from 14 to 5. This decrease in thickness of the barrier layer may potentiate the penetration of other topical agents.

   a. **Instructions for use**

   (1) Erythema and peeling—a mild flush—are the objects of therapy. More severe dryness is to be avoided. It is the achievement of a mild facial flush that is important, not specific adherence to a predetermined course of therapy.

   (2) Fair-complexioned patients with easily irritated skin should start with the 0.05% cream or gel; others may use the 0.1% cream, or solution.

   (3) All other topical acne agents must be stopped prior to initiating retinoic acid therapy. Use mild, gentle soaps no more than twice daily.

   (4) Apply once daily lightly to all areas except around the eyes and lips. Apply approximately 1 hr before bedtime on thoroughly dry skin—wait for at least 15 min after the face has been washed.

   (5) Avoid excessive exposure to sun. There is some experimental evidence that exposure to ultraviolet light in tretinoin-treated animals leads to an increased incidence of skin cancers, but this question is not yet resolved.

   (6) Expect redness and peeling within a week, lasting 3–4 weeks,

and a flare-up in the acne during the first 2–4 weeks. This is explained as the surfacing of lesions onto the skin.

(7) Clearing requires approximately 3 months. Inflammatory lesions improve more rapidly, but comedones take longer. Effectiveness cannot be judged before 8 weeks and is best assessed at 12 weeks.

(8) Water-based cosmetics can be used.

(9) If a patient cannot tolerate the solution, use the 0.05% cream or 0.01% gel. Also, application can be less frequent—every other night, or skipping every third night, etc.

(10) Tretinoin application should be continued after the lesions clear.

b. Tretinoin products. Retin-A cream, 0.1% or 0.05%; Retin-A liquid, 0.05%; Retin-A gel, 0.01% or 0.025%.

3. Combined tretinoin-bacteriostatic therapy. With this mode of therapy the tretinoin prevents or removes comedones, while the benzoyl peroxide or topical antibiotic eradicates *P. acnes*. The tretinoin also enhances absorption of the other products. Irritation reactions limit the use of this combination therapy but some claim that the two agents used together are less irritating than tretinoin alone.

a. Instructions for use

(1) Apply tretinoin cream or solution in the evening as with tretinoin alone.

(2) Apply benzoyl peroxide gel or topical antibiotic in the morning.

(3) After clearing, decrease frequency of therapy and concentration of medication.

(4) These agents must be applied at different times, **not** simultaneously. Mixing the highly unsaturated tretinoin with reactive oxidants such as benzoyl peroxide destroys both chemicals.

C. Moderate or severe involvement (inflammatory papules, pustules, cysts, abscesses, and/or scarring). Use topical therapy as discussed above, plus antibiotics.

1. Antibiotics. Some systemic antimicrobials suppress the growth of normal cutaneous flora (primarily *P. acnes*). As bacteria are decreased and the FFA level slowly diminishes, inflammatory lesions decrease and new lesions stop appearing within 2–6 weeks. The beneficial effects of antibiotics may be multifold. Not only are the number of bacteria and FFA levels decreased, but certain antibiotics useful in acne therapy may directly interfere with local chemical and cellular inflammatory mechanisms. Tetracycline, erythromycin, and clindamycin have been shown to inhibit leukocyte chemotaxis, and may also directly inhibit extracellular lipases responsible for the generation of inflammatory compounds. Antibiotic therapy cannot be truly evaluated until 6–8 weeks after starting. Antibiotic levels in sebum are not detectable until about 7 days after treatment has started, and in addition, lipid formed in basal cells of sebaceous follicles may require 1 month to reach the skin surface. While sebum composition changes, the secretory rate remains constant. Therapy may need to be continued for months to years.

a. Tetracycline is the drug of choice. It is the least expensive, has the fewest side effects, and is best tolerated for long periods of time. Several studies have clearly shown no adverse effects after long-term oral administration. Tetracycline is effective in low doses because high concentrations are achieved within sebaceous follicles, especially when inflammation is present.

Aside from minor gastrointestinal tract irritation, *Candida* vaginitis is the only common complication. Although tetracyclines can cause enamel hyperplasia and hence tooth discoloration, by age 12 growth of teeth is essentially complete. Tetracycline should not be used in younger children nor administered during pregnancy. There is drug interaction with the metallic ions Al^{3+}, Mg^{2+}, and Ca^{2+} present in antacid preparations and dairy products; these products should never be taken at the same time as tetracycline.

Initiate therapy at 250 mg 4id (or 500 mg 2id) taken on an empty stomach (half hour before meals or 2 hr after) until there is clear improvement; then decrease the dosage to a maintenance level (250–500 mg/day) or eliminate it. If inflammatory lesions have not subsided after 4–6 weeks, increase the dose to 1.5 gm/day for 2 weeks, and if necessary to 2 gm/day for the subsequent 2 weeks. Occasionally it is of benefit to use 2–3 gm/day for several weeks in order to induce remission in otherwise unresponsive patients. Once remission is achieved, it is almost always possible to decrease the dosage to a lower level.

b. Erythromycin, 1 gm/day, is the usual second drug of choice. The same dose and time responses noted for tetracycline also apply to this drug.

c. Minocycline (Minocin, Vectrin) is very effective in patients unresponsive to other antibiotics. This antibiotic is very lipid-soluble and penetrates the sebaceous follicle more effectively. There appears to be no cross resistance with tetracycline. Dizziness, nausea, and vomiting may be a problem if full doses are administered initially. Start at 50 mg/day and slowly increase to as much as 100 mg 2id. Some patients may eventually achieve complete control on 50 mg/day.

d. Clindamycin (Cleocin) 300–450 mg/day is an extremely effective agent for acne. However, the risk of pseudomembranous colitis limits its systemic use to only very severe cases unresponsive to all other modes of therapy.

e. Trimethoprim/sulfamethoxazole (Bactrim, Septra) has also been shown to decrease FFA levels and inhibit inflammatory acne. Trimethoprim is very lipophilic, which enhances follicle penetration. Start with one regular strength tablet 2id; up to 4 tablets/day may be used.

f. Cephalosporins may be useful in patients resistant to other antibiotics.

2. **Sebaceous gland suppression**

   a. **Estrogens** (given as anovulatory agents) may be of use in very severe or otherwise unresponsive cases in young women, but should not be used unless more conventional regimens prescribed and overseen by a dermatologist fail after an adequate trial. Furthermore, if an acne patient is already taking anovulatory agents for contraception, an effort should be made to utilize a formulation known to improve, rather than exacerbate, acne. Most or all of the estrogen effect is the result of adrenal androgen inhibition rather than local suppression at the gland site; small doses of androgen can overcome the sebum-suppressive effects of large doses of estrogen in women as well as in men. There is a direct correlation between the degree of sebaceous gland inhibition and acne improvement. The gland, however, responds variably to estrogen suppression. On the average there will be a decrease of 25% in sebum production on administration of 0.1 mg of ethinyl estradiol. This drug and its 3-methyl ether, mestranol (which has two-thirds the potency of ethinyl estradiol), are the estrogens present in oral contraceptives. With combination therapy it is important to use a pill with adequate estrogenic effect linked with nonandrogenic progestogens such as norethynodrel and ethynodiol diacetate.

      (1) The preferable pills are Enovid E (0.1 mg mestranol, 2.5 mg norethynodrel), Enovid 5 (0.075 mestranol, 5.0 mg norethynodrel), Ovulen (0.1 mg mestranol, 10 mg ethynodiol diacetate), or Demulin (0.05 mg ethinyl estradiol, 1.0 mg ethynodiol diacetate), in decreasing order of effectiveness. Improvement in acne should be noted within 3 months and marked improvement within 4 months of administration. Ovral and the progestational agent norgestrel should be avoided. Estrogen therapy is rarely needed before age 16, after which time there will be no problem with growth retardation.

      (2) Concomitant administration of estrogen and prednisone (5.0–7.5 mg, PM administration) may act synergistically in suppressing sebum production by inhibiting both adrenal and ovarian androgen production. Many patients with severe cystic acne may have elevated androgen levels, and a woman with severe acne may have this associated with polycystic ovarian syndrome or partial hydroxylase deficiency. Sebum excretion rate in women with severe acne may fall 50% with a concomitant improvement in their acne.

   b. Patients with severe recalcitrant cystic acne unresponsive to aggressive conventional therapies may be considered for treatment with **isotretinoin** (13-*cis*-retinoic acid; Accutane). Oral administration of this retinoid will inhibit sebaceous gland function and induce a decrease in sebum production to as low as 10% of pretreatment values. The response rate may be as high as 90% with 1 to 2 courses of therapy. About 30% of patients require a second course, which may be repeated after a drug-free interval of 8 weeks. The skin will often continue to clear after drug administration has been stopped, and some patients may note prolonged remission of cyst formation. Decrease in sebum secretion is temporary, is related to the dose and duration of treatment, and reflects both a reduction in sebaceous gland size and inhibition of sebaceous gland differentiation.

Isotretinoin is teratogenic in animals and has significant adverse reactions, some occurring in more than 90% of patients. Dosage, indications and side effects, and prescribing information are found on page 237.

c. **Vitamin A** (Aquasol A), in doses ranging from 50,000–500,000 units/day in divided doses, has been advocated for the treatment of severe nodulocystic acne that does not respond to other modalities. This treatment has yet to be evaluated in an adequately controlled, prospective clinical trial and is not an approved indication for the drug. The extent of potential long-term toxicity, especially to the liver, and potential teratogenicity, which may persist after the drug has been discontinued, have yet to be fully evaluated. However, vitamin A is available without prescription, and patients may take it on the advice of friends or the lay press. The toxic dose for adults is usually at least 50,000 IU/day over a period of a year or longer. Normal diets contain about 7500–10,000 IU/day. Physicians should be aware of the signs and symptoms of chronic hypervitaminosis A, as patients may take an excess of the vitamin without their knowledge or approval. Signs and symptoms include dry, coarse, scaly skin, hair loss, fissures of the lips, pruritus, sore tongue or mouth, and low-grade fever. Normal serum vitamin A levels do not rule out a diagnosis of hypervitaminosis A.

D. Adjunctive therapy

1. Acne surgery

a. **Comedo expression.** Gentle removal of comedones by pressing over the lesion with a comedo extractor or the opening of an eye dropper not only relieves the patient of unsightly lesions but also may prevent progression to more inflammatory lesions. Occasionally it may be necessary to incise the follicular opening carefully with a No. 11 scalpel blade or 25-, 27-, or 30-gauge needle. Over-rigorous attempts to express comedones may result in an increased inflammatory response.

Recurrence of comedones after removal is common. Open comedones have been shown to recur within 24–40 days, and closed comedones within 30–50 days. Fewer than 10% of comedo extractions are a complete success. Nevertheless this mode of therapy, carefully done, is useful in the appropriate case.

b. **Draining of cysts.** Careful and judicious incision and drainage of cysts and/or abscesses may initiate healing and shorten the duration of lesions.

2. Intralesional corticosteroids.
The therapy of choice for cystic lesions and acne abscesses is the intralesional injection of small amounts of corticosteroid preparations (triamcinolone acetonide or diacetate, 2.5 mg/ml). The high local concentration of corticosteroid injected leads to rapid involution of these nonpyogenic, sterile, inflammatory lesions.

The stock 10-, 25-, or 40-mg/ml steroid suspension should be diluted with lidocaine and only enough injected through a 1-ml syringe with a 27- or 30-gauge needle to distend the cyst slightly (usually 0.025–0.1 ml). Use of undiluted solutions or injections of too large an amount may lead to temporary atrophic depressions in the skin (see p. 272). Most lesions, particularly early ones, will flatten and disappear within 48 hr after injection.

3. **Cryosurgery.** Desquamation and involution of lesions will often occur after use of a slush made of precipitated sulfur, powdered dry ice, and acetone; or the use of solid carbon dioxide dipped in acetone; or liquid nitrogen spray for 5–10 sec.

4. **Vleminckx's solution.** Hot compresses with Vleminckx's solution (sulfurated lime, available as Vlem-Dome) used for 10–20 min 1–2id are useful in very active, cystic disease. Vleminckx's solution has also just become available in a drying clay mask (Vlemasque) that can be applied daily for 20–25 min and then washed off.

5. **Ultraviolet light (UVL).** Exposure to sunlight or UVB sunlamps may be moderately effective in some patients. Administer enough UVL to cause a mild erythema (see p. 219). Patients also using tretinoin may show a heightened sensitivity to UVL.

E. **Patient education about long-standing misconceptions.** Neither changes in diet nor use of vitamins or vaccines has been shown to affect sebaceous gland function or acne activity. If a patient finds that certain foods aggravate the eruption, those items alone should be avoided. Strict diets, on the other hand, lead to a great deal of intrafamilial conflict and personal grief, but no improvement in the skin.

References

Barranco, V. P. Effect of androgen-dominant and estrogen-dominant oral contraceptives on acne. *Cutis* 14:384–386, 1974.

Becker, L. E., et al. Topical clindamycin therapy for acne vulgaris. *Arch. Dermatol.* 117:482–485, 1981.

Chakmakjian, Z. H., McCaffree, D., and Herndon, J. H., Jr. Severe cystic acne: A spectrum of treatable endocrinopathies. Read at the 63rd Annual Meeting of the Endocrine Society, Dallas, June 17–19, 1981.

Dahl, N. G. C., and McGibbon, D. H. Complement C_3 and immunoglobulin in inflammatory acne vulgaris. *Br. J. Dermatol.* 101:633–640, 1979.

Dobson, R. L., and Belknap, B. S. Topical erythromycin solution in acne. *J. Am. Acad. Derm.* 3:478–482, 1980.

Esterly, N. B., Fureg, N. L., and Flanagan, L. E. The effect of antimicrobial agents on leukocyte chemotaxis. *J. Invest. Dermatol.* 70:51–55, 1978.

Farrell, L. N., Strauss, J. S., and Stranleri, A. M. The treatment of severe cystic acne with 13-cis-retinoic acid: Evaluation of sebum production and the clinical response in a multiple-dose trial. *J. Am. Acad. Derm.* 3:602–611, 1980.

Fulton, J. E., Jr., and Pablo, G. Topical antibacterial therapy for acne. *Arch. Dermatol.* 110:83–86, 1974.

Gowland, G., Ward, R. M., Holland, K. T., and Cunliffe, W. T. Cellular immunity to *P. acnes* in the population and patients with acne vulgaris. *Br. J. Dermatol.* 99:43–47, 1978.

Hurley, J. H., and Shelley, W. B.   Special topical approach to the treatment of acne: Suppression of sweating with aluminum chloride in an anhydrous formulation. *Cutis* 22:696–698, 1948.

Kaidbey, K. H., and Kligman, A. M.   The pathogenesis of steroid acne. *J. Invest. Dermatol.* 62:31–36, 1974.

Kaidbey, K. H., and Kligman, A. M.   Effectiveness of peeling agents on experimental open comedones. *Cutis* 16:53–56, 1975.

Kligman, A. M., et al.   Oral vitamin A in acne vulgaris: Preliminary report. *Int. J. Dermatol.* 20:278–285, 1981.

Kligman, L. H., and Kligman, A. M.   The effect on Rhino mouse skin of agents which influence keratinization and exfoliation. *J. Invest. Derm.* 73:354–358, 1979.

Leyden, J. J., et al.   Gram-negative folliculitis–a complication of antibiotic therapy in acne vulgaris. *Br. J. Dermatol.* 88:533–538, 1973.

Melski, J. W., and Arndt, K. A.   Topical therapy for acne. *N. Engl. J. Med.* 302:503–506, 1980.

Montagna, W., Bell, M., and Strauss, J. S. (eds.).   Sebaceous Glands and Acne Vulgaris. Proceedings of the 22nd Annual Symposium on the Biology of Skin. *J. Invest. Dermatol.* 62:119–339, 1974.

Plewig, G., and Kligman, A. M.   *Acne Morphogenesis and Treatment* (3rd ed.). New York: Springer-Verlag, 1975.

Pochi, P. E.   Antibiotics in acne. *N. Engl. J. Med.* 294:43–44, 1976.

Pochi, P. E., and Strauss, J. S.   Sebaceous gland suppression with ethinyl estradiol and diethylstilbestrol. *Arch. Dermatol.* 108:210–214, 1973.

Steinberger, E., et al.   The menstrual cycle and plasma testosterone levels in women with acne. *J. Am. Acad. Derm.* 4:54–58, 1981.

Stoughton, R. B.   Topical antibiotics for acne vulgaris: Current usage. *Arch. Dermatol.* 115:486–489, 1979.

Stoughton, R. B., and Aly, R.   Topical antibiotic therapy of acne: Laboratory investigation of vehicles, various antibiotics, and stability characteristics. *Cutis* 25:216–220, 1980.

Strauss, J. S., Windhorst, D. B., and Weinstein, G. D. (eds.).   Oral retinoids: A workshop. *J. Am. Acad. Dermatol.* 6(2):573–832, 1982.

Taaffe, A., Cunliffe, W. J., Cove, J., Eady, A., and Holland, K. T.   Topical erythromycin in acne: A double-blind study. *Br. J. Dermatol.* 105(Suppl. 19):19–20, 1981.

The Therapeutic Use of Vitamin A Acid.   G. Stüttgen, Conference Chairman. *Acta Derm. Venereol.* (Stockh.) 55(Suppl. 74):1975.

Tucker, S. B., et al.   Inflammation in acne vulgaris: Leukocyte attraction and cytotoxicity by comedonal material. *J. Invest. Dermatol.* 74:21–25, 1980.

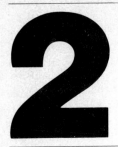

Alopecia areata

I. **Definition and pathophysiology.** Alopecia areata is a unique, often self-limited disorder characterized by plaques of asymptomatic, noninflammatory, nonscarring, complete hair loss most commonly involving the scalp. Children and young adults are most frequently affected and there is a positive family history in 10–25% of cases. The cause is unknown but it seems likely that it is related to immune mechanisms. Some studies demonstrate the presence of C_3 and occasionally IgG and IgM in hair follicles of more than 90% of alopecia areata patients; T cell number and function may be reduced, particularly in those with circulating autoantibodies. The histopathology is similar to that of presumed autoimmune diseases such as Hashimoto's thyroiditis; the disease responds to anti-inflammatory medications, and there appears to be an increased incidence of other autoimmune diseases and circulating antibodies to other tissues, particularly thyroid. Vitiligo is present in approximately 4% of cases. Emotional stress is often mentioned as another precipitating factor.

The course of alopecia areata is erratic and impossible to predict. In general, the younger age of the patient at onset and the more widespread the disease, the poorer the prognosis. Cases developing before puberty have a particularly dismal regrowth rate. One patient in 10 has hair loss only in sites other than the scalp—eyelashes, eyebrows, beard, general body hair—and approximately 10% of patients progress to loss of all scalp hair (alopecia totalis). Regrowth of hair during the first attack takes place within 6 months in 30% of cases, within 1 year in 50%, and within 5 years in 75%; complete recovery occurs in approximately 30%; in up to 33% the hair never regrows. New lesions reappear within months to years in up to 50% of cases. A prolonged and difficult course with poor outlook is associated with total loss of hair from scalp and body (alopecia universalis); with rapid progression of disease; with eyebrow, eyelash, or beard involvement, and with severe associated nail changes.

II. **Subjective data.** The hair loss is usually without discomfort; rarely, there may be paresthesias in affected areas.

III. **Objective data**

A. Lesions are well defined, single or multiple, round or oval areas of total hair loss in which the skin seems very smooth and soft. Any hair-bearing area can be affected.

B. In active lesions the "exclamation point hair" may be seen around the margins. These loose hairs protrude about 3–10 mm above the scalp surface and have a dark, rough, brushlike tip, a narrower, less pigmented shaft, and an atrophic root. These hairs reflect the disturbed keratinization seen after injury to the growing hair follicle and with transition to a resting follicle; they are pathognomonic of expanding alopecia areata.

C. Regrowing hairs appear first as fine, downy, vellus strands that are gradually replaced by normal terminal hair. These new hairs are often lusterless, may break easily, and may be white.

D. Nail changes, present in 10–20% of cases, consist of discrete pits in the nail surface usually arranged in horizontal or vertical rows, longitudinal ridging and thickening, or severe dystrophy.

IV. Assessment

A. Careful examination will show no evidence of scarring or inflammation. In tinea capitis, hair loss is not total in the involved areas, hairs present are dull and lusterless, and erythema and scaling are present. Traumatic or self-induced hair loss (trichotillomania) is characterized by only partial hair thinning and hairs that are twisted, broken, and of varying lengths. A mass or traces of preceding inflammation accompany subjacent furuncles or inflamed cysts. Other differential diagnostic considerations include secondary syphilis and lupus erythematosus. If the diagnosis is in question, a biopsy will be useful; typical findings of alopecia areata include a lymphocytic infiltrate around an affected hair bulb and lower one-third of the follicle, and atrophic hairs.

B. Patients with alopecia areata are generally healthy and do not require investigative laboratory studies.

V. Therapy

A. Reassurance about the likelihood of spontaneous regrowth and a simple explanation covering the nature and course of the disease, as well as the poor results of most treatments, are usually all that is necessary. When hair loss is extensive or when there is total or universal alopecia, an honest discussion of the chronic nature of alopecia areata is necessary. A wig is useful in extensive cases.

B. Topical medications usually induce changes that are no more than a placebo effect. Occasionally, use of occlusive topical corticosteroids leads to some regrowth.

C. Intralesional corticosteroid injections can be considered for small areas that are cosmetically disfiguring and persistent, particularly on the scalp or occasionally on the eyebrows. Some regrowth should be evident 4–6 weeks after injections. Up to 33% of patients will not regrow hair; failures occur primarily in new and rapidly expanding plaques, or in areas of long-standing hair loss.

1. Inject plaques at 1- –2-cm intervals with a tuberculin syringe and a 27- or 30-gauge needle, or with a needleless jet injector.

2. Dilute triamcinolone acetonide suspension to 5 mg/ml; 0.05–0.1 ml should be placed in each site.

3. Reinject at 4- –6-week intervals. If no growth is present at 3 months, it is not worth continuing the procedure.

4. Areas of corticosteroid-related regrowth may begin to thin after 3–6 months and can be injected again if necessary. Spontaneous regrowth frequently occurs during this interval.

D. Treatment with systemic corticosteroids will often stimulate hair regrowth but infrequently alters the basic course and is rarely if ever warranted.

E. Repeated applications of topical sensitizers such as dinitrochlorobenzene (DNCB) and squaric acid dibutylester have been found to induce regrowth of scalp hair in 70–90% of those treated. Allergic contact sensitization may enhance the T lymphocyte pool or, according to one hypothesis, may induce "antigenic competition" that inhibits autoimmune reactions. Therapy with allergic contactants must be prolonged (months), has many side effects (constant mild rash, pruritus, adenopathy, possibility of autosensitization reaction), and may be hazardous (DNCB is a potential mutagen).

F. Nonantigenic irritant dermatitis induced by anthralin may also cause regrowth of scalp hair in the majority of patients treated. 0.2%–0.8% anthralin ointment applied daily led to beginning regrowth in 5–8 weeks in 21 of 24 patients with moderate hair loss. However, treatment with another irritant, croton oil, has recently been shown to be ineffective in patients who later responded to DNCB. In the latter study only the proven contact allergen was effective.

G. Prolonged photochemotherapy (PUVA) may induce regrowth of scalp and body hair in 70% of those treated. Hair regrowth seems related to total energy delivered. Initial response is seen after 85–120 joule/sq cm; satisfactory results may require 350 joule/sq cm for alopecia areata and 730 joule/sq cm for alopecia totalis. PUVA decreases a subset of T lymphocytes and may affect alopecia areata by altering immune mechanisms.

References

Abell, E., and Munro, D. D.   Intralesional treatment of alopecia areata with triamcinolone acetonide by jet injector. *Br. J. Dermatol.* 88:55–59, 1973.

Bystryn, J. C., Orentreich, N., and Stengel, F.   Direct immunofluorescence studies in alopecia areata and male pattern alopecia. *J. Invest. Dermatol.* 73:317–320, 1979.

Claudy, A. L., and Gagnaire, D.   Photochemotherapy for alopecia areata. *Acta Derm. Venereol.* (Stockh.) 60:171–172, 1979.

Daman, L. A., Rosenberg, E. W., and Drake, L.   Treatment of alopecia areata with DNCB. *Arch. Dermatol.* 114:1036–1038, 1978.

Ebling, F. J., and Rook, A.   Hair. In A. Rook, D. S. Wilkinson, and F. J. G. Ebling (eds.), *Textbook of Dermatology* (3rd ed.). Oxford: Blackwell, 1979. Pp. 1777–1784.

Friedman, P. S.   Decreased lymphocyte reactivity and auto-immunity in alopecia areata. *Br. J. Dermatol.* 105:145–151, 1981.

Friedman, P. S.   Alopecia areata and auto-immunity. *Br. J. Dermatol.* 105:153–157, 1981.

Friedman, P. S.   Response of alopecia areata to DNCB: Influence of auto-antibodies and route of sensitization. *Br. J. Dermatol.* 105:285–289, 1981.

Happle, R., Cebulla, K., and Echternacht-Happle, K.   Dinitrochlorobenzene therapy for alopecia areata. *Arch. Dermatol.* 114:1629–1631, 1978.

Kern, F., et al.   Alopecia areata: Immunologic studies and treatment with prednisone. *Arch. Dermatol.* 107:407–412, 1973.

Mehlman, R. D., and Griesemer, R. D.   Alopecia areata in the very young. *Am. J. Psychiatry* 125:605–614, 1968.

Muller, S. A.   Alopecia: Syndromes of genetic significance. *J. Invest. Dermatol.* 60:475–492, 1973.

Safai, B.   Alopecia Areata. In B. Safai and R. A. Good (eds.), *Immunodermatology.* New York: Plenum, 1981. Pp. 355–360.

Schmoeckel, C., et al.   Treatment of alopecia areata by anthralin-induced dermatitis. *Arch. Dermatol.* 115:1254–1255, 1979.

Swanson, N. A., et al.   Topical treatment of alopecia areata. *Arch. Dermatol.* 117:384–387, 1981.

Winter, R. J., Kern, F., and Blizzard, R. M.   Prednisone therapy for alopecia areata. *Arch. Dermatol.* 112:1549–1552, 1976.

3

Aphthous stomatitis (canker sores)

I. **Definition and pathophysiology.** Canker sores are recurrent, painful, mucosal erosions that appear on the inner cheeks, lips, gums, tongue, palate, and pharynx. The prevalence of aphthous ulcerations in the general population is about 20%, and although they may be found at any age they occur most commonly between 10 and 40 years. Multiple local and systemic triggering factors such as food and drug allergy and physical and emotional stress have been implicated in the pathogenesis, but the data are conflicting and the etiology of this syndrome has not been firmly established. Dental trauma is the most common inducing factor in recurrent aphthous stomatitis. Herpes simplex virus has never been isolated from aphthae. Premenstrual flare-ups and remissions during the third trimester of pregnancy are common.

Recurrent lesions of aphthous stomatitis may be divided into four stages. The premonitory stage lasts up to 24 hr and is characterized by tingling, tense, burning, painful, or hyperesthetic sensations in the absence of any clinical changes. The preulcerative stage may last 18 hr to 3 days with variable but often moderately severe pain. Flat or raised indurated areas surrounded by a red halo are present and are gradually covered by a gray or yellow membrane in the ulcerative stage. This third phase usually lasts 1–16 days and lesions are severely painful until 2–3 days after the ulcer has formed. The healing stage lasts from 4–35 days with the natural history one of eventual remission. Two of three patients with recurrent lesions will go into remission within 15 days, while one of these will continue to have lesions for up to 40 years. Patients with superficial (minor) lesions remit earlier than those with deeper, more destructive (major) lesions.

Evidence for an immunopathogenesis of aphthous stomatitis related to lymphocyte-epithelial cell interaction is based on the pathologic features of early lesions, positive lymphocyte transformation, lymphocytotoxicity, and leukocyte migration tests. The presence of antimucosal antibodies indicates an immunologic reaction to damaged epithelial tissue.

One regular finding is the isolation of a pleomorphic alpha-hemolytic streptococcus, *S. sanguis,* from aphthous lesions. These organisms or their cell wall material can produce lesions in animals that are histologically similar to those found in sections of human lesions, and they may produce a hypersensitivity reaction of a delayed type in animals and humans with recurrent aphthae. Streptococcal cell wall material may be pathogenic in aphthous stomatitis, with the cell wall lacking L-form present during remissions. Whether cross reactions between streptococcal antigens and oral mucosal antigens occur and are central to the pathogenesis of aphthous stomatitis remains to be seen.

II. Subjective data. Tingling or burning may antedate the appearance of the lesions by 24 hr. During the first 2–3 days the lesions are extremely painful and may interfere with eating and speaking.

III. Objective data. Aphthae appear as single or multiple, small (1- –10-mm diameter) shallow erosions with clearly defined borders covered by a gray membrane and surrounded by an intense erythematous halo. Rarely, extremely large or exceedingly numerous lesions appear.

IV. Assessment. Morphologically similar lesions can be seen with: (1) acute herpes simplex gingivostomatitis (see p. 94), (2) candidiasis (see p. 82), (3) Vincent's angina, (4) traumatic ulcers, (5) ulcers in patients with agranulocytosis or cyclic neutropenia, (6) B_{12} or folate-deficient macrocytic anemia, and (7) iron deficiency. Differential diagnosis from erythema multiforme, erosive lichen planus, pemphigus, pemphigoid, and herpangina should not be difficult. Aphthae may be associated with chronic ulcerative colitis, Crohn's disease, and malsorption syndromes. The erosions of Behçet's syndrome (oral and genital ulceration associated with iritis) may be identical, and it is possible that this syndrome is a severe form of the same entity as aphthous stomatitis.

V. Therapy. Therapy of aphthous stomatitis is aimed at: (1) controlling the pain, (2) shortening the duration of lesions already present, and (3) aborting new lesions. Those objectives may often be attained.

A. Controlling pain

  1. Topical anesthetics. Apply dyclonine HCl solution (Dyclone) to ulcers as often as needed. Onset of anesthesia is rapid, and duration of numbing is up to 1 hr. Lidocaine (Xylocaine, ointment 5% or viscous) or diphenhydramine HCl (Benadryl elixir) may be used in the same way. Avoid extensive spread of topical medications. If local anesthetics are used over too wide an area, a disturbing "cotton-mouth" feeling and total loss of taste results; these symptoms frequently are worse than those of the original problem.

   a. An anesthetic in a denture-adhesivelike base is Benzodent. This product contains 20% benzocaine (see p. 244), 0.4% eugenol (see p. 291), and 0.1% hydroxyquinoline sulfate. It is applied directly to aphthous ulcers. Ora-Jel-D is a similar product.

  2. Silver nitrate stick application destroys nerve endings and may provide relief from pain for the duration of the eruption, but the ulcers may enlarge slightly and heal more slowly.

B. Aborting lesions and shortening course

  1. Suppression of oral streptococci by topical antibiotics is a logical approach to therapy and is often successful.

   a. The application of tetracycline compresses is the method of choice. Saturate gauze pledgets with 250 mg of tetracycline dissolved in 30 ml of water and apply for 10–20 min 4–6 times a day. Nothing should be taken by mouth for the following 30 min. Continue therapy for 5–7 days. In many patients this treatment effectively shortens the duration of lesions, decreases pain, and aborts early lesions, although, unfortunately, some lesions do not respond to this regimen. Patients with recurrent lesions should be instructed to initiate therapy as early as possible.

b. Some patients acquire resistance to tetracycline. In those instances use a 1% cephalexin monohydrate compress made by dissolving a 250-mg capsule of cephalexin (Keflex) in 30 ml of water and apply for 10–20 min 4–6 times a day.

2. **Topical steroids** also can be useful, especially if applied during the prodromal stages. Triamcinolone acetonide 0.1% in a base that adheres to mucous membrane (Kenalog in Orabase) or other corticosteroid agents (e.g., Lidex ointment or compounded in Orabase) should be applied at least 4id. Others advocate use of 2.5-mg tablets of hydrocortisone sodium succinate, or 0.1-mg tablets of betamethasone 17-valerate, allowed to dissolve slowly near the lesion, 3–4 times a day.

3. **Administration of systemic corticosteroids** can abort attacks if taken for 4 days during the prodromal period, and it will usually induce healing of lesions in patients with severe erosive lesions.

4. **Levamisole,** an investigational drug thought to act through potentiation of cell-mediated immune mechanisms, seems effective in some patients with recurrent aphthae.

References

Brody, H. A., and Silverman, S., Jr.   Studies on recurrent oral aphthae: I. Clinical and laboratory comparisons. *Oral Surg.* 27:27–34, 1969.

Dolby, A. E.   Management of recurrent oral ulcerations. *Practitioner* 210:403–408, 1973.

Editorial: Recurrent oral ulceration. *Br. Med. J.* 3:757–758, 1974.

Graykowski, E. A., et al.   Recurrent aphthous stomatitis: Clinical, therapeutic, histopathologic, and hypersensitivity aspects. *J.A.M.A.* 196:637–644, 1966.

Lehner, T., Wilton, J. M. A., and Ivanyi, L.   Double blind crossover trial of levamisole in recurrent aphthous ulceration. *Lancet* 2:926–929, 1976.

Lennette, E. H., and Magoffin, R. L.   Virologic and immunologic aspects of major oral ulcerations. *J. Am. Dent. Assoc.* 87:1055–1073, 1973.

Lozada, F., and Silverman, S.   Topically applied fluocinonide in an adhesive base in the treatment of vesiculoerosive diseases. *Arch. Dermatol.* 116:898–901, 1980.

Rogers, R. S., III.   Recurrent aphthous stomatitis: Clinical characteristics and evidence for an immunopathogenesis. *J. Invest. Dermatol.* 69:499–509, 1977.

Rogers, R. S., III.   Recurrent Aphthous Stomatitis and Behçet's Syndrome. In B. Safai and R. A. Good (eds.), *Immunodermatology.* New York: Plenum, 1981. Pp. 345–353.

Rogers, R. S., Sams, W. M., and Shorter, R. G.   Lymphocytotoxicity in recurrent aphthous stomatitis: Lymphotoxicity for oral epithelial cells in recurrent aphthous stomatitis and Behçet's syndrome. *Arch. Dermatol.* 109:361–363, 1974.

Rostas, A., McLean, D. I., and Wilkinson, R. D.   Management of recurrent aphthous stomatitis: A review. *Cutis* 22:183–189, 1978.

Ship, I. I., and Galili, D. A.   Systemic significance of mouth ulcers. *Postgrad. Med.* 49:67–77, 1971.

Shore, R. N., and Shelley, W. B.   Treatment of aphthous stomatitis by suppression of intralesional streptococci. *Arch. Dermatol.* 109:400–402, 1974.

Weathers, D. R., and Griffin, J. W.   Intraoral ulcerations of recurrent herpes simplex and recurrent aphthae: Two distinct clinical entities. *J. Am. Dent. Assoc.* 81:81–88, 1970.

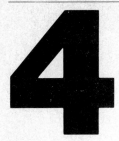

Bacterial skin infections

I. Definition and pathophysiology

A. Pyodermas

1. A pyoderma is a purulent infection of the skin. Most are caused by streptococci or staphylococci. Pyodermas occur in up to 10% of children in the southeastern United States, in 80% of children in endemic areas, and are also very common in adults. Impetigo and folliculitis are the primary bacterial skin infections. Folliculitis may lead to the production of furuncles or carbuncles. Preceding cutaneous lesions, obesity, treatment with steroids and chemotherapeutic agents, dysglobulinemia, white cell dysfunction in leukemia or chronic granulomatous disease, and probably diabetes—all predispose to the development of these infections.

   a. **Nonbullous streptococcal impetigo** is found most often on the face and other exposed areas. It is very contagious among infants and young children but much less so in older persons. Predisposing factors include poor health and hygiene, malnutrition, and a warm climate, as well as antecedent scabies, chicken pox, contact and atopic dermatitis, and other eruptions. Group A streptococci are unable to survive on intact skin and require at least superficial damage to the stratum corneum in order to take hold and proliferate. The primary lesion is a fragile subcorneal pustule that most frequently contains group A beta-hemolytic streptococci and, less commonly and later in the course of the disease, secondarily colonizing coagulase-positive staphylococci. In patients who ultimately develop impetigo, streptococci may be cultured first from normal skin, then from lesions, and much later from the respiratory tract; staphylococci are initially in the respiratory tract, then on normal skin, and finally in skin lesions. Untreated streptococcal impetigo spontaneously clears both clinically and bacteriologically in about 10 days.

   The overall incidence of postpyodermal acute glomerulonephritis is about 2%. In tropical climates, nephritogenic strains of streptococci commonly cause impetigo, and in some southern areas of the United States 85% of all cases of acute nephritis in preschool children are preceded by cutaneous streptococcal infection.

   b. **Bullous staphylococcal impetigo** is seen primarily in children and is caused by group II phage type 71 staphylococci. These organisms elaborate an exfoliative toxin that induces an intraepidermal, subgranular cleavage plane, resulting in blister formation.

This organism can also be responsible for an exfoliative dermatitis in infants **(Ritter's disease)** and for toxic epidermal necrolysis **(staphylococcal scalded-skin syndrome)** in infants and children.

c. **Folliculitis** is a staphylococcal infection starting around hair follicles. Superficial folliculitis usually does not represent a serious problem, but deep and/or recurrent lesions of the scalp, nose, and eyelid cilia (sties) are far more distressing.

d. **Furuncles,** or boils, usually develop from a preceding superficial staphylococcal folliculitis. They are most frequently found in areas of hair-bearing skin subject to friction and maceration, especially the face, scalp, buttocks, and axillae. **Recurrent furunculosis** inexplicably develops in an unfortunate few who seem unable to rid themselves permanently of the staphylococcus. There is no evidence that these patients harbor any specific staphylococcal strains or have any definable deficiency in their host defense mechanisms.

e. **Carbuncles** are staphylococcal abscesses that are larger and deeper than boils and develop in thick inelastic skin. They usually drain at multiple points and are found commonly on the back of the neck, the back, and the thighs.

B. **Erythrasma,** a mild, chronic, localized, superficial bacterial infection involving intertriginous areas of skin, is caused by *Corynebacterium minutissimum*. This organism is often part of the normal flora, and some change in host-parasite relationship, such as increased heat or humidity, results in the development of the clinical disorder.

II. **Subjective data**

A. Impetigo is usually pruritic.

B. All forms of deep folliculitis hurt; sties, boils, and carbuncles may become exquisitely painful.

C. Erythrasma lesions are usually asymptomatic.

III. **Objective data (See color insert.)**

A. **Nonbullous streptococcal impetigo** begins as a small erythematous macule that rapidly develops into a fragile vesicle with an erythematous areola. The vesicopustule breaks and leaves a red, oozing erosion capped with a thick, golden yellow crust that appears "stuck on." Satellite pustules and lesions are usual. The presenting lesions of bullous staphylococcal impetigo are flaccid bullae that are first filled with clear, then cloudy, fluid and then quickly replaced by a thin, varnishlike crust.

B. **Folliculitis** lesions consist of superficial or deep pustules, or follicular nodules. The face is a common site for deep folliculitis.

C. **Sties** are erythematous swellings around eyelid cilia.

D. **Furuncles** start as firm, red, tender nodules that become fluctuant, point, and rupture, discharging a core of necrotic tissue.

E. **Carbuncles** appear similar to furuncles, but drain at multiple points.

F. **Erythrasma** may be seen as dry, smooth to slightly creased or scaly, sharply marginated, red brown plaques in the inguinal, axillary, or inframammary folds; as mild scaling or fissuring between the 3–4 or 4–5 toe webs; or in generalized scaly patches. Lesions are easily mistaken for those of superficial fungal infection.

IV. Assessment

A. Factors predisposing to infection should be identified, evaluated, and treated or eliminated.

B. Most cases of impetigo or folliculitis need not be routinely cultured; recalcitrant or unusual cases deserve a Gram's stain and culture of the exudate.

C. Ninety percent of patients with acute glomerulonephritis secondary to pyoderma will have an elevated serum titer of anti-DNase B; only 50% of similar patients will have elevated levels of antistreptolysin O.

D. Erythrasma is diagnosed by the characteristic coral red fluorescence of lesions when viewed under the Wood's light. Fluorescence is caused by a water-soluble porphyrin, and hence may be lacking if the patient has bathed recently. The organisms appear as gram-positive rodlike filamentous and coccoid forms and are best viewed under $45\times$ magnification or oil immersion after Gram's or Giemsa's stain of affected scales. Culture is rarely required and needs special media.

V. Therapy

A. Impetigo caused by both streptococci and staphylococci should be treated with systemic antibiotics; such treatment is valid despite the fact that the disease is often self-limited, and that there is no convincing evidence that treating pyodermas will prevent subsequent glomerulonephritis. Systemic treatment is justified for several reasons: (1) impetigo sometimes does not resolve for a very long time and may become widespread before it does; (2) systemic antibiotics can shorten the healing time and decrease the number of recurrences; (3) benzathine penicillin will decrease streptococcal carrier rates for at least 4 weeks, and is thus useful both therapeutically as well as prophylactically; (4) data now accumulated document the ineffectiveness of topical antibiotics in reliably eliminating either staphylococci or streptococci from lesions of streptococcal impetigo. Studies from the southern United States have shown a cure rate of 39% for streptococcal impetigo after 2 weeks of therapy with topical hexachlorophene and bacitracin, compared to 99% after IM benzathine penicillin or a 10-day course of oral erythromycin, or 98% after 10 days of oral phenoxymethyl penicillin.

1. Treat with one injection of IM benzathine penicillin (600,000 units in children 6 years or younger, 1.2 million units if 7 or older) or 10 days of erythromycin (250 mg 4id) or phenoxymethyl penicillin (250 mg 4id). Bullous staphylococcal impetigo should be treated with a semisynthetic penicillin (dicloxacillin, 250 mg 4id) or erythromycin if organisms are sensitive (5–15% of staphylococci are now resistant to erythromycin and methicillin-resistant strains are also emerging).

2. The lesions should be soaked 3–4 times a day in warm tap water, saline, or a soap solution to remove the crusts. In addition, it might be useful to have both patient and family bathe at least once daily with a bacteriocidal iodine (e.g., Betadine skin cleanser) or bacteriostatic soap or solution containing hexachlorophene or chlorhexidine (Hibiclens) (see also p. 254).

3. Apply an iodine ointment (Betadine) or simple bland emollient to the base of cleansed lesions after crust has been removed.

B. **Superficial folliculitis** may respond to aggressive topical hygiene and local antibiotics. Folliculitis on the male beard area is unusually recalcitrant and recurrent and should be treated with systemic antibiotics. Simple **furunculosis** needs to be treated only with moist heat. Local ophthalmic antibiotics should be instilled into the eye for sties. Larger boils should be carefully and conservatively incised and drained after they point; after the incision only topical antibiotics are needed. Furuncles or carbuncles associated with a surrounding cellulitis or those associated with fever or located on the upper lip, nose, cheeks, or forehead also are treated with a semisynthetic penicillin, erythromycin, or clindamycin. Chronic folliculitis of certain areas, particularly the buttocks, may respond to the application of 6.25% aluminum chloride hexahydrate in absolute ethyl alcohol (Xerac AC) once daily at bedtime (see also p. 253). This compound probably acts through a combination of direct antibacterial and antiperspirant effects.

C. **Recurrent furunculosis** represents a difficult therapeutic problem, one which should be approached as follows:

1. Assess the organism's antibiotic sensitivity and start on the appropriate drug (most often a semisynthetic penicillin). Continue treatment for 1–3 months and then later as necessary. Long-term systemic therapy will keep new lesions from erupting and sometimes induces the problem to disappear completely.

2. Methods for maintaining rigorous topical hygiene are noted below. However, the use of such programs alone often does not inhibit recurrent furunculosis, and it is now not clear whether topical treatment substantially adds anything of benefit to the care of such patients.

   a. Patient and family should bathe and shampoo 1–2 times daily. Nails should be clipped short and scrubbed as in a surgical prep. Avoid occupational situations that result in occlusion or maceration of skin appendages (dirt, oils, impermeable clothing).

   b. Instill an antibiotic cream or ointment into the anterior nares daily (e.g., Betadine ointment, Neosporin ointment).

   c. Precautions before and during shaving must be maintained whenever there are facial lesions. The beard should be soaked with hot water for 5 min prior to shaving. Blades should be discarded daily. As an aftershave, 70% alcohol should be used. The razor should be left in alcohol between shaves or boiled for 5–10 min prior to shaving; similarly, electric razor heads are soaked in alcohol for 1–2 hr between shaves. Use a brushless shaving cream or soap alone.

   d. Separate towels, washcloths, sheets, and clothing should be used; they should be laundered in boiling water and changed daily.

   e. Dressings must be changed frequently and disposed of immediately. Paper tissues should be used instead of handkerchiefs.

   f. Consider bacterial interference treatment when all else fails. In this method a nonpathogenic staphylococcus is inoculated onto multiple sites on the patient's skin after the pathogenic strain has been eliminated by intensive antibiotic administration. After the new organism colonizes the skin, furuncles may cease.

D. Erythrasma may be treated with miconazole or clotrimazole creams or with keratolytic compounds such as Keralyt Gel or 3% or 6% sulfur and salicylic acid ointment 2id for 1–2 weeks. It may also be treated by topical application of 1.5–2.0% hydroalcoholic erythromycin solutions 2id for 2 weeks or by oral administration of erythromycin 250 mg 4id for 2 weeks.

References

Dajani, A. S., Ferrieri, P., and Wannamaker, L.   Endemic superficial pyoderma in children. *Arch. Dermatol.* 108:517–522, 1973.

Dillon, H. C.   Streptococcal Infections of the Skin and Their Complications: Impetigo and Nephritis. In L. W. Wannamaker and J. M. Masten (eds.), *Streptococci and Streptococcal Diseases: Recognition, Understanding and Management.* New York: Academic, 1972. Pp. 571–587.

Dillon, H. C.   Topical and systemic therapy for pyodermas. *Int. J. Dermatol.* 19:443–451, 1980.

Dillon, H. C., Jr., and Reeves, M. S. A.   Streptococcal immune responses in nephritis after skin infection. *Am. J. Med.* 56:333–346, 1974.

Elias, P. M., Fritsch, P., and Epstein, E. H.   Staphylococcal scalded skin syndrome: Clinical features, pathogenesis, and recent microbiological and biochemical developments. *Arch. Dermatol.* 113:207–219, 1977.

Leyden, J. J., Stewart, R., and Kligman, A. M.   Experimental infections with group A streptococci in humans. *J. Invest. Dermatol.* 75:196–201, 1980.

Maibach, H. I., and Hildick-Smith, G.   *Skin Bacteria and Their Role in Infection.* New York: McGraw-Hill, 1964.

Noble, W. C. (ed.).   Microbial skin disease. *Br. J. Dermatol.* 86 (Suppl. 8):1, 1972.

Pitcher, D. G., Noble, W. C., and Seville, R. H.   Treatment of erythrasma with miconazole. *Clin. Exper. Dermatol.* 4:453–456, 1979.

Rasmussen, J. E.   Topical antibiotics. *J. Dermatol. Surg.* 2:69–71, 1976.

Sarkany, I., Taplin, D., and Blank, H.   Incidence and bacteriology of erythrasma. *Arch. Dermatol.* 85:578–582, 1962.

Shelley, W. B., and Hurley, H. J.   Anhydrous formulation of aluminum chloride for chronic folliculitis. *J. Am. Med. Assn.* 244:1956–1957, 1980.

Steele, R. W.   Recurrent staphylococcal infection in families. *Arch. Dermatol.* 116:189–190, 1980.

Storrs, F. J.   Treatment of nonbullous impetigo. *Cutis* 16:886–891, 1975.

Wannamaker, L. W.   Impetigo contagiosa. *Prog. Dermatol.* 7:11–14, 1973.

5

Bites and stings (spiders, snakes, insects)

I. **Definition and pathophysiology.** Reaction to bites and stings is initiated by either a toxin or allergen injected by the offending arthropod (spider, tick, scorpion, mite) or snake. The direct toxic mechanisms include contact with venoms, irritating hairs, salivary secretions, or vesicant fluids; indirect contact may result from inhalation or ingestion of debris, particles, body parts, or excretions. Spiders and snakes inject venoms that may be hemolytic or may disturb the clotting system or act as neurotoxins. Intravascular coagulation may account for the clinical picture seen after the recluse spider bite; sphingomyelinase D is the fraction of spider venom responsible for the most damage. The vast majority of serious reactions to biting insects, including bees, hornets, wasps, yellow jackets, fleas, mosquitoes, fire ants, and bedbugs, are caused by an acquired hypersensitivity; over 80% of deaths result from anaphylactic reactions and occur within an hour of the sting. Many patients who develop generalized reactions to insect stings have no history of previous systemic or local reaction to a sting. Of about 45,000 snake bites in the United States each year, only about 20% are by poisonous snakes. Approximately 50% of deaths attributed to venomous animals result from Hymenoptera (bee or wasp) stings; rattlesnake bites account for 20% of fatalities, and poisonous spiders, 14%. At least 30–50 people in the United States die each year from systemic reactions to stings. Venom from Hymenoptera contains serotonin, kinins, acetylcholine, lecithinase, hyaluronidase, and phospholipase; exposure to this venom has been shown to release histamine from leukocytes of Hymenoptera-allergic patients.

II. **Subjective data**

A. **Spiders.** The spiders that cause serious reactions in humans in the United States most commonly are the black widow (*Latrodectus mactans*) and the brown recluse spider (*Loxosceles reclusa*). After a short, sharp pain at the site of a black widow spider bite, systemic symptoms, including chills, vomiting, pain in abdomen and legs, sweating, and cramps, begin in 15–60 min and usually subside within several hours. Reactions to about 90% of recluse spider bites is trivial. However, sometimes severe local pain associated with local swelling occurs between 4–8 hr after a bite. Viscerocutaneous loxoscelism, with severe chills, vomiting, arthralgias, and hematologic abnormalities, is rare.

B. **Snakes.** The pit vipers (rattlesnake, moccasin, and copperhead) are the most dangerous snakes in the United States. Local reactions to bites are pain, swelling, ecchymosis, and lymphadenopathy, which may be accompanied by a tingling sensation around the lips, vertigo, muscular twitching, or bleeding (hematuria, hematemesis).

C. **Insects.** The **normal reaction** to the sting of a bee, wasp, hornet, or yellow jacket is itching and pain, both of which subside within a few hours. Severe **local reactions** result in itching, pain, and in an unusual amount of swelling around the site of the sting. **Toxic reactions,** which occur after 10 or more simultaneous stings, are characterized by gastrointestinal symptoms, vertigo, headache, and fever. **Immediate systemic allergic reactions** show the usual manifestations of anaphylaxis: urticaria, laryngeal edema, bronchospasm, abdominal cramps, and shock. **Delayed allergic reactions** occur within hours to 2 weeks following the sting and have symptoms similar to those of serum sickness.

The harvester ant and fire ant cause most ant-sting reactions in humans. Both are associated with "fire" because of the intense burning and pain associated with their stings. Some patients may develop immediate systemic allergic reactions to fire ant stings.

The immediate allergic reaction to the injected salivary fluids of mosquitoes is itching; the delayed reaction, occurring several hours later, is accompanied by a more severe, intense, burning itch. Flies do not actually bite but pierce through the skin, thus allowing salivary gland fluids to enter and cause toxic and allergic reactions. The little (1 x 5 mm) black fly is renowned for inducing an extremely painful and long-lasting reaction. Flea bites itch.

III. Objective data

A. **Spiders.** The local reaction to a black widow spider bite is unremarkable. Severely ill patients will have the symptoms described, which may be accompanied by a morbilliform erythema. The bite of the recluse spider is relatively painless; the more serious but uncommon bite reactions go through stages, beginning with edema, progressing to bulla formation (0–2 hr), then to surrounding ischemia (2–6 hr), blue black cyanosis (5–12 hr), and then to extensive necrosis and gangrene (12 hr on).

B. **Snakes.** The bite will usually consist of two fang marks surrounded by intense edema, ecchymosis, and sometimes bullae.

C. **Insects**

1. **Bees, wasps, hornets, yellow jackets**

   a. **Normal:** red area with a central punctum gradually surrounded by a white zone and red flare. Later a wheal forms and disappears within hours.

   b. **Local reaction:** intense edema around the sting area.

   c. **Toxic reactions:** cutaneous signs are usually edema without urticaria.

   d. **Immediate systemic allergic reactions:** signs of anaphylaxis.

   e. **Delayed systemic allergic reactions:** urticaria, accompanied by lymphadenopathy and polyarthritis.

2. **Ants.** Fire ant stings develop as a wheal surmounted by two hemorrhagic puncta and evolve into vesicles and, 8–10 hr later, umbilicated pustules. Crusts and scar tissue gradually form over the next week.

3. **Mosquitoes.** The immediate reaction is production of a wheal; a swollen papular lesion may appear as a delayed reaction several hours later.

4. **Flies.** The blackfly sting causes either nodular vesicular lesions or firm, rough pruritic nodules. Both reactions may last weeks to months.

5. **Fleas.** These bites are typically grouped urticarial papules, some with a central punctum.

IV. Assessment. Patients with severe systemic reactions should be cared for in facilities prepared to handle acute respiratory and cardiovascular emergencies.

V. Therapy

A. **Spiders.** Mild local reactions to black widow spider bites should be treated by cool compresses or application of an ice cube, calamine lotion, and/or a topical corticosteroid. When there is a severe reaction to a black widow spider bite, treatment should be immediate and include a tight proximal tourniquet to occlude venous return, incision of the sting area, suction to remove the venom, opiates for pain, and specific horse serum antivenom effective against bites of all spiders of the genus *Latrodectus* (Lyovac). Mild cutaneous loxoscelism heals well with no specific therapy aside from splinting protection and reassurance. High-dose systemic corticosteroids are appropriate for most large (>2 cm diameter) bites and always at the first indication of systemic loxoscelism. In the case of large, deep bites over the fat pads in children or for bites on the more fatty areas of the skin of adults, treat with 100 mg prednisone for 4 days and observe for renal injury or hemolysis. Dialysis may be required in patients with acute renal failure, anuria, and azotemia. Early surgical excision of these spider bites is not warranted (see Anderson, 1978). Tetanus prophylaxis must be considered. See Table 1 for recommendations on tetanus prophylaxis.

B. **Snakes.** The best first aid measures for snake bites are: (1) Immobilize the injured part. Tourniquets should not be used as they will not prevent death, can cause extensive necrosis, and loosening may produce shock. A constricting band may be applied proximal to the bite tightly enough to occlude veins but loosely enough to preserve a distal pulse. Apply a firm constrictive bandage around as much of the limb as possible and then a splint. (2) Although incision and suction can remove venom, most clinicians feel that this procedure is not generally effective and causes permanent damage. Only if the interval between bite and treatment is going to be prolonged should the bite be cooled by applying ice. (3) Get the victim to a physician or hospital as soon as possible. At that time start an IV in the contralateral arm; type and cross match blood early, before venom action makes this impossible; and check for the presence of coagulopathy. (4) In severely envenomized patients, administer horse-based antiserum. Two types of antivenom are commercially available, one for bites by rattlesnakes and other pit vipers, and the other for coral snake bites. Antivenom reactions are common. Pit viper envenomation causes local platelet consumption, which can be ameliorated somewhat by antivenom but is worsened by steroids. Platelet and clotting factors should be re-

Table 1. Guide to tetanus prophylaxis in wound management

History of tetanus immunization (dose)	Clean minor wounds		All other wounds	
	Td	TIG	Td	TIG
Uncertain	Yes	No	Yes	Yes
0–1	Yes	No	Yes	Yes
2	Yes	No	Yes	No***
3 or more	No*	No	No**	No

Key: Td = Tetanus and diphtheria toxoids absorbed. For children less than 7 years old, DPT is preferred. TIG = Tetanus immune globulin.
* = Yes, if more than 10 years since last dose.
** = Yes, if more than 5 years since last dose.
*** = None, if wound is more than 24 hr old.
Source: *Morbidity and Mortality Weekly Reports* 30:404, 1981.

stored by blood component therapy as indicated. Tissue necrosis and injury should be limited by debridement and mechanical removal of venom and local necrotic tissue. Other treatment methods as well as sources of antivenom are detailed in Arnold (1973). Locations of antivenoms for rare species of poisonous snakes, and names and phone numbers of experts on venomous bites can be obtained 24 hr a day from the Oklahoma City Poison Control Center (405-271-5454).

C. Insects

1. Flick (do not squeeze) the insect off the skin. This should also remove the venom sac. If the stinger is left in the skin remove it carefully with tweezers.

2. Cold applications (ice, cold compresses) at the sting site may retard absorption and reduce chemical activity of the venom.

3. **Local reactions**

   a. Cold open wet compresses for 1 hr 3id.

   b. Calamine lotion alone or with 0.25% menthol and 1% phenol will be soothing. Solutions that contain phenol should not be given to pregnant women.

   c. A topical corticosteroid may be useful for the pruritus and inflammation.

   d. Systemic antihistamines.

4. **Systemic allergic reactions and treatment for anaphylaxis**

   a. Inject 0.3–0.5 mg epinephrine HCl (0.3–0.5 ml of a 1:1000 dilution) IM and repeat every 15–30 min as needed. Rub the injection site to hasten absorption. Lower doses should be used in the elderly and in patients with cardiovascular problems. Only in profound anaphylaxis with hypotension and poor peripheral circulation should intravenous administration be necessary. In such cases use epinephrine in a 1:10,000 dilution (1 mg = 10 ml) and give 0.1 mg boluses until symptoms improve.

b. Apply a tourniquet proximal to a sting on an extremity. The tourniquet should not be so tight as to cut off arterial circulation. Relax the occlusion 1 min every 3 min. Inject 0.2 mg epinephrine HCl 1:1000 subcutaneously into the reaction site. Carefully remove the stinger stylet. Do not pinch the venom sac.

c. Begin an intravenous line as soon as possible with a saline drip. If patients are not responsive to initial measures, critical care with fluids, oxygen, and pressors may become necessary. Cases of severe laryngeal edema may require intubation or tracheostomy.

d. Persistent bronchospasm should be treated with intravenous aminophylline and inhaled bronchodilators such as albuterol, isoetharine, or isoproterenol. The recommended dose of aminophylline is a loading dose of 3–5 mg/kg followed by a drip of 0.5–0.9 mg/kg/hr. The dose should be lowered in elderly patients and in those with congestive heart failure or liver disease. Smokers may require higher doses.

e. Antihistamines should be administered to block the effects of histamine on receptor sites. Their usefulness is greatest in blocking reactions of the mucous membranes and skin. There is little or no effect with respect to preventing bronchoconstriction. Antihistamines should be used as an adjunct to epinephrine as their effect is not immediate. Use diphenhydramine 50 mg PO or IM depending on the severity of the reaction. Treatment should continue as long as symptoms persist. Reactions generally are over in 2–3 days.

f. Steroids have a delayed onset of action and are not first-line drugs for treating a severe systemic reaction. However, unless medically contraindicated, they should be used to prevent continued reaction in all but the most mild allergic reactions. Begin with hydrocortisone 100 mg IV q6h and discharge on prednisone 30 mg/day tapering over 3–7 days as symptoms dictate. Reactions usually subside within 1–2 days.

5. Prophylaxis

a. Sensitive patients should carry medications such as an epinephrine inhalation spray, ephedrine, and antihistamine tablets with them at all times. Commercial kits are available containing a syringe loaded with epinephrine, and a tourniquet and antihistamine tablets (Ana-Kit). Patients should also always carry an aerosol insecticide spray and avoid walking without shoes. They should dress in protective clothing, and avoid wearing the following items, all of which attract flying insects:

(1) Perfumes and other scented preparations (hair spray, aftershave lotion, deodorant); (2) Brightly colored objects such as clothing or jewelery (white is said to be the least insect-attracting color); (3) Wool, suede, and leatherlike apparel.

b. Desensitization (hyposensitization, immunotherapy) is effective and **should be considered mandatory** for patients who have had an immediate systemic reaction to an insect sting such as respiratory difficulty, hypotension, and generalized urticaria. Whether patients who have had large local reactions to a sting should be tested and desensitized has not been determined. Successful desensitization is accompanied by a decrease in basophil histamine release and an increase in blocking (IgG) antibody level. The material of choice for desensitization is Hymenoptera venom alone, rather than whole body extract.

c. Insect repellents (see also p. 302).

(1) Repellents containing diethyltoluamide (deet) are the agents of choice for protection against mosquitoes, flies, fleas, mites, and ticks. Ethyl hexanediol, dimethyl phthalate, dimethyl carbate butopyronoxyl are also effective, but do not cover the wide spectrum that deet does. A combination of two or more of these repellents is more effective than one alone. No product will protect against spiders, wasps, or bees.

(2) Factors that attract mosquitoes to skin include warmth, sweat, moisture, CO_2, and other body emanations found in the convective air currents above or downwind of humans.

(3) Repellents do not mask these attractive stimuli but seem to form a barrier against penetration that extends to less than 4 cm away from the skin on which the repellent has been freshly applied. Deet blocks the ability of the mosquito to track the human's CO_2 vapor trail. This means that nontreated areas only a few centimeters away from those protected may be bitten. At room temperature, protection time may last 10–12 hr. About 10% of applied deet evaporates from the skin in the first hour after application. There are many factors that will decrease the protection time, including warmer temperatures, high wind velocities, loss of repellent from rubbing against clothing, and washoff with water or sweat.

(4) If mosquitoes are dense, a high dose of repellent must be applied. The volume will depend on the amount of active ingredient in the repellent mixture. One should apply at least 1 mg/sq cm of exposed skin, which means applying liberally and, under most outdoor conditions, frequently (every half to 2 hr).

(5) Repellent-treated nets and clothing not only prevent mosquitoes from biting through clothes, but also prevent them from biting adjacent areas. Repellents may remain effective for several days on fabric.

(6) Diethyltoluamide-containing products include Mosquitone lotion, OFF products, and Cutter insect repellent. Ethyl hexanediol is present in 6–12 lotion, stick, or towelettes.

References

Anderson, P. C.   Brown recluse spider bites: An update. *J. Ky. Med. Assn.* 76:172–173, 1978.

Arnold, R. E.   *What to Do About Bites and Stings of Venomous Animals.* New York: Macmillan, 1973.

Barr, S. E.   Insect sting allergy. *Cutis* 17:1069–1074, 1976.

Berger, R. S., Adelstein, E. H., and Anderson, P. C.   Intravenous coagulation: The cause of necrotic arachnidism. *J. Invest. Dermatol.* 61:142–150, 1973.

Frazier, C. A.   *Insect Allergy: Allergic and Toxic Reactions to Insects and Other Arthropods.* St. Louis: Green, 1969.

Frazier, C. A.   Cutaneous manifestations of insect allergy. *Cutis* 13:1038–1047, 1974.

Frazier, C. A. (ed.).   Insect Allergy (special issue). *Cultis* 19:749–802, 1977.

Harves, A. D., and Millikan, L. E.   Current concepts of therapy and pathophysiology in arthropod bites and stings: I. Arthropods: II. Insects. *Int. J. Dermatol.* 14:543–562, 621–634, 1975.

Hunt, K. J., Valentine, M. D., Sobotka, A. K., Benten, A. W., Anodeo, F. J., and Lichtenstein, L. M.   A controlled trial of immunotherapy in insect hypersensitivity. *N. Engl. J. Med.* 299:157–161, 1978.

Immunization Practices Advisory Committee (ACIP). Diphtheria, tetanus, and pertussis: Guidelines for vaccine prophylaxis and other preventive measures. *Morbidity and Mortality Weekly Reports* 30:392–407, 1981.

Kelly, J. F., and Patterson, R.   Anaphylaxis. Course, mechanisms and treatment. *J. A. M. A.* 227:1431–1436, 1974.

Lichtenstein, L. M., Valentine, M. D., and Sobotka, A. K.   A case for venom treatment in anaphylactic sensitivity to Hymenoptera sting. *N. Engl. J. Med.* 290:1223–1227, 1974.

Lichtenstein, L. M., Valentine, M. D., and Sobotka, A. K.   Insect allergy: The state of the art. *J. Allergy Clin. Immunol.* 64:5–12, 1979.

Maibach, H. I., Khan, A. A., and Akers, W.   Use of insect repellents for maximum efficacy. *Arch. Dermatol.* 109:32–35, 1974.

Parrish, H. M., and Wiechmann, G. H.   Rattlesnake bites in the eastern United States. *South. Med. J.* 61:118–126, 1968.

Reisman, R. E., and Arbesman, C. E.   Stinging insect allergy: Current concepts and problems. *Pediatr. Clin. North Am.* 22:185–192, 1975.

Simon, T. L., and Grace, T. G.   Envenomation coagulopathy in wounds from pit vipers, *N. Engl. J. Med.* 305:443–447, 1981.

Sobotka, A. K., Valentine, M. D., Benton, A. W., and Lichtenstein, L. M.   Allergy to insect stings: I. Diagnosis of IgE-mediated Hymenoptera sensitivity by venom-induced histamine release. *J. Allergy Clin. Immunol.* 53:170–184, 1974.

Spencer, T. S., Hill, J. A., Feldmann, R. J., and Maibach, H. I.   Evaporation of diethyltoluamide from human skin *in vivo* and *in vitro*. *J. Invest. Dermatol.* 72:317–319, 1979.

Treatment of snakebite in the USA. *Med. Lett. Drugs Ther.* 24:87–89, 1982.

Wright, R. H.   Why mosquito repellents repel. *Sci. Am.* 233:104–111, 1975.

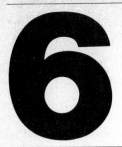

Burns

I. Definition and pathophysiology. More than 2 million individuals in the United States suffer burns each year, of which 100,000 require hospitalization and 12,000 die. The incidence of burns is high among the very young and very old, among nonwhites and members of lower socioeconomic groups, and in rural areas where space heaters or fireplaces are used for heat. The degree of cutaneous damage caused by thermal injury to the skin is related directly to the duration and intensity of exposure to heat. The types of burns may be summarized as follows:

A. First-degree burn

1. Histopathology

   a. Epidermis: loss of intercellular cohesiveness with cleft formation.

   b. Dermis: vasodilatation and edema.

2. Clinical condition: red, swollen skin.

3. Course: heals within 3–4 days without scarring.

B. Second-degree burn (partial-thickness burn)

1. Histopathology

   a. Epidermis: coagulative necrosis with bulla formation at dermoepidermal junction.

   b. Dermis: marked vasodilatation and edema.

2. Clinical condition: red, blistered skin with maintenance of epidermal integrity.

3. Course: reepithelialization takes place from epidermal appendages and, if left undisturbed, will heal within 2–3 weeks without scarring.

C. Third-degree burn (full-thickness burn)

1. Histopathology: necrosis of variable amounts of epidermis, dermis, and subcutaneous tissue.

2. Clinical condition: ulcerated wound with extensive tissue necrosis.

3. Course: heals slowly (in months) with scarring.

The depth of the burn may be related to its cause. Scalds from hot liquids are usually partial thickness, while injuries from contact with flames, hot metal, or electrical current are usually full thickness in depth. Chemical burn damage depends on the agent, and injury may progress for several days. In practice, it is often difficult to determine the depth of injury during the first 2 weeks of healing.

II. **Subjective data.** First- and second-degree burns are extremely painful, whereas deeper damage destroys nerves and renders the tissues insensitive to pain.

III. **Objective data**

A. First-degree burns are erythematous and edematous and heal rapidly; there is mild epidermal desquamation and postinflammatory hyperpigmentation.

B. Second-degree burns demonstrate blistering; evidence of continued capillary circulation may be observed.

C. With deeper burns, coagulated blood vessels are present, and the skin appears dry and mahogany-colored. In damaged skin that appears marble-white, the depth of damage is difficult to assess. These wounds may be full thickness, but at times they heal spontaneously and are then best termed deep, partial-thickness injury.

IV. **Assessment.** Partial-thickness burns that involve less than 15% of the body surface and spare the face, hands, feet, and perineum, and full-thickness burns of less than 2% of the body surface are classified as minor burns. Such burns can almost always be managed on an ambulatory basis.

V. **Therapy.** The pathophysiology and therapy of moderate and severe burns will not be discussed here. Such burns require intensive specialized care in hospitals for expert management of the wound and of the severe fluid and electrolyte changes associated with extensive cutaneous damage.

A. **Immediate therapy.** Apply wet towels soaked in ice water or cold water, or ice itself, or immerse the burned area in static cold tap water (72–77°F). This is effective because burned skin retains enough heat to extend coagulation to surrounding tissues. Treatment should be started as soon as possible (within the first hour after injury) after the area has been cleansed with soap and water. Application of cold relieves pain, reduces edema and reactive hyperemia, and probably diminishes the extent of injury. The burned area should be kept in water until it is free of pain both in and out of water; this may take up to 45 min. Warm blankets should be put on uninvolved areas to prevent systemic hypothermia.

B. **Postemergency therapy**

1. **Very superficial burns** require no dressing or medications, although the application of an emollient such as petrolatum may be soothing. Burn wounds should be washed gently with a bland soap and water and dirt removed. Patients should receive tetanus immunization as indicated and be given analgesics as required (see Table 1 on p. 32 for recommendations on tetanus prophylaxis). Topical anesthetics containing more than 5% benzocaine base (see p. 243) may dull the immediate discomfort but will add the risk of allergic contact sensitization. There are no clinical studies that demonstrate the efficacy of antibiotics after their topical application to the superficial burn and their use is contraindicated. A topical corticosteroid will inhibit inflammation and may also decrease pain.

2. **Second-degree burns** should be cleansed and a dressing applied. In general, it is best to remove blisters or dead tissue. Almost all burns treated on an ambulatory basis do better when treated with dressings. The dressing should occlude the wound, splint the part, be easily removed, and be comfortable. If oozing or weeping is present, application of a water-soluble ointment or ointment gauze next to the wound will keep the dressing from sticking. Absorptive material such as fluffed gauze pads should be placed over the initial gauze layer, and a final layer of elastic bandage should be put on with even compression. Dressings should remain in place for about 5 days unless there is much weeping, in which case they may need to be changed more often. If dressings are stuck, they should be moistened or the affected part soaked in warm water before the dressings are removed. If there is any question of infection, a topical antibacterial preparation, such as povidone-iodine ointment, solution, or spray (Betadine or generic products), silver sulfadiazine (Silvadene), or mafenide (Sulfamylon) should be applied.

3. **Chemical burns** require immediate and prolonged irrigation with water. The depth of the injury may be reduced by 2–4 hr or more of washing. Do not rinse acid burns with alkali and vice versa; doing this causes an exothermic reaction, which leads to further tissue damage. Industrial toxicity texts should be consulted concerning specific therapy for offending chemicals.

References

Abston, S.   Burns in children. *Ciba Clin. Symp.* 28:4, 1976.

Artz, C. P., and Moncrief, J. A.   *The Treatment of Burns* (2nd ed.). Philadelphia: Saunders, 1969.

Bloch, M.   Cold water for burns and scalds. *Lancet* 1:695, 1968.

Bollin, J. C.   Evaluation of a new topical agent for burn therapy: Silver sulfadiazine (Silvadene). *J.A.M.A.* 230:1184–1185, 1974.

Dalili, H., and Adriani, J.   The efficacy of local anesthetics in blocking the sensations of itch, burning, and pain in normal and "sunburned" skin. *Clin. Pharmacol. Ther.* 12:913–919, 1971.

Moncrief, J. A.   Burns. *N. Engl. J. Med.* 288:444–454, 1973.

Moncrief, J. A. (ed.).   Topical antibacterial therapy of the burn wound. *Clin. Plast. Surg.* 1:563–576, 1974.

Nance, F. C., Lewis, V. L., Jr., Hines, J. L., Barnett, D. P., and O'Neill, J. A.   Aggressive outpatient care of burns. *J. Trauma* 12:144–146, 1972.

Pearson, R. W.   Response of human epidermis to graded thermal stress: A morphologic comparison of burns, cold-induced blisters and pemphigus vulgaris. *Arch. Environ. Health* 11:498–507, 1965.

Sørensen, B.   First aid in burn injuries: Treatment at home with cold water. *Mod. Treat.* 4:1199–1202, 1967.

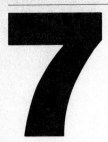

Corns and calluses

I. **Definition and pathophysiology.** Corns (clavi) and calluses are acquired areas of thickened skin that appear over sites of repeated or prolonged trauma to the epithelium. Neither soft corns nor hard corns occur in normal feet. These lesions arise as a result of pressure, friction, and shearing forces of bone (through the overlying skin) against adjacent digits, metatarsal heads, or footwear. The severity and type of growth are related to the degree and chronicity of the local irritation. The formation of the center (nucleus, radix) of a corn is secondary to vascular changes and fibrosis underlying the point of maximum stress. In both conditions there is marked hyperkeratosis of the stratum corneum overlying an epidermis that is otherwise the same thickness as adjacent skin.

Some studies show that the structure of keratin in callus differs from that of the normal stratum corneum. The individual cells are thicker, much more highly interdigitated, and the intercellular spaces are occupied by a dense cement material. All signs of desquamation are absent. The keratin appears to be similar in structure to that of finger pad and nail.

Corns are more symptomatic and better demarcated than calluses. They appear most frequently over the dorsolateral aspect of the fifth toes, but may be seen commonly at any point under the metatarsal ends. Small "seed corns" may be found anywhere on the plantar surface. Poorly fitting shoes are the most frequent cause of corns. Soft corns that result from pressure of the head of the proximal phalanx of the fifth toe on the base of the proximal phalanx of the fourth toe, or those that result from interdigital maceration, are most often located in the fourth interdigital web.

Calluses are more diffuse hyperkeratotic areas present most commonly under the first and/or fifth metatarsal heads. They are seen also as occupational marks, e.g., the callused palms of a laborer or the callused fingers of a violinist.

II. **Subjective data.** Corns may cause a constant dull discomfort or a severe knifelike pain on downward pressure. Calluses are either asymptomatic or are painful on pressure, causing a feeling somewhat akin to walking with a pebble in one's shoe. Lateral pressure elicits pain in a wart; direct pressure produces pain in a corn.

III. **Objective data**

   A. Corns are sharply delineated, hyperkeratotic, small (several millimeters in diameter or smaller) areas with a central translucent area. They are conical in shape, with the apex pointing into the tissue. Soft corns are less discrete, whitish thickenings found in the interdigital webs. If one palpates these lesions, an underlying bony prominence will always be found.

B. Calluses are large (millimeters to centimeters in diameter) diffuse areas of thickened skin with indefinite borders.

IV. Assessment. If a suspect lesion is pared down (debrided), a number of differential features become apparent.

A. Corns. A central nucleus becomes evident; with continued debridement this clear area becomes smaller and eventually disappears, at which point the normal skin markings can again be followed through the lesion.

B. Soft corns. These are often confused with simple maceration or an interdigital fungal infection. Paring the lesion will reveal a central nucleus and at times a small sinus tract at the base of the interdigital web. This sinus may close intermittently and result in recurrent bouts of bacterial infection.

C. Calluses. The normal skin markings remain evident, and no nucleus is found.

D. Plantar warts (see also p. 191). A central area composed of red and black dots, punctate bleeding, and obliteration of skin marking will be revealed on debridement. The dots represent thrombosed capillaries in the highly vascularized wart. A callus will commonly overlie a wart and be responsible for the associated discomfort.

V. Therapy

A. Therapy to allay symptoms

1. With both corns and calluses the cause of pain is thickened hyperkeratotic areas of skin. The pain caused by such a mass may be completely eradicated simply by reducing the lesion by debridement with a No. 15 blade or a No. 86 Beaver or No. 313 Gillette chisel blade. To ensure satisfactory results with a corn, it is often advisable to anesthetize the area (to remove the entire central nucleus). The following instructions will enable the patient to carry out intermittent debridement:

   a. Cut out a piece of 40% salicylic acid plaster slightly larger than the lesion and apply it to the skin, sticky side down.

   b. Apply felt pad fashioned to fit around the lesion to relieve the pressure.

   c. Leave overnight, or for as long as 5–7 days for very thick lesions.

   d. Remove the dressing and soak the foot in water.

   e. Remove whitened, soft, and macerated skin with a rough towel, pumice stone, or callus file.

   f. Reapply plaster as often as necessary to keep the lesion flat.

   g. As a corn thins, protective felt padding is all that is necessary.

2. At times, injection of a small amount of corticosteroid (Aristocort, Celestone, Kenalog) beneath a painful corn will result in dramatic relief of symptoms.

B. Definitive therapy. Removal of the lesion treats only the result and not the cause of the difficulty. Poorly fitting footwear, anatomic malformations, faulty weight distribution, or similar factors must be corrected or the hyperkeratoses will rapidly recur. Both corns and calluses will disappear after the causative factors have been removed. Corrective shoe supports, x-ray studies for anatomic defects, and referral to a podiatrist or orthopedic surgeon are warranted in difficult cases.

References

Carney, R. G. Confusing keratotic lesions of the sole. *Cutis* 7:32–34, 1971.

Montgomery, R. M. Corns, calluses and warts. Differential diagnosis. *N.Y. State J. Med.* 63:1532–1534, 1963.

Orfanos, C. E., Mahrle, G., and Ruska, H. Callus and its keratin before and after treatment with sodium thioglycolate: A study by scanning and conventional electron microscopy. *Br. J. Dermatol.* 85:437–449, 1971.

Potter, G. K. Histopathology of clavi. *J. Am. Podiatry Assoc.* 63:57–66, 1973.

Root, M. L., Orien, W. P., and Weed, J. H. *Normal and Abnormal Function of the Foot: Clinical Biomechanics* (vol. 2). Los Angeles: Clinical Biomechanics Corp., 1977.

Woodland, L. J. Corns, callosities and footwear. *Med. J. Aust.* 39:638–641, 1952.

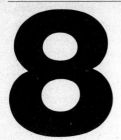

Dermatitis (eczema)

I. Definition and pathophysiology. The different forms of superficial inflammatory diseases of the skin represent the most common reaction pattern seen by the dermatologist. The morphologic and histopathologic changes in all forms of dermatitis and eczema, terms that are used interchangeably, are similar. The earliest and mildest changes are erythema and edema. These early changes may progress to vesiculation and oozing and then to crusting and scaling. Finally, if the process becomes chronic, the skin will become lichenified (thickened, with prominent skin markings), excoriated, and either hypopigmented or hyperpigmented.

The microscopic changes in this process show: (1) early, intercellular and intracellular fluid accumulation, with resultant vesicle formation and associated dermal vasodilatation and infiltration with chronic inflammatory cells; and (2) later, thickening of the epidermis and altered keratinization patterns, with retention of nuclei in the stratum corneum.

The factors that may initiate dermatitis are numerous, and the patterns of the dermatitis will dictate both the clinical classification and therapy.

The following categories of dermatitis will be discussed separately:

Atopic dermatitis, p. 45
Circumscribed chronic dermatitis, p. 49
Contact dermatitis, p. 50
Hand dermatitis, p. 53
Nummular dermatitis, p. 54

Atopic dermatitis

I. Definition and pathophysiology. Atopic dermatitis is an intensely pruritic, chronic eruption. It is the most common type of infantile eczema and is also seen in characteristic patterns in children, adolescents, and adults. Ninety percent of affected children manifest their disease by 5 years of age. Approximately 70% of patients with atopic dermatitis have a family history of atopy, about 3% of infants have some evidence of atopic dermatitis during the first few months of life, and about 50% of children with atopic dermatitis develop either rhinitis or asthma. Atopic dermatitis appears to be of polygenic or multifactional inheritance. Severe, easily triggered itching is the outstanding feature of this entity. Many of the clinical signs seen are secondary to scratching and rubbing of the skin. Atopic dermatitis may be particularly devastating in its effects on the patient's mental well-being and emotional development, as it is frequently present during the most critical periods of life. In infancy it interferes with a healthy mother-child relationship; in adolescence and early adulthood it plagues and disfigures patients during a crucial formative period. Emotional stress and altered family interactions play an important role in its course.

Patients with atopic dermatitis often have elevated levels of IgE skin-sensitizing antibodies (reagin), and there is usually a correlation between IgE serum level and the severity, duration, and amount of body surface affected by dermatitis. There are, however, many facts that argue against IgE's playing an important role in the causation of this entity. About 20 percent of adults with atopic dermatitis have normal or low IgE, and others have no IgE at all, while there are some patients with enormous elevations of IgE who have no dermatitis. Further, in infantile eczema IgE levels are consistently low or normal. Also, IgE does not mediate delayed hypersensitivity reactions of which eczema/dermatitis is considered an exemplary type. It has never been shown that reaginic antibodies, with their associated allergens, can actually incite clinical atopic skin disease. Skin testing, hyposensitization, and special diets are usually unrewarding.

A lower clinical incidence of allergic contact dermatitis is seen in patients with atopic dermatitis than in patients with some other dermatoses; it has been shown that the incidence of poison ivy allergy is 10 times less frequent in patients with atopic dermatitis than in the general population. Evidence of defective leukocyte phagocytosis, decreased absolute numbers and percentage of T lymphocytes, and depressed or absent T-cell response to *Candida,* phytohemagglutinin, and streptokinase-streptodornase in patients with atopic dermatitis suggests that this disorder may represent a state of cellular immunodeficiency rather than one of heightened allergy. There is also evidence that there is an abnormal balance between alpha- and beta-receptors in the skin, resulting, in a physiologic sense, in a blockade of the beta-receptors on the surface of atopic epidermal cells. Atopic patients react in an aberrant fashion to many environmental and physiologic factors: they demonstrate heightened and prolonged pruritus in response to normally sub-threshold stimuli and an altered vascular response to pressure and injections of histamine, serotonin, cholinergic and sympathomimetic agents, as well as abnormal reactions to heat and cold.

II. **Subjective data.** The primary and predominant symptom of atopic dermatitis is itching. This often sets up a vicious cycle: itching leads to scratching, scratching causes lichenification and other changes, and lichenification lowers the threshold for renewed itching.

III. **Objective data**

   A. In the **infantile phase** of atopic dermatitis (age 2 months–2 years) there is involvement primarily of the chest, face, scalp, neck, and extensor extremities with erythematous papulovesicles and oozing. Some infants also have very dry skin that predisposes them to itching and recurrent inflammation.

   B. In the **childhood phase** (between the ages of 4 and 10 years) the lesions are less acute and exudative, more scattered, and often localized in the flexor folds of the neck, elbows, wrists, and knees. Dry papules, excoriations, lichenification, and periorbital erythema and edema are common.

   C. In the **adolescent and adult phase** (from the early teens to the early twenties) the lesions are primarily dry, lichenified, hyperpigmented plaques in flexor areas and about the eyes. Persistent hand dermatitis may be the only remnant of an atopic diathesis.

D. These three phases may imperceptibly blend together, or any of the changes may be seen at any time.

Although atopic dermatitis may disappear with time, it is estimated that 30–80% of atopic patients will continue to have intermittent episodes of exacerbation throughout life, often when under physical or emotional stress.

IV. Assessment

A. A detailed personal, family, environmental, and psychologic history is mandatory for delivering proper care.

B. Factors that often trigger pruritus include the following: extreme heat or cold, rapid changes in temperature, sweating, irritating or occlusive medications or clothing (especially wool and silk), greases, oils, soaps and detergents, and, at times, inhalants or other environmental allergens.

C. Concomitants of atopic dermatitis include pathologic changes in the eye (posterior cataract, keratoconus, and retinal detachment) and lowered resistance to viral infections—especially with herpes simplex and vaccinia viruses—resulting in dissemination of usually localized infections. Patients with atopic dermatitis should not be vaccinated nor be near family or friends who have had recent vaccinations or have active herpes simplex infections. If vaccination is mandatory, it should take place immediately after administering vaccinia immune globulin (0.3 ml/kg IM), or should utilize newer strains of vaccinia virus that reduce the risk of eczema vaccinatum.

V. Therapy. The aims of therapy are to decrease trigger factors and pruritus, suppress inflammation, lubricate the skin, and alleviate anxiety.

A. Preventive measures

1. The environment should be kept at a constant temperature, and excess humidity should be avoided. Clothing worn next to the skin should be absorbent and nonirritating (cotton), laundered with bland soaps, and thoroughly rinsed. A vacation in a warm, dry climate is often beneficial. Adequate rest and relaxation are important.

2. Eliminate excessive bathing and other factors that promote xerosis. Keep the skin moist and supple (see Dry Skin, p. 68). Use a bland nonirritating soap or just a bath oil.

3. Emollients or medications should be applied immediately after bathing in order to "trap" water in the skin. Frequent application of bland lubricants both soothes and physically protects the skin and is the most important single measure in the therapy of atopic dermatitis.

4. Scratch and intradermal allergy tests are not useful. Patch tests for contact allergies may be productive. A decrease in environmental allergens and trial elimination diets might be considered if the more usual therapeutic measures fail, but these measures are usually not helpful.

5. The patient's emotional stability is essential. Continued contact with

an optimistic and reassuring physician will allay much anxiety. Occasionally, formal psychiatric therapy will be of benefit.

6. Short-term hospitalization is often efficacious, and improvement in the skin may appear before medications are applied. This complete but temporary environmental and emotional rearrangement will often suffice to break the itch-scratch cycle.

B. Treatment for active dermatitis

1. Exudative areas should be compressed with aluminum acetate (Burow's) or aluminum chloride solution (see p. 313), 20 min 4–6 times a day, or the patient placed in a tub with antipruritic and/or emollient additives such as oatmeal (Aveeno or Oilated Aveeno) or lubricating bath additives (see p. 315).

2. The primary and most important therapeutic tool in eczema is the frequent use of **topical corticosteroids.** They should be applied in small amounts 2–3 times a day and with occlusion if this is tolerated (see p. 273). If the skin remains dry, use emollients between steroid applications. This therapy will suppress inflammation and stop pruritus, thus interrupting the inflammation-itch-scratch-inflammation cycle. Treatment should be initiated with a fluorinated steroid in order to quickly quell inflammation and pruritus. If maintenance therapy is needed, 1% hydrocortisone or a low-strength fluorinated steroid are more appropriate. Ointments are better lubricants for dry skin and are often the base of choice for chronic lesions. Alternate application of corticosteroids with lubricants in order to avoid prolonged steroid use with concomitant adverse topical effects and tachyphylaxis (see p. 273).

3. **Tar compounds** (Estar gel; Zetar emulsion; T gel; liquor carbonis detergens 5–10% in hydrophilic ointment; or others [see p. 307]) are useful as adjunctive therapy in patients with chronic dermatitis. Their use may be alternated with the corticosteroids (i.e., tars overnight, corticosteroids during the day), or they may be applied at the same time to affected skin, or used in the bath.

4. **Antihistamines** by mouth will often suppress pruritus, allay anxiety, and allow sleep. These drugs are particularly useful in treating infants and children with widespread or very pruritic disease. The dose administered should be gradually increased to an effective level (see p. 246). In acute cases these drugs should be given on a continuous basis. Hydroxyzine is often the drug of choice.

5. Long-term administration of systemic corticosteroids plays no part in the therapy of atopic dermatitis. Acute flare-ups may be suppressed by a short-term course of prednisone (40–60 mg PO every day to 0 in 10–14 days) or one injection of 6 mg betamethasone sodium phosphate and betamethasone acetate suspension (Celestone), or 40–80 mg of methylprednisolone (Depo-Medrol), or 40 mg triamcinolone acetonide (Kenalog), or triamcinolone diacetate (Aristocort). Occasionally the dermatitis will flare up after cessation of steroids, but usually the eczematous disease will not reappear for months after one such course.

6. Photochemotherapy (PUVA) (see p. 220) can induce remission in selected patients with recalcitrant chronic atopic dermatitis. UBV phototherapy used along with emollients or tars is also very effective.

Circumscribed chronic dermatitis (lichen simplex chronicus)

I. **Definition and pathophysiology.** Circumscribed chronic dermatitis (lichen simplex chronicus) is a localized, chronic pruritic disorder resulting from repeated scratching and rubbing. Patients with this disease often have other atopic manifestations (asthma, allergic rhinitis) and frequently have a positive personal and family history of atopic disorders. The original pruritogenic stimulus usually remains undefined; it could have been an insect bite, constricting clothing, contact or seborrheic dermatitis, or psoriasis. Once the itch-scratch-lichenification cycle is established, it makes little difference what initially incited the problem. Scratching in these patients seems to be a conditioned response, one that becomes a fixed pattern and has a relative specificity for certain areas of skin, all in areas easily accessible to the patient. Lichenified skin tends to be more itchy than normal skin following minor stimuli, thus leading to further scratching. It must be emphasized that the scratching of these lichenified areas is not always unpleasant—it is sometimes almost erotic—and this secondary gain may interfere with conscientious application of therapy by the patient. Scratching is often vigorously accomplished with the heels, nails, combs, or other implements. This repeated trauma to the skin results in an increased number of cells undergoing mitosis, an increased transepidermal transit time, and hyperplasia involving all components of the epidermis. Within nodular lesions there may also be thickened nerve fibers, axon and Schwann cell proliferation, neuroma-schwannoma formation, and axon swelling. The extreme pruritus in chronic lesions may be related to the increased number of dermal nerves.

II. **Subjective data.** Continuous, spasmodic, or paroxysmal pruritus is the only symptom.

III. **Objective data.** These well-circumscribed, lichenified plaques, at times with psoriasiform scaling, are located most frequently on the ankles and anterior tibial and nuchal areas. The inner thighs, sides of the neck, extensor surfaces of the forearms, and anogenital areas may also be affected. Dry keratotic papules and giant "scratch papules" or prurigo nodules are also a response to repeated scratching. Patients will usually have only one area of involvement.

IV. **Assessment.** Detailed questioning regarding the itch stimulus is worthwhile but often fruitless. Psychogenic factors are important. Secondary infection or sensitization to topical therapeutic agents is not uncommon.

V. **Therapy.** In spite of the chronicity of these lesions, effective therapy will usually induce remission of the pruritus and the lichenification within 1–2 weeks.

    A. **Fluorinated topical corticosteroids,** usually applied under occlusion, are extremely effective. Cordran tape applied repeatedly for 24-hr periods is also a most useful modality.

    B. **Intralesional injection** of corticosteroids will induce involution most rapidly and is often the therapy of choice (see pp. 272 and 285).

    C. **Topical photochemotherapy** may induce remission in those responding poorly to other forms of treatment.

    D. **Antihistamines** or ataractic agents occasionally are of value, especially before bed.

E. Emollients containing antipruritic agents (menthol, phenol) or tar can also be useful (see p. 289). Agents with phenol should not be given to pregnant women.

Contact dermatitis

I. **Definition and pathophysiology.** Contact dermatitis may be produced by primary irritants or allergic sensitizers. **Primary irritant contact dermatitis** is a nonallergic reaction of the skin caused by exposure to irritating substances. Any substance can act as an irritant provided the concentration and duration of contact are sufficient. Most primary irritants are chemical substances, although physical and biologic (infectious) agents may produce the same picture. Irritants account for 80% of occupational contact dermatitis and also cause the most frequent type of nonindustrial contact reaction. The two types of irritants are: (1) mild, relative, or marginal irritants, which require repeated and/or prolonged contact to produce inflammation and include soaps, detergents, and most solvents; and (2) strong or absolute irritants, which are such damaging substances that they will injure skin immediately on contact (strong acids and alkalis). If daily exposure to mild irritants is continued, normal skin may become "hardened" or tolerant to this trauma, and contact may be continued without further evidence of irritation.

Allergic contact dermatitis is a manifestation of delayed hypersensitivity and results from the exposure of sensitized individuals to contact allergens. The sequence leading to inflammation is initiated by the binding of relatively simple chemical group(s) to an epidermal protein on or in the vicinity of Langerhans cells to form a complete antigen, which then reacts with sensitized T lymphocytes independent of free antibody or complement (type 4 reaction). These lymphocytes then release mediators that attract an inflammatory infiltrate including macrophages, neutrophils, basophils, and eosinophils that are involved in the eczematous response. Most contact allergens produce sensitization in only a small percentage of those exposed. Poison oak and ivy, which induce sensitization in more than 70% of the population, are marked exceptions to this rule. The incubation period after initial sensitization to an antigen is 5–21 days, while the reaction time after subsequent reexposure is 12–48 hr. Mild exposure of a sensitized person to poison oak or ivy, for example, will result in appearance of the rash in 2–3 days and clearing within the following 1–2 weeks; with massive exposure, lesions will appear more quickly (6–12 hr) and heal more slowly (2–3 weeks). Factors that contribute to the development of contact dermatitis include genetic predisposition, local concentration of antigen, duration of exposure, site variation in cutaneous permeability, and the development of immune tolerance. Other contributing factors may be friction, pressure, occlusion, maceration, heat and cold, and the presence of other skin diseases.

II. **Subjective data.** Primary irritants will cause an inelastic and stiff-feeling skin, discomfort related to dryness, pruritus secondary to inflammation, and pain related to fissures, blisters, and ulcers. As with other forms of acute and chronic dermatitis, the primary symptom of allergic contact dermatitis is pruritus.

III. Objective data (See color insert.)

A. Mild irritants produce erythema, microvesiculation, and oozing that may be indistinguishable from allergic contact dermatitis. Chronic exposure to mild irritants or allergens results in dry, thickened, and fissured skin.

B. Strong irritants cause blistering, erosion, and ulcers.

C. Mild allergic contact dermatitis is similar in appearance to the irritant eruption. A more typical allergic contact reaction will consist of grouped or linear tense vesicles and blisters. If involvement is severe there may be marked edema, particularly on the face, periorbital, and genital areas. The allergen is frequently transferred from hands to other areas of the body, where the rash then appears. Palms, soles, and scalp, however, are relatively resistant to contact reactions because of thicker stratum corneum and greater barrier function. The gradual appearance of the allergic contact eruption over a period of several days reflects the amount of antigen deposited on the skin and the reactivity of the individual site. Vesicle fluid, as in poison ivy, is a transudate and will not spread the eruption elsewhere on the body or to other people.

It is not the specific morphology of lesions that clinically distinguishes contact dermatitis from other types of eczema, but their distribution and configuration. The eruption is in exposed or contact areas and typically has a bizarre or artificial pattern, with sharp, straight margins, acute angles, and straight lines. Any eruption with such an unusual appearance should suggest contact dermatitis.

IV. Assessment.
Exact diagnosis is very important, since successful therapy depends on avoidance of contact with irritants and elimination of contact with allergens. The patient must be questioned about his or her total environment: home, work, hobbies, medications, clothing, cosmetics, and any other contactants. Inquiry must be detailed, imaginative, and frequently repetitive if the necessary details are to be elicited. Sensitization to components of topical medications is not uncommon and must be considered when an eruption is slow to disappear while being treated with what appears to be appropriate therapy.

Patch testing for contact allergens is essential for specific identification of causative agents (see p. 216). This test, in effect, attempts to reproduce the disease in diminutive form. There are no clinically useful methods available to evaluate patients thought to have an irritant dermatitis.

V. Therapy

A. Preventive measures—for primary irritant or hand dermatitis

1. **Decrease exposure to household and work irritants** such as soaps, detergents, solvents, bleaches, ammonia, and moist vegetables such as onions or garlic.

2. **Avoid abrasive soaps.** Remove all rings that occlude the underlying skin before doing any work. Waterless hand cleansers will remove stubborn soils and greases without significant damage to the skin. (Use of solvents to cleanse the skin is one of the most frequent predisposing factors.)

3. **Lubricate the skin** frequently with a bland cream or lotion such as Eucerin (see p. 297).

4. If possible, **wear heavy-duty vinyl gloves** or plastic gloves while working. Bluettes cotton knit lined gloves, Super Ebonettes Flock lined gloves, and Nimble Fingers gloves contain no rubber. Lined rubber gloves (Playtex) are acceptable, but occasionally patients become allergic to the rubber. Gloves provide excellent protection against mild irritants, but some antigens such as nickel may penetrate rubber-base gloves. High concentrations of irritants such as 10% potassium hydroxide will also penetrate. Gloves should be carefully chosen and frequently changed. Tru-Touch plastic gloves are very helpful, for they permit freer use of the hands while working. Thin white cotton liners (Dermal gloves) should be worn next to the skin to absorb sweat and prevent maceration.

5. **Barrier protective creams** designed to be used against aqueous compounds (Kerodex No. 71, SBS-44; West No. 311), solvents (Kerodex No. 51, SBS-46; West No. 411), or dusts (West No. 211) will be moderately useful. They should be applied in the morning and then reapplied at lunchtime and at work breaks.

B. Preventive measures—for allergic contact dermatitis

1. Wash thoroughly as soon as possible after exposure to antigens.

2. The results of hyposensitization to allergic contact antigens such as poison oak and ivy are usually of negligible, if any, benefit. Unpleasant and dangerous adverse effects can occur with currently available preparations.

C. Treatment for active dermatitis

1. Acute, mild-to-moderate, exudative, and vesicular

a. Aluminum acetate (Burow's solution) (diluted 1:20) or aluminum chloride (AluWets) cold compresses 20–30 min 4–6 times a day.

b. Soothing shake lotions, e.g., calamine.

c. After vesiculation subsides, a topical corticosteroid aerosol, cream, or lotion will help.

d. Antihistamines PO.

2. Acute, absolute irritant

a. Forceful and prolonged irrigation with water.

b. Then treat as for a burn (see p. 38).

3. Acute, severe, marked edema and bullae

a. Topical therapy as in **C.1.a.**

b. Tepid tub baths with Aveeno, 1 cup to ½ tub, 2–3 times a day, or cornstarch (see p. 315).

c. Early and aggressive treatment with systemic corticosteroids: Initial prednisone dosage should be at least 60 mg every day; the course should be no shorter than 2–3 weeks (see p. 280). Alternatives to oral prednisone include: ACTH gel 80 units q12h × 2, 6 mg betamethasone sodium phosphate and betamethasone acetate suspension (Celestone), 40–80 mg methylprednisolone (Depo-Medrol), 40 mg triamcinolone acetonide (Kenalog), or 40 mg triamcinolone diacetate (Aristocort), which are equally effective. Treatment with inadequate amounts of steroid for inadequate periods of time is unfortunately too common. Systemic corticosteroids should be withdrawn gradually to prevent a flare-up or rebound reaction. If the process is suppressed for too short a time, a generalized exacerbation of rash and symptoms may result when steroids are stopped. Inhibition of the rash and symptoms will be seen within 48 hr after therapy is initiated. It is essential that secondary infection such as impetigo, cellulitis, or erysipelas be diagnosed and treated before corticosteroid therapy is initiated. The clinical picture of erysipelas can at times be quite similar to that of an allergic contact dermatitis.

4. **Chronic contact or hand dermatitis**

   a. Soak the hands or other affected area for 5 min in water; then immediately apply a hydrophobic emollient (e.g., petrolatum) and/or topical corticosteroid **ointment** with or without occlusion.

   b. High-potency fluorinated corticosteroids are needed in the treatment of chronic hand dermatitis (see p. 274).

   Occasionally a preparation more concentrated than those commercially available is needed. A pharmacist can prepare 1% triamcinolone acetonide in propylene glycol by pouring off the liquid from a 5-ml vial of triamcinolone acetonide 40 mg/ml (Kenalog 40 injection) and then dissolving the sediment in 25 ml propylene glycol.

   c. Tar and/or iodochlorhydroxyquin preparations (see pp. 307 and 268) are useful adjuncts in chronic cases.

   d. UVB phototherapy or even photochemotherapy can be extremely useful in cases of chronic hand dermatitis.

5. Bacterial superinfection is not uncommon and should be treated with topical and systemic antibiotics.

Hand dermatitis

I. **Definition and pathophysiology.** Hand dermatitis is a common, chronic pruritic disorder that is perplexing and frustrating to patient and physician alike. The clinical changes are not specific and may be a manifestation of one or several precipitating or predisposing factors. It is most commonly a reaction to repeated contact with mild primary irritants such as soap and water, detergents, and solvents. The eruption itself is common in housewives, food handlers, bartenders, nurses, dentists, and surgeons. It is often called "housewife's eczema," "dishpan hands," and other colorful names, and it is the most frequent dermatitis seen in industry.

Chronic hand dermatitis is often a remnant or part of **atopic** or **nummular dermatitis.**

Allergic contact dermatitis will tend to involve the sides of the fingers and the dorsa of the hands more than the palms and show a more bizarre configuration.

Primary fungal infection or dermatophytid (id) reactions to **Tinea pedis** must always be considered in the differential diagnosis, and fungal scrapings and cultures obtained.

Dyshidrosiform eruptions involve the sides of fingers and palms preferentially and may also affect the soles of the feet as well. Hyperhidrosis may be seen in such patients, but no abnormality of sweating or of the eccrine apparatus is present.

Pustular psoriasis and hand involvement with other cutaneous eruptions, such as drug reactions, may also appear as hand dermatitis.

It is often impossible to find a specific etiology for chronic hand dermatitis.

II. **Subjective data.** Pruritus is the primary symptom, but dryness, fissuring, inelasticity, and superinfection often lead to inability to use the hands at all. Hand dermatitis is the cause of much social, personal, and financial grief.

III. **Objective data**

   A. Erythema, dryness, and chapping are the mildest changes.

   B. The most characteristic lesions are myriads of small "bubbles"— intraepidermal spongiotic vesicles—scattered on the sides of the fingers and, less often, throughout the palms.

   C. More severe changes include bulla formation and extreme hardening and inelasticity of the skin, with deep fissures.

   D. Hyperhidrosis and secondary bacterial infections are common.

IV. **Assessment.** A detailed history and physical examination must include inquiry about a personal or family history of atopy or psoriasis or other cutaneous disease; factors that precipitate and alleviate the dermatitis; and occupational, household, and hobby contactants. Patch testing, using a screening tray as well as properly diluted occupational or other agents that the patient has supplied, may identify a causative agent.

V. **Therapy.** See Contact Dermatitis, p. 51

Nummular dermatitis

I. **Definition and pathophysiology.** Nummular dermatitis, characterized by coin-shaped eczematous plaques, is a chronic, often very pruritic, but nonspecific reaction pattern found most commonly in older patients. It may also be a manifestation of atopic dermatitis in children, a reaction to topical irritants, or a manifestation of xerosis, particularly in wintertime. IgE levels are usually not elevated. Emotional stress has been emphasized as a contributing factor. The course tends to be chronic, with remission occurring frequently during the summer.

II. **Subjective data.** Pruritus is the primary symptom.

III. **Objective data.** Dry to inflammatory papular, vesicular, exudative, and/or crusted, round plaques 1–5 cm in diameter are located most commonly on the dorsa of the hands and forearms, lower legs, and buttocks.

IV. **Assessment.** Questioning should be directed toward eliciting a history of predisposing environmental factors (i.e., dryness), occupational or household work habits, other cutaneous diseases, and any recent or chronic emotionally stressful situation.

V. Therapy

A. Decrease exposure to irritants. If dryness is a factor, see the items outlined under Dry Skin, p. 67. Decrease amount of bathing and add bath oils and emollients.

B. For acute dermatitis, Burow's solution compresses, 20 min 3id, followed by:

C. Topical corticosteroids 1–3 times a day. Ointments are often preferable. Overnight application under occlusion is very effective, coupled with use of emollients during the day.

D. Intralesional corticosteroid injection will rapidly eliminate lesions.

E. Tar compounds (Estar; 10% liquor carbonis detergens in hydrophilic ointment; tar ointments; also see p. 307) and iodochlorhydroxyquin are occasionally useful. Daily application of topical corticosteroids and nightly use of the tar compounds and/or iodochlorhydroxyquin may work when either medication used alone is not wholly effective.

F. Phototherapy may be effective in nummular dermatitis as it is in other chronic inflammatory dermatoses.

G. Antihistamines, particularly hydroxyzine (Atarax, Vistaril), will diminish itch and anxiety.

References

CONTACT DERMATITIS

Adams, R. M. *Occupational Contact Dermatitis*. Philadelphia: Lippincott, 1969.

Baer, R. L., and Bickers, D. R. Allergic Contact Dermatitis, Photoallergic Contact Dermatitis and Phototoxic Dermatitis. In B. Safai and R. A. Good (eds.), *Immunodermatology*. New York: Plenum, 1981. Pp. 259–271.

Bettley, F. R. Management and treatment of contact eczema. *Br. Med. J.* 2:1245–1246.

Cronin, E. *Contact Dermatitis*. Edinburgh: Churchill Livingstone, 1981.

Epstein, W. Poison oak hyposensitization. *Arch. Dermatol.* 109:356–360, 1974.

Fisher, A. A. *Contact Dermatitis* (2nd ed.). Philadelphia: Lea & Febiger, 1973.

Fregert, S. *Manual of Contact Dermatitis*. Chicago: Year Book, 1974.

Hjorth, N. Contact dermatitis: 1980. *Br. J. Dermatol.* (Suppl. 18) 103:19–20, 1980.

Hjorth, N., and Wilkinson, D. W. Contact dermatitis. *Br. J. Dermatol.* 88:103–104, 1973.

Kligman, A. M. Poison ivy (*Rhus*) dermatitis. *Arch. Dermatol.* 77:149–180, 1958.

Rajka, G. *Atopic Dermatitis. Major Problems in Dermatology* (vol. 3). Philadelphia: Saunders, 1975.

Rostenberg, A., Jr. Primary irritant and allergic eczematous reactions: Their interactions. *Arch. Dermatol.* 75:547–558, 1957.

Roth, H. L., and Kierland, R. R. The natural history of atopic dermatitis. A 20-year follow-up study. *Arch. Dermatol.* 89:209–214, 1964.

Sax, N. I. *Dangerous Properties of Industrial Materials* (5th ed.). New York: Van Nostrand Reinhold, 1979.

Winkelmann, R. K.   Nonallergic factors in atopic dermatitis. *J. Allergy* 37:29–37, 1966.

CIRCUMSCRIBED CHRONIC DERMATITIS

Feuerman, E. J., and Sandbank, M.   Prurigo nodularis: Histological and electron microscopical study. *Arch. Dermatol.* 111:1472–1477, 1975.

Marks, R., and Wells, G. C.   Lichen simplex: Morphodynamic correlates. *Br. J. Dermatol.* 88:249–256, 1973.

Robertson, I. M., Jordon, J. M., and Whitlock, F. A.   Emotions and skin: II. The conditioning of scratch response in cases of lichen simplex. *Br. J. Dermatol.* 92:407–412, 1975.

Runne, U., and Orfanos, C. E.   Cutaneous neural proliferation in highly pruritic lesions of chronic prurigo. *Arch. Dermatol.* 113:787–791, 1977.

Shaffer, B., and Beerman, H.   Lichen simplex chronicus and its variants: A discussion of certain psychodynamic mechanisms and clinical and histopathologic correlations. *Arch. Dermatol. Syphilol.* 64:340–351, 1951.

Singh, G.   Atopy in lichen simplex (neurodermatitis circumscripta). *Br. J. Dermatol.* 89:625–627, 1973.

Vaatainen, N., Hannuksela, M., and Karvonen, J.   Local photochemotherapy in nodular prurigo. *Acta Dermatol. Venereol.* (Stockh.) 59:544–547, 1979.

ATOPIC DERMATITIS

Elliott, S. T., and Hanifan, J. M.   Delayed cutaneous hypersensitivity and lymphocyte transformation: Dissociation of atopic dermatitis. *Arch. Dermatol.* 115:36–39, 1979.

Finlay, A. Y., Nicholls, S., King, C. S., and Marks, R.   The "dry" non-eczematous skin associated with atopic eczema. *Br. J. Dermatol.* 102:249–256, 1980.

Hanifan, J. M.   Atopic dermatitis. *J. Am. Acad. Dermatol.* 6:1–13, 1982.

Hanifan, J. M., and Lobitz, W. C.   Newer concepts in atopic dermatitis. *Arch. Dermatol.* 113:663–370, 1977.

Horsmanheimo, M., Horsmanheimo, A., Banov, C. H., Ainsworth, S. K., and Feidenberg, H. H.   Cell-mediated immunity in vitro in atopic dermatitis. *Arch. Dermatol.* 115:161–164, 1979.

Jones, H. E., Lewis, C. W., and McMarlin, S. L.   Allergic contact sensitivity in atopic dermatitis. *Arch. Dermatol.* 107:217–222, 1973.

Jordon, J. M., and Whitlock, F. A.   Emotions and the skin: The conditioning of scratch responses in cases of atopic dermatitis. *Br. J. Dermatol.* 86:574–585, 1972.

Karel, I., Myska, V., and Kuicalova, E.   Ophthalmological changes in atopic dermatitis. *Acta Dermatol. Venereol.* (Stockh.) 45:381–386, 1965.

Morison, W. L., Parrish, J. A., and Fitzpatrick, T. B.   Oral psoralen photochemotherapy of atopic eczema. *Br. J. Dermatol.* 98:25–28, 1978.

Morison, W. L., Parrish, J. A., and Fitzpatrick, T. B.   Oral methoxsalen photochemotherapy of recalcitrant dermatoses of the palms and soles. *Br. J. Dermatol.* 99:297–302, 1978.

Silberberg-Sinakin, I., and Thorbecke, G. J.   Contact hypersensitivity and Langerhans cells. *J. Invest. Dermatol.* 75:61–64, 1980.

HAND DERMATITIS

Epstein, E.   Therapy of recalcitrant hand dermatitis. *Cutis* 15:346–376, 1975.

Epstein, E.   Hand dermatitis: Weekly report. *Dermatology* 11:1–7, 1979.

Jordan, W. P.   Allergic contact dermatitis in hand eczema. *Arch. Dermatol.* 110:567–569, 1974.

Shelley, W. B.   Dyshidrosis (pompholyx). *Arch. Dermatol. Syphilogr.* (Paris) 68:314–319, 1953.

Simmons, R. D. G. Ph.   Eczema of the Hands. In *Investigation into Dyshidrosiform Eruptions*. St. Louis: Green, 1966.

NUMMULAR DERMATITIS

Cowan, M. A.   Nummular eczema: A review, follow-up and analysis of 325 cases. *Arch. Dermatol. Venereol.* (Stockh.) 41:453–460, 1961.

Hellgren, L., and Mobacken, H.   Nummular eczema: Clinical and statistical data. *Arch. Dermatol. Venereol.* (Stockh.) 49:189–196, 1969.

Krueger, C. G., Kahn, G., Weston, W. L., and Mandel, M. J.   IgE levels in nummular eczema and ichthyosis. *Arch. Dermatol.* 107:56–58, 1975.

Weidman, A. I., and Sawicky, H. H.   Nummular eczema: Review of the literature: Survey of 516 case records and follow-up of 125 patients. *Arch. Dermatol.* 73:58–65, 1956.

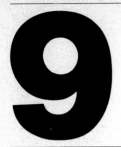

Diaper rash

I. Definition and pathophysiology. Diaper rash is the end result of constant exposure to an adverse local environment. Multiple factors may initiate or aggravate this eruption but the most important is overhydration. Other factors include: constant dampness, irritant chemicals, intestinal enzymes, stool, and contact reaction to rubber, plastic, diaper detergents, and disinfectants. Diarrhea, high environmental heat and humidity, infrequent change of diapers, inadequate skin cleansing, and occlusive, impermeable diapers also contribute to this primary irritant contact dermatitis. Ammonia plays no role in induction of common diaper dermatitis. Once established, diaper dermatitis may be colonized by organisms (*Staphlococcus aureus, Candida*) that induce secondary changes. Diaper rash is unusual during the first month of life and most common between the second and fourth months, but may continue until diapers are no longer needed. Underlying atopic, seborrheic, or psoriatic diathesis may predispose to this eruption.

II. Subjective data. The baby feels itchy and uncomfortable and is irritable.

III. Objective data

A. The usual mild diaper rash is a primary irritant reaction and appears as simple, shiny erythema. The eruption is located over the convex contact areas, i.e., buttocks, genitalia, lower abdomen, and upper thighs, sparing the flexural folds. Legs and heels may be affected from contact with the wet diaper.

B. With more intense involvement there will be erythematous papules, vesicles or erosions, oozing, and ulceration.

C. An erosive and crusted urethral meatitis is often seen in males, and spots of blood may appear on the diaper.

D. A chronic eruption, or one that is slowly healing, appears as a glazed erythema.

E. Erythematous papules and pustules scattered within and outside the eruption suggest *C. albicans* superinfection.

F. The explosive, widespread appearance of psoriasiform scaling papules and plaques, usually preceded by inflammation in the diaper area (or scalp), is not uncommon. These infants often have a family history of psoriasis and up to 25% later develop true psoriasis.

IV. Assessment

A. A detailed history concerning skin and diaper care is necessary to discover the immediate predisposing factors.

B. The entire child should be inspected to see if there is any evidence of infantile eczema or other skin disease.

C. Erosive lesions must be differentiated from those of congenital syphilis.

D. Pustule contents should be examined by Gram's stain and/or fungal stain and cultured on blood agar plates and/or fungal media for bacterial pathogens or *C. albicans*. Gram-negative rods may play a collaborative role with *C. albicans* in pustular eruptions; this is important to remember both in assessing the lesions and in choosing therapeutic agents.

V. Therapy

A. Preventive. The primary aim of long-term management of diaper dermatitis is prevention. A number of measures must be kept in mind:

1. The area must be kept free of irritants and as dry as possible. This entails frequent diaper changes. Excessively bulky or multilayered diapers should not be used.

2. Cleanse the diaper area after each change with tepid to warm water, or with pledgets soaked in baby oil, mineral oil, Balneol lotion, or Cetaphil lotion. Avoid excessive use of soaps and water. Disposable paper diapers are useful.

3. Talcum or baby powder (not cornstarch, which may be metabolized by microorganisms) or a bland protective ointment (Desitin, Diaparene) or adherent paste (1 part Burow's solution, 2 parts Aquaphor, 3 parts zinc oxide ointment) may prevent maceration and irritation.

4. Discontinue use of occlusive pants.

5. Try to keep the baby's room from becoming excessively hot and humid.

6. Thorough rinsing of diapers is necessary to reduce the alkalinity imparted by soap and detergent residues. A final rinse in dilute acetic acid (30 ml [1 oz] vinegar to 1 gallon water) will help.

B. Treatment of a preexisting inflammatory eruption

1. If mild, apply a topical corticosteroid, such as 1% hydrocortisone cream. This can be followed by application of zinc oxide ointment, adherent paste (as described in **A.3**) or petrolatum, all of which may increase steroid penetration and keep the steroid from being washed off by urine.

2. If *C. albicans* infection is present, add an antiyeast agent to the steroid (1% hydrocortisone–3% iodochlorhydroxyquin [Vioform-Hydrocortisone]; corticosteroid cream plus antiyeast agent such as clotrimazole [Lotrimin, Mycelex], Miconazole [Monistat-Derm], or nystatin [Nilstat, Mycostatin]). An antiyeast medication may be used alone but the inflammation will subside very slowly. Take care to use the lowest potency corticosteroid cream that is effective, and for the shortest time possible. Nystatin powder is a convenient medication both for treating yeast infection and for decreasing maceration and friction. Oral nystatin suspension (1 ml [100,000 units] 4 times a day) should be given to infants with severe or recurrent eruptions.

    a. Triamcinolone-neomycin-gramicidin-nystatin cream (Mycolog) should not be used because of the potential for sensitization to its ingredients and the possibility of corticosteroid-induced-atrophy. Mycolog ointment lacks the most potent sensitizer (ethylenediamine) but others remain (neomycin) and adverse reaction to topical steroids must still be kept in mind.

3. Psoriasiform generalized lesions respond slowly (weeks to months) to topical corticosteroids and emollients. It is imperative also to treat any inflammatory lesions in the diaper area.

4. Local bacterial infection should be treated with an antibiotic cream or thinly applied ointment: polymyxin B-neomycin-gramicidin (Neosporin-G) cream, or ointment (Neosporin), or polymyxin B-bacitracin ointment (Polysporin), bacitracin ointment, or povidone-iodine ointment.

5. If more severe inflammation or vesiculation and oozing are present, Burow's solution compresses should also be used, 20 min 3id. Avoid greasy occlusive medications at this stage.

6. For urethral meatitis, remove crusts with water, saline, or Burow's compresses and apply topical antibiotic ointment.

References

Andersen, S. L., and Thomsen, K. Psoriasiform napkin dermatitis. *Br. J. Dermatol.* 84:316–319, 1971.

Burgoon, C. F., Jr., Urbach, F., and Grover, W. D. Diaper dermatitis. *Pediatr. Clin. North Am.* 8:835–856, 1961.

Dixon, P. N., Warin, R. P., and English, M. P. Alimentary *Candida albicans* and napkin rashes. *Br. J. Dermatol.* 86:458–462, 1972.

Jacobs, A. H. Eruptions in the diaper area. *Pediatr. Clin. North Am.* 25:209–224, 1978.

Koblenzer, P. J. Diaper dermatitis: An overview with emphasis on rational therapy based on etiology and pathogenesis. *Clin. Pediatr.* (Phila.) 12:386–392, 1973.

Leyden, J. J., Katz, S., Stewart, R., and Kligman, A. M. Urinary ammonia and ammonia-producing microorganisms in infants with and without diaper dermatitis. *Arch. Dermatol.* 113:1678–1680, 1977.

Leyden, J. J., and Kligman, A. M. The role of microorganisms in diaper dermatitis. *Arch. Dermatol.* 114:56–59, 1978.

Neville, E., and Finn, O. Psoriasiform napkin dermatitis: A follow-up study. *Br. J. Dermatol.* 92:279–285, 1975.

Rebora, A., and Leyden, J. J. Napkin (diaper) dermatitis and gastrointestinal carriage of *Candida albicans*. *Br. J. Dermatol.* 105:551–555, 1981.

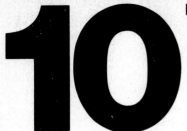

Drug eruptions, allergic

I. **Definition and pathophysiology.** Drug reactions may take numerous forms. The most common of these are hypersensitivity reactions, most frequently caused by mediators released after exposure to sensitizing molecules.

    A. Immediate allergic reactions occur within 1 hr and consist of pruritus, urticaria, flushing, or other manifestations of anaphylaxis.

    B. Accelerated reactions take place within 1–72 hr of drug administration and also consist primarily of itching and hives, but laryngeal edema may also be seen.

    C. Late reactions start more than 3 days after initiation of drug therapy and may be urticarial, serum-sickness-like, or exanthematous. In addition, drug reactions may be manifested as fever or as abnormal reactions of one or many organ systems (e.g., hemolysis, thrombocytopenia, renal damage).

    D. Exanthematous eruptions, the most common type of reaction, usually appear within 1 week after the causative drug has been started; sensitization may occur after the first exposure or may develop to an antigen that the patient has been intermittently exposed to for years. Rash may also start within 4–7 days after the offending drug has been stopped. Whenever the eruption starts, whether it is while the patient is taking the drug or after its discontinuation, the cutaneous lesions will become more severe and widespread over the following several days to a week and then will clear over the following 7–14 days. This slow and constant evolution of the eruption makes it difficult to single out the offending agent from among numerous drugs, and whether or not the correct one has been stopped, the rash will go through its 2- –3-week course.

    E. Erythema multiforme and erythema nodosum may also be caused by drugs and are discussed in separate chapters. Less common forms of drug reactions, which will not be discussed in detail, include toxic epidermal necrolysis, leukocytoclastic vasculitis, fixed drug eruptions, bullous and pustular drug eruptions, lichen planus-like eruptions, abnormal pigmentary reactions, and exfoliative dermatitis. Toxic epidermal necrolysis, with extensive sheetlike shearing off of epidermis, may be life-threatening, as may drug-induced vasculitis.

II. **Subjective data.** Mild to severe pruritus is the predominant symptom of late exanthematous eruptions.

III. **Objective data**

    A. The typical exanthematous eruption will begin as faint pink macules, which gradually enlarge to bright red macular areas or edematous plaques.

B. At times there is mild central clearing within an erythematous plaque.

C. The eruption may mimic the pinpoint redness of scarlet fever, the blotchy pattern of measles, or the generalized distribution of a viral exanthem.

D. Lesions most often start first and clear first from the head and upper extremities. Lesions of the trunk and lower legs often follow in succession.

E. Palms, soles, and mucous membranes may be involved.

F. Mild petechiae or frank purpura on the lower extremities are commonly associated with a vigorous eruption, but this does not mean that vasculitis or thrombocytopenia is present.

G. More serious and violent reactions may include bullae, erosions, extensive purpura, or exfoliation. Palpable purpuric lesions that do not blanch on pressure (diascopy) suggest vasculitis.

H. Many types of drugs can produce identical eruptions; the morphology of the rash usually gives no clue as to the causative agent.

IV. Assessment

A. Questioning about offending drugs must be detailed and direct. Any substance that enters any body orifice, with the exception of most foods and water, is suspect. Specific questioning concerning eye or ear drops, nasal sprays, suppositories, injections, immunization, nerve pills, vitamins, laxatives, sedatives, and analgesics, including even aspirin, must be pursued. Nonmedical items such as preservatives, tonics, toothpaste, and topical lotions must also be considered. Penicillin is present in small amounts in some biologic products (such as poliomyelitis vaccine) and in dairy products from cows treated for mastitis. The possibility of illicit drugs must be considered.

Penicillin drugs, sulfonamides, and blood products are the most common causes of cutaneous reactions to drugs (see Table 2). Ampicillin, for instance, can be expected to incite an eruption in approximately 5% of courses of drug therapy. Drug-specific quantitative data are available to help evaluate which agents are the most likely causes of drug-induced rash, itching, or hives. This information gives reaction rates for all commonly used drugs and allows one to calculate which drug might (as well as might not) have caused an adverse reaction (see Arndt and Jick, 1976).

B. If palpable purpuric lesions are present a complete physical and laboratory examination is required with an eye toward ruling out vasculitic involvement of other organ systems and toward ruling out other causes of vasculitis such as infection or collagen vascular disease. A skin biopsy should be considered to confirm the diagnosis.

C. Erythema multiforme and erythema nodosum are discussed in separate chapters (see pp. 71 and 75).

D. Skin testing with penicilloyl-polylysine (PPL, Pre-Pen) and a "minor determinant mixture" (usually diluted aqueous penicillin G) can accurately predict reactions to all penicillins. RAST tests on serum for penicillin

Table 2. Drugs with reaction rates > 1%

Drug	Reaction rate (reactions/1000 recipients)
Trimethoprim-sulfamethoxazole	59
Ampicillin	52
Semisynthetic penicillins	36
Whole blood	35
Corticotropin	28
Blood platelets	28
Erythromycin	23
Sulfisoxazole	17
Penicillin G	16
Gentamicin sulfate	16
Cephalosporins	13
Quinidine	12
Plasma protein fraction	12

Source: Arndt and Jick, 1976.

allergy will give similar data without the danger of injecting an allergenic drug. No other in vivo or in vitro tests are currently available or routinely used for ascertaining the cause of drug eruptions or screening potentially allergic individuals. Penicillin skin testing is indicated only in special circumstances and should be performed by experienced personnel in a hospital.

V. Therapy

A. Antihistamines PO.

B. Soothing tepid water baths with Aveeno or cornstarch and/or cool compresses may be useful.

C. A drying antipruritic lotion (calamine with or without 0.25% menthol and/or 1% phenol) or lubricating antipruritic emollients (Eucerin or Keri Lotion with 0.25% menthol and 1% phenol) applied prn will help relieve the pruritis. Lotions with phenol should not be given to pregnant women.

D. If signs and symptoms are severe, a 2-week course of systemic corticosteroids (prednisone, starting at 60 mg) or injection of a repository corticosteroid preparation (see Contact Dermatitis, p. 52) will usually stop the symptoms and prevent further progression of the eruption within 48 hr of the onset of therapy.

References

Arndt, K. A., and Jick, H.   Rates of cutaneous reactions to drugs. *J. A. M. A.* 235:918–923, 1976.

Bruinsma, W.   *A Guide to Drug Eruptions.* De Zwaluw, P. O. Box 2, Oostuizen, The Netherlands, 1982.

Cluff, L. E., Caranasos, G. J., and Stewart, R. B.   *Clinical Problems with Drugs.* Philadelphia: Saunders, 1975.

Demis, J. D.   Allergy and drug sensitivity of skin. *Annu. Rev. Pharmacol.* 9:457–482, 1969.

Felix, R. H., and Comaish, J. S.   Value of patch and other skin tests in drug eruptions. *Lancet* 1:1017–1019, 1974.

Levine, B. B.   Immunochemical mechanisms of drug allergy. *Annu. Rev. Med.* 17:23–38, 1966.

Miller, R. R., and Greenblatt, D. J. (eds.).   *Drug Effects in Hospitalized Patients.* New York: Wiley, 1976.

Wintroub, B. U., Shiffman, N. J., and Arndt, K. A.   Adverse Cutaneous Reactions to Drugs. In T. B. Fitzpatrick et al. (eds.), *Dermatology in General Medicine* (2nd ed.). New York: McGraw-Hill, 1979.

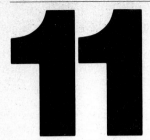

Dry skin (chapping, xerosis) and ichthyosis vulgaris

I. Definition and pathophysiology. Dry skin and ichthyosis vulgaris are often indistinguishable, and since the clinical findings blend together it is useful to discuss the two entities together. Dry skin, a dehydration of the stratum corneum, is a very common condition especially prevalent among the elderly. It is also found to be associated with diverse other developmental and acquired cutaneous conditions such as ichthyosis and atopic and contact dermatitis. When it is severe enough to be associated with inflammation and pruritus, it has also been termed *asteatotic eczema* and *winter itch*. The sequence leading to dry skin varies considerably from person to person and in many cases remains obscure. Some individuals will have always noticed a familial tendency to excessive dryness and chapping. Others will state that this problem appeared only with increasing age or illness and that it has tended to be seasonal.

Environmental factors are extremely important: Repeated exposure to solvents, soaps, and disinfectants will remove lipid from the skin, thus damaging the cutaneous barrier and increasing water loss up to 75 times normal; decreasing relative humidity and exposure to dry, cold winds will lead to water loss from the stratum corneum and will literally "pull" water from the skin. Factors that act to decrease relative humidity include increasing room heat and ventilating with cold, dry, winter air, which holds little moisture when cool and thus becomes drier when warmed inside the house.

The typical patient is an elderly person who comes in with localized or generalized pruritus. Dryness and itching of the lower extremities may be particularly notable. Symptoms start in early winter soon after the heat goes on, the relative humidity indoors decreases, and exposure to cold, dry winds increases. Rubbing and scratching cause increased irritation, thus leading to more pruritus and inflammation. If untreated, the symptoms subside spontaneously the following spring.

Ichthyosis vulgaris is a dominantly inherited disorder of keratinization that is estimated to occur in 1:100 individuals. Skin changes, usually not present at birth, may be noted from early infancy to the teens; dry skin and prominent keratotic follicles are usually present by ages 5–10. Those with ichthyosis vulgaris also have a high incidence of atopic diseases (atopic dermatitis, rhinitis, asthma) and keratosis pilaris.

II. Subjective data. Lesions are usually asymptomatic. If symptoms are present, the chief complaint is always pruritus, at times severe.

III. Objective data

    A. Dry skin covered with a fine scale is seen most often on the anterior tibial areas, dorsa of the hands, and on the forearms. The distribution may be both diffuse and in round patches. With more severe involvement the skin loses its suppleness, cracks, and becomes fissured. The superficial reticulated cracking takes on an uneven diamond pattern similar to that of cracked porcelain and erythema appears in and around involved areas (eczema or erythema craquelé). Nummular plaques of eczema also may be present.

B. In **ichthyosis vulgaris** scaling is most prominent over the extensor aspects of the extremities. Flexural areas are spared. Milder forms appear as dryness present only during winter months. More severe lesions, particularly those seen on the lower legs in winter, may resemble the "fish skin" from which the term ichthyosis is derived. Follicular accentuation **(keratosis pilaris)** may be prominent over arms, thighs, and buttocks. The palms and soles have accentuation of the dermatoglyphic lines and appear to be wrinkled.

IV. **Assessment.** A detailed family history and history of the home and work environment are needed, both to help make an educated etiologic diagnosis and to outline a therapeutic program that will eliminate or counteract any causative factors. Hypothyroidism may be associated with xerosis, and this possibility should be investigated.

V. **Therapy.** Skin is dry not because it lacks grease or skin oils, but because it lacks water. All therapeutic efforts are aimed at replacing the water in the skin and in the immediate environment.

A. **Preventive**

1. Room temperature should be kept as low as is consistent with comfort.

2. The use of humidifiers is to be encouraged. These may be either portable or installed in the ducts of forced-air heating systems. However, unless the house is relatively airtight with proper insulation, the moisture will either disperse rapidly to the outside or be caught within the walls and cause eventual damage to the house or paint.

3. Bathing should not be excessive (once every 1–2 days), and the bath water should be warm but not hot. Bath oils may be added (Alpha Keri, Lubrex, or others [see p. 315]). These will, however, make the bathtub slippery and difficult to clean. An alternative instruction to the patient is to add 1 teaspoon of bath oil to ¼ cup warm water and to use the mixture as a rubdown either after the bath or as a substitute for a bath.

4. Excessive exposure to soap and water, solvents, or other drying compounds should be eliminated. Use a mild soap such as Dove (see p. 294). It is the very mild irritants, often used casually and without thinking, that cause most of the trouble. Mechanical trauma from rough (often wool) or constricting clothing must be avoided.

5. Frequent use of emollients should be encouraged. The lubricating agents may range from lotions (Keri, Lubrex, Lubriderm, U-Lactin) and creams (Keri, Nivea) to thicker preparations (Aquaphor, Eucerin, hydrated petrolatum, petrolatum [see p. 297]). They are best applied when the skin is moist. Many elderly patients seem to tolerate petrolatum better than some of the more elegant preparations.

6. The patient should consider moving to a subtropical environment, especially for the winter.

B. Treatment of preexisting dryness

1. The primary means of correcting dryness is first to add water to the skin and then to apply a hydrophobic substance to keep it there. In vitro, the stratum corneum can absorb as much as 5–6 times its own weight and increase its volume threefold when soaked in water. In vivo, this is accomplished by either soaking the affected area or bathing for 5–10 min and then immediately applying water-in-oil or fatty hydrophobic medications (Aquaphor, Eucerin, lanolin, petrolatum). Use of the latter ointments alone is only moderately effective; they would then hydrate the skin simply by preventing the normal transepidermal water loss.

2. Topical corticosteroid ointments used with occlusive dressings are the most effective and rapid therapy for symptomatic xerosis with associated eczematous changes.

3. Maximum hydration can be accomplished by the use of 40–60% propylene glycol in water applied under plastic occlusion overnight. If 6% salicylic acid is added to this formula (Keralyt gel), an extremely effective keratolytic and hydrating gel is formed (see p. 306). Used overnight once or twice weekly initially and then only as often as needed thereafter, this product is the therapy of choice for the dry, scaly skin of ichthyosis vulgaris.

4. Urea-containing creams (Aquacare [2% urea], Aquacare/HP [10% urea], Carmol [20% urea]) and those containing alpha-hydroxy acids such as lactic acid (LactiCare lotion [5% lactic acid, 2.5% sodium pyrrolidone carboxylate] and Purpose Dry Skin Cream [3.5% lactic acid]) are claimed to produce prolonged hydration and help remove scales and crusts (see p. 308). U-Lactin lotion contains both urea and lactic acid and may be particularly effective. These are hydrophilic substances that enhance the ability of the stratum corneum to hold water and counteract the tendency of the skin to dry out.

5. Some patients with ichthyosis vulgaris and many affected with more severe types (lamellar, X-linked) may respond to oral isotretonoin (see p. 237).

References

Anderson, R. L., Cassidy, J. M., Hansen, J. R., and Yellin, W.   The effect of in vivo occlusion on human stratum corneum hydration-dehydration in vitro. *J. Invest. Dermatol.* 61:375–379, 1973.

Baden, H. P., and Alper, J. C.   A keratolytic gel containing salicylic acid in propylene glycol. *J. Invest. Dermatol.* 61:330–333, 1973.

Blair, C.   The action of a urea-lactic acid ointment in ichthyosis with particular reference to the thickness of the horny layer. *Br. J. Dermatol.* 94:145–153, 1976.

Blank, I. H.   Action of emollient creams and their additives. *J. A. M. A.* 164:412–415, 1959.

Chernosky, M. E.   Dry skin and its consequences. *J. Am. Med. Wom. Assoc.* 27:133–135, 1972.

Frost, P.   Ichthyosiform dermatoses. *J. Invest. Dermatol.* 60:541–552, 1973.

Goldsmith, L. A.   The ichthyosis. *Prog. Med. Gen.* 1:185–211, 1976.

Goldsmith, L. A., and Baden, H. P. Management and treatment of ichthyosis. *N. Engl. J. Med.* 286:821–823, 1972.

Marks, R., and Dykes, P. J. (eds.), *The Ichthyosis*. New York: Spectrum, 1978.

Middleton, J. O. The effects of temperature on extensibility of isolated corneum and its relation to skin chapping. *Br. J. Dermatol.* 81:717–721, 1969.

Tagami, H. Evaluation of the skin surface hydration in vivo by electrical measurement. *J. Invest. Dermatol.* 75:500–507, 1980.

Van Scott, E. J., and Yu, R. J. Control of keratinization with alpha-hydroxy acids and related compounds: I. Topical treatment of ichthyotic disorders. *Arch. Dermatol.* 110:586–590, 1974.

Warin, A. P. Eczema craquelé as the presenting feature of myxoedema. *Br. J. Dermatol.* 89:289–291, 1973.

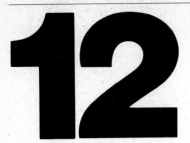

Erythema multiforme

I. Definition and pathophysiology. Erythema multiforme is a reaction pattern of the skin represented clinically by a variety of lesions, including the characteristic iris or target lesion. It is characterized histologically first by endothelial cell swelling, dermal papillary edema, and a perivascular lymphohistiocytic infiltrate. Later, epidermal necrosis, dermal-epidermal interface alteration, and subepidermal, or less frequently, intraepidermal separation and bulla formation occur. The condition is thought to be a hypersensitivity reaction based on an immune mechanism of unclear type. Several reports have now documented the presence of complement and immunoglobulin in the superficial cutaneous microvasculature in early lesions, as well as circulating immune complexes in serum. These studies suggest that deposition of immune complexes in vessel walls plays a role in the pathogenesis of erythema multiforme. This acute, self-limited, frequently recurrent disorder occurs most commonly in winter and early spring in children and young adults.

Multiple precipitating factors have been found, including infections, drugs, endocrine changes, and underlying malignancy. Herpes simplex infections are the most frequent antecedent infectious cause and direct links with this virus and with *Mycoplasma pneumoniae* have been most thoroughly documented. Many other viral, bacterial, and mycobacterial agents also have been implicated. Penicillin, barbiturates, sulfonamides, and many other drugs may initiate the same picture. In about 50% of cases, no provocative factor can be identified. Recurrences of varying severity occur in 10–20% of patients, especially in those with mucous membrane involvement.

The mild form of erythema multiforme heals spontaneously in 2–3 weeks; the severe form, with widespread mucosal involvement, referred to by many as the Stevens-Johnson syndrome, may last 6–8 weeks and is a life-threatening disease.

II. Subjective data. Mild prodromal symptoms of malaise and sore throat often precede the eruption, and drugs given for these symptoms are often inadvertently blamed for the erythema multiforme. Individual lesions may sting or burn, and large bullae may be painful. In severely ill patients there is high fever, malaise, and severe pain in mucosal areas with secondary photophobia and inability to ingest food or fluids.

III. Objective data (See color insert.)

   A. In the mild and typical case the patient will usually have lesions distributed symmetrically on extensor surfaces, distal limbs, palms and soles, and face. Bright red purple annular, macular, and papular areas and some urticarialike lesions may be seen. The iris or target lesion is seen most often on the hands and consists of a central vesicle or livid erythema surrounded by a concentric pale and then red ring. Iris lesions need not be present in order to make a diagnosis of erythema multiforme. Mucosal lesions are present in 20–45% of cases. At times only mucous membrane lesions may be seen.

B. With severe erythema multiforme there are usually generalized lesions (with and without bullae or hemorrhage) with severe involvement of ocular, oral, and other mucous membranes. A copious and often purulent discharge from the eyes and mouth may be present.

C. There are many variations in morphology and extent of the eruption.

IV. Assessment

A. Workup. Antecedent infection, drug administration, or illness for up to 3 weeks prior to the rash should be detailed. For a complete workup the following should be considered:

1. Cultures for streptococci, *Mycoplasma,* and deep fungi (e.g., histoplasmosis, coccidioidomycosis).

2. Serologic studies for hepatitis-associated antigens, histoplasmosis, mononucleosis, *Mycoplasma* infection.

3. Skin tests, chest x ray (to rule out *Mycoplasma* pneumonia, deep fungal infection, or tuberculosis).

4. Skin biopsy will demonstrate a characteristic histopathologic picture. This is a worthwhile test, particularly when the clinical presentation is not typical.

5. Has the patient been vaccinated recently, had a "cold sore," had x-ray therapy for a tumor? Is she pregnant or has she been taking birth control pills? The causes of erythema multiforme are so numerous that they cannot all be listed here, and the direct cause may escape detection.

B. Differential diagnosis includes: (1) other vascular reaction pattern diseases (urticaria, erythema nodosum, vasculitis); (2) blistering eruptions (pemphigus, bullous pemphigoid, toxic epidermal necrolysis); (3) mucocutaneous syndromes (Behçet's syndrome, hand-foot-and-mouth disease, aphthous stomatitis, acute herpetic gingivostomatitis); (4) drug reactions; and (5) Kawasaki's disease.

V. Therapy

A. Mild involvement

1. Antihistamines PO.

2. Antibiotics (tetracycline or erythromycin, 1 gm/day) if there is suspected *Mycoplasma* infection.

3. Open wet compresses for bullous or erosive lesions (see p. 313).

4. Mouth care

   a. Hydrogen peroxide (3%) mouthwash for cleanliness 2–5 times a day.

   b. Dyclone solution applied directly to the lesions for pain prn.

c. Chloraseptic mouthwash may be utilized for both purposes as needed 3id.

5. Bland foods are preferable.

6. Analgesics (aspirin, 600 mg q4h).

B. Severe involvement

1. Immediate hospitalization and institution of intravenous fluid administration.

2. Prednisone PO or prednisolone IM 80–120 mg every day should be given until the disease responds, then tapered off over 2–3 weeks. The usefulness of systemic corticosteroids is still controversial but severe erythema multiforme often responds to these medications.

3. Local care as previously described for mild involvement; bullae may be drained, but the blister roof is left intact.

References

Ackerman, A. B., Penneys, N. S., and Clark, W. H. Erythema multiforme exudativum: Distinctive pathological process. *Br. J. Dermatol.* 84:554–566, 1971.

Bianchine, J. R., Macaraeg, P. U. J., Lasagna, L., Azarnoff, D. L., Brunk, S. F., Hvidberg, E. F., and Owen, J. A. Drugs as etiologic factors in the Stevens-Johnson syndrome. *Am. J. Med.* 44:390–405, 1968.

Bushkell, L. L., Mackel, S. E., and Jordan, R. E. Erythema multiforme: Direct immunofluorescence studies and detection of circulating immune complexes. *J. Invest. Dermatol.* 74:372–374, 1980.

Lyell, A. Erythema multiforme: Manifestations and management. *Curr. Med. Drugs* 8:3–14, 1968.

Orfanos, L. E., Schaumburg-Lever, G., and Lever, W. Dermal and epidermal types of erythema multiforme: A histopathologic study of 24 cases. *Arch. Dermatol.* 109:682–688, 1974.

Shelley, W. B. Herpes simplex virus as a cause of erythema multiforme. *J. A. M. A.* 201:153–156, 1967.

Southeimer, R. D., Goribaldi, R. A., and Krueger, G. G. Stevens-Johnson syndrome associated with *Mycoplasma pneumoniae* infections. *Arch. Dermatol.* 114:241–244, 1978.

Tonneson, M. G., and Soter, N. A. Erythema multiforme. *J. Am. Acad. Dermatol.* 1:357–363, 1979.

Weupper, K. D., Watson, P. A., and Kazmierowski, J. A. Immune complexes in erythema multiforme and the Stevens-Johnson syndrome. *J. Invest. Dermatol.* 74:368–371, 1980.

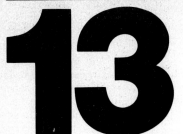

13

Erythema nodosum

I. **Definition and pathophysiology.** Erythema nodosum, a cutaneous reaction pattern, consists of tender red nodules on the legs and occasionally elsewhere. It represents a hypersensitivity response, perhaps involving immune complex formation, to any of numerous factors. Erythema nodosum appears most commonly in young women, but may be seen in patients of any age. It indicates a need for an investigation of underlying precipitating disorders and should not be viewed as a disease in itself.

The most common cause of erythema nodosum in the United States is a preceding streptococcal infection. Reactions to medications, particularly sulfonamides and birth control pills, and concurrent sarcoidosis are also frequent causes. Other etiologic considerations should include primary infection tuberculosis, viral and deep fungal infections (coccidioidomycosis, histoplasmosis), and inflammatory bowel diseases (ulcerative colitis, regional enteritis).

Erythema nodosum usually will subside spontaneously in 3–6 weeks, temporarily leaving an area resembling a deep bruise. Chronic erythema nodosum or erythema nodosum migrans refers to a syndrome differing from acute erythema nodosum because of persistent course, peripherally expanding lesions, tendency to unilateral distribution, and a lesser degree of tenderness.

II. **Subjective data.** A 1- –2-week period of malaise and arthralgias with or without fever may precede the outbreak of lesions. The overriding characteristic of these nodose lesions is their exquisite sensitivity, so severe that even contact with bed clothing or sheets may be intolerable.

III. **Objective data (See color insert.)** Single to numerous, bright red, hot, oval or round, slightly raised nodules, several centimeters in diameter, with diffuse borders and surrounding edema, are seen distributed unilaterally or bilaterally, although not necessarily symmetrically, on the pretibial surfaces. Other sites may include the thighs, arms, face, and neck. The extent of the lesions is easier to determine by palpation than by inspection. After 1–2 weeks the redness will become blue and then yellow green as the nodules subside. Mild scaling will be seen as the lesions heal. Ulceration or scarring is never a part of the syndrome.

IV. **Assessment**

    A. **Workup**

        1. A detailed history concerning travel, present illness, and drug administration.

        2. A thorough physical examination.

3. Laboratory studies should include a CBC, ESR, urinalysis, chest x ray, throat culture, antistreptolysin-O (ASLO) titer, and TB and deep fungal skin tests.

B. Differential diagnosis. Other entities that may resemble the nodose lesions of erythema nodosum include erythema induratum, superficial thrombophlebitis, Weber-Christian disease, fungal granuloma, bite reactions, or fat necrosis produced by lipolytic enzymes liberated in acute or chronic pancreatic disease.

C. Histopathology. Biopsy of erythema nodosum will reveal a septal panniculitis. Although a specific histologic diagnosis may not be possible in all instances, many of the foregoing conditions have consistent clinicopathologic patterns. An adequate deep incisional biopsy should be considered part of a thorough investigation. Punch biopsies frequently provide insufficient information to make a diagnosis and should be avoided.

V. Therapy

A. Treat the underlying disease as indicated.

B. Bed rest with elevation of the patient's legs will gradually reduce pain and edema. A bed cradle will keep sheets and blankets from direct skin contact.

C. Analgesics (aspirin, 600 mg q4h). Naproxen has been reported to benefit chronic erythema nodosum.

D. Very symptomatic patients may be treated with potassium iodide 360–900 mg (or saturated solution of potassium iodide 0.36–0.90 ml [6–15 drops] in fruit juice) daily for 3–4 weeks. Decrease in pain and swelling should occur within 24–48 hr and complete resolution within 2 weeks. Early cessation of therapy may result in relapse.

E. In chronic or recurrent cases unresponsive to these treatments, there is often a therapeutic dilemma. The most detailed investigation may not uncover the cause in the majority of cases, and yet some patients may be disabled, in pain, and unable to work. In such instances, the injection of small amounts of a corticosteroid suspension into the middle of each nodule will cause involution of the lesion within 48–72 hr. A 1- –2-week course of oral corticosteroids is also effective; the possibility of an underlying primary tuberculous infection must never be overlooked.

References

Arndt, K. A., and Harrist, T. Fever and subcutaneous masses in an elderly man (Case records of the Massachusetts General Hospital). *N. Engl. J. Med.* 306:1035–1043, 1982.

Editorial. "Nodules-on-the-leg" syndrome. *N. Engl. J. Med.* 274:463–464, 1966.

Fine, R. M., and Meltzer, H. D. Chronic erythema nodosum. *Arch. Dermatol.* 100:33–38, 1969.

Forstrom, L., and Winkelmann, R. K. Acute panniculitis: A clinical and histopathologic study of 34 cases. *Arch. Dermatol.* 113:909–917, 1977.

Gordon, H. Erythema nodosum: A review of 115 cases. *Br. J. Dermatol.* 73:393–409, 1979.

Horio, T., Imamura, S., Danno, K., and Ofuji, S.   Potassium iodide in the treatment of erythema nodosum and nodular vasculitis. *Arch. Dermatol.* 117:29–31, 1981.

Hughes, P. S. H., Apisarnthanarax, P., and Mullins, J. F.   Subcutaneous fat necrosis associated with pancreatic disease. *Arch. Dermatol.* 111:506–510, 1975.

Kanarek, D. J., and Mark, E. J.   A 60 year old woman with erythema nodosum and lymphadenopathy: Case records of the Massachusetts General Hospital. *N. Engl. J. Med.* 305:89–94, 1981.

Lehman, C. W.   Control of erythema nodosum with naproxen. *Cutis* 26:66–67, 1980.

Medeiros, A. A., Marty, S. D., Tosh, F. E., and Chin, T. D.   Erythema nodosum and erythema multiforme as clinical manifestations of histoplasmosis in a community outbreak. *N. Engl. J. Med.* 274:415–420, 1966.

Reed, R. J., Clark, W. H., and Mihm, M. C.   Disorders of the panniculus adiposus. *Hum. Pathol.* 4:219–229, 1973.

Rostas, A., Lowe, D., and Smout, M. S.   Erythema nodosum migrans in a young woman. *Arch. Dermatol.* 116:325–326, 1980.

Salvatore, M. A., and Lynch, P. J.   Erythema nodosum, estrogens, and pregnancy. *Arch. Dermatol.* 116:557–558, 1980.

Schultz, E. F., and Whiting, D. A.   Treatment of erythema nodosum and nodular vasculitis with potassium iodide. *Br. J. Dermatol.* 94:75–78, 1976.

Soderstrom, R. M., and Krull, E. A.   Erythema nodosum: A review. *Cutis* 21:806–810, 1978.

Weinstein, L.   Erythema nodosum. *DM*, June 1969.

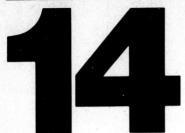

Fungal infections

Candidiasis

I. Definition and pathophysiology. The yeastlike fungus *Candida albicans* can normally be found on mucous membranes, skin, in the gastrointestinal tract, and in the vaginal vault. It can, under certain circumstances, change from a commensal organism to a pathogen and cause localized or generalized mucocutaneous disease.

Factors that predispose to infection include: (1) a local environment of moisture, warmth, maceration, and/or occlusion; (2) the systemic administration of antibiotics, corticosteroids, or birth control pills; (3) pregnancy; (4) diabetes; (5) Cushing's disease; and (6) debilitated states. Further, immune reactivity to *Candida* is reduced in infants up to 6 months of age; in patients with certain neoplastic diseases of the blood and reticuloendothelial systems; and in patients on immunosuppressive therapy resulting in an increased incidence of *Candida* infections. The resident bacteria on skin, mainly cocci, presumably inhibit proliferation of *C. albicans;* it is often difficult to establish experimental *C. albicans* infection unless the bacterial population is reduced.

Cell-mediated immunity plays a major role in the defense against chronic superficial fungal infections including candidiasis. In addition, *C. albicans* can activate complement via the alternative pathway and induce epidermal neutrophilic microabscesses in acute experimental infections in humans and animals. The host defense mechanisms respond at least in part to mannin, a *C. albicans* cell wall polysaccharide.

II. Subjective data. In chronic paronychia the area surrounding the nail is tender on pressure, and the associated onychia is cosmetically and mechanically embarrassing. *Candida* intertrigo, perlèche, and vulvovaginitis are often pruritic and at times very uncomfortable. The lesions of thrush may be painful and may interfere with the normal ingestion of food.

III. Objective data

    A. Paronychial lesions show rounding and lifting of the posterior nail fold and erythema and swelling of the distal digit (usually without overt purulence). Often the nail becomes ridged and may have a green or brown discoloration.

    B. Intertriginous lesions (inframammary, axillary, groin, perianal, interdigital) are moist and red, with occasional scaling, and are often macerated in the folds. Well-defined, peeling borders surrounded by **satellite erythematous papules or pustules** are characteristic of *Candida* infections.

C. **Thrush** appears as white plaques loosely attached to oral or vaginal mucous membrane. The underlying mucosa is bright red and moist. Lesions start as pinpoint spots and may extend to the corners of the mouth or into the esophagus.

D. **Perlèche** appears as a cracked and fissured erythematous and moist area in the corners of the mouth.

E. The lesions of **vulvovaginitis** are frequently, but not always, associated with a vaginal discharge. The degree of vulvar erythema and edema parallels the severity of the symptoms. Primary vulvar candidiasis appears similar to other intertriginous *Candida* involvement.

IV. Assessment

A. Direct examination with potassium hydroxide (KOH) or Swartz-Medrik stain (SMS) will reveal budding yeasts with or without hyphae or pseudohyphae. For technique of fungal scraping and KOH examination see page 214. The presence of hyphal forms is pathognomonic of infection on mucous membranes, but they are usually not seen with infection on skin. On Gram's stain, fungi appear as gram-positive organisms larger than bacteria.

B. *C. albicans* grows readily within 48–72 hr on fungal or bacterial media. Specific identification is based on the presence of chlamydospores when the organism is subcultured on chlamydospore or cornmeal agar.

C. Gram-negative rods may play a synergistic role in infection of intertriginous areas; appropriate Gram's stain and culture are important.

D. A change in the predisposing environment, or evaluation and treatment of underlying medical conditions, is necessary for a successful and lasting cure. Diminution of factors that lead to accumulation of moisture is most important.

V. Therapy.
There are four agents available for the topical therapy of fungal infections: an alkylaryl ether, haloprogin (Halotex); two synthetic imidazole compounds, miconazole (Monistat-Derm) and clotrimazole (Lotrimin, Mycelex); and nystatin (see also p. 258). The first three have the advantage of being effective both for dermatophyte fungi and *C. albicans*. The middle two compounds are at least as effective as nystatin for treating cutaneous candidiasis, and miconazole and clotrimazole vaginal cream may be more effective than nystatin in treatment of vulvovaginal candidiasis. Tolnaftate (Tinactin, see p. 265) is not effective against *Candida* infections.

The polyene antifungal antibiotic nystatin is also a useful therapeutic agent for most forms of candidiasis (see p. 262). The use of nystatin tablets (500,000 units PO 3–4 times a day) is beneficial in many circumstances. Recurrent or recalcitrant perianal, vulvar, or diaper-area involvement may represent reinfections from gut organisms and often can be controlled when oral medication is added to topical care. Often, women who have experienced vaginal candidiasis hesitate to take antibacterial antibiotics for control of conditions such as acne for fear of reactivation of disease. Recurrent infection can almost always be prevented by giving 1–2 weeks of oral nystatin and vaginal miconazole, clotrimazole, or nystatin therapy preceding antibiotic administration and continuing the PO nystatin along with the other antibiotic. This regimen appears to rid the gut and vagina of sufficient *Candida* organisms to prevent clinical symptoms and also keeps them inhibited during concurrent antibiotic therapy. Nystatin or amphotericin B PO is not otherwise needed along with broad-spectrum antibiotics in the therapy of young healthy women.

Oral ketoconazole (Nizoral) is an effective treatment for chronic mucocutaneous candidiasis but has no role in the therapy of the usual superficial *Candida* infections (see p. 261).

A. Paronychia

1. All wet work must be stopped. Gloves and cotton liners must be worn to protect the hands. If this is not possible, it is unlikely that any active therapy will be successful. Even successful treatment of a chronic paronychia is slow and requires weeks to months before remission occurs.

2. Apply clotrimazole (Lotrimin, Mycelex) or haloprogin (Halotex) or miconazole (Monistat-Derm) cream or solution, or nystatin cream to nail folds frequently. If there is associated pain or edema, a steroid-nystatin ointment (e.g., Mycolog) is used. Overnight application of medication under a finger cot may increase effectiveness. If paronychia is severe, oral nystatin and miconazole or clotrimazole under occlusion, with or without topical steroids, is often helpful.

3. Amphotericin B (Fungizone) lotion or cream or 1% alcoholic solution of gentian violet may also be of value. Do not use amphotericin B along with imidazole agents as their effects may counteract each other.

4. The paradoxical approach of interdicting wet work yet applying aqueous medications may be circumvented by the use of 2–4% thymol in chloroform (or absolute alcohol). This nonaqueous preparation reaches the paronychial area by capillary action and should be applied 2–3 times a day. It often works when other remedies have failed.

5. Nails will grow out normally within 3–6 months after the paronychial area has healed.

B. Intertriginous lesions (inframammary, axillary, groin, perianal, interdigital)

1. Conditions leading to moisture and maceration must be eliminated or countered. Inframammary or groin lesions should be exposed several times daily to the drying warmth of an electric light bulb or the drying breeze from a fan. Supportive clothing is useful, as is weight reduction. Air conditioning in warm environments may become a necessity. After lesions subside, continued application of a drying powder or nystatin powder should be emphasized.

2. If lesions are inflammatory, compress 3–4 times a day with water or Burow's solution to cool and soothe as well as to remove the irritant endotoxin substance.

3. After compresses and thorough drying with a towel, bulb, or fan, apply one of the topical antifungal creams given for paronychia or steroid-nystatin cream (or nystatin powder) to affected areas.

4. Amphotericin B (Fungizone) lotion or cream also may be useful.

5. Gentian violet 0.25–2.0% or Castellani's paint (fuchsin, phenol, and resorcinol) are also effective but often sting and are messy, and they will stain clothing, bed linen, and skin (see p. 265).

C. Thrush

1. Nystatin oral suspension (4–6 ml [400,000–600,000 units] 4 id) should be held in the mouth for several minutes before swallowing. The dosage for infants is 2 ml (200,000 units) 4id.

2. Ten mg clotrimazole buccal troches taken 5id for 2 weeks are highly effective for chronic oral candidiasis.

3. Amphotericin B (80 mg/ml) used as a rinse is also effective.

4. Gentian violet solution 1–2% is probably the most useful agent available, but is aesthetically unappealing. With difficult or recurrent cases it is the therapy of choice.

D. Vulvovaginitis

1. Treatment may be aided by wearing cotton underwear and avoiding tight clothing such as pantyhose or jeans.

2. Clotrimazole tablets or cream (Gyne-Lotrimin), Mycelex G, or miconazole (Monistat) should be inserted intravaginally once daily for 7 days.

3. Nystatin vaginal suppositories (100,000 units) may be slightly less effective; when used they should be inserted high into the vagina twice daily for 7–14 days, then nightly for an additional 2–3 weeks.

4. Canicidin (Candeptin, Vanobid) tablets or chlordantoin (Sporostacin) cream may be used in the same fashion.

5. In severe *Candida* vulvitis, addition of a topical corticosteroid for the first 3–4 days will speed resolution.

Dermatophyte infections

I. **Definition and pathophysiology.** The dermatophyte (or ringworm) fungi are a distinct and unique class of fungi, both botanically and pathologically. Humans may acquire dermatophyte infection from three sources: organisms that live in soil, animal fungi, or, most commonly, pathogens that will infect only humans and cannot survive elsewhere. Dermatophyte fungi live in the superficial layers of the epidermis, in nails, and in hair. They do not invade living epidermis but will, however, grow readily on excised tissue from many organs, including skin. It has become apparent that dermatophyte fungi grow only within keratin layers because there is a serum fungal inhibitory factor that enters the extravascular space and protects living tissue against deep penetration of fungal elements.

Poor nutrition and hygiene, a tropical climate, debilitating diseases, and contact with infected animals, persons, or fomites all increase the likelihood of fungal infection. Pathogenic fungi of all kinds are common in our environment, yet the overall incidence of infection is low; host resistance factors would seem to be the most important determinants of susceptibility to clinical fungal infection. Acute infection tends to be associated with the rapid development of a delayed hypersensitivity to intracutaneously injected trichophyton antigen. Reinfection in such patients requires a greater inoculum, and lesions heal more rapidly. Protective cell-mediated immunity is acquired by 80% of patients after primary infection. Chronic infection develops in approximately 20% of those infected; in these patients, often atopics, injection of trichophyton elicits only an immediate wheal response. This may well indicate a specific immunologic defect in such patients who, presumably for genetic reasons, develop a predominantly B cell response and produce antibodies. If the infection can be eradicated with therapy, however, delayed hypersensitivity can emerge that may be effective in preventing reinfection. Potent therapeutic agents may exert their effects not only by killing fungi but by permitting appropriate host defenses to develop.

Although some species of dermatophyte tend to produce a specific clinical picture, it may be difficult to ascertain the causative organism from the clinical characteristics of the eruption.

II. Clinical types of infection

A. **Tinea capitis,** or ringworm of the scalp, after affecting children for over 2000 years is now readily controlled by systemic antifungal antibiotics. Epidemic ringworm is transmitted by contact from child to child. Organisms have been cultured from such objects as barbers' instruments, hairbrushes, theater seats, and hats. Minor trauma with a break in the cutaneous barrier is necessary to initiate infection. Children up to puberty are more susceptible, and boys are infected more often than girls.

1. **Subjective data.** Scalp ringworm is usually asymptomatic. A kerion, which is a deep, boggy swelling caused by infection with certain fungi, is painful.

2. **Objective data.** Patchy hair loss and broken hairs, inflammation, and scaling are characteristic. Such findings in children should be presumed to be ringworm until proved otherwise. A kerion appears as a pustular folliculitis within an area of purulence and swelling. The inflammation is often vigorous and scarring can result.

B. **Tinea barbae,** or ringworm infection of the beard and moustache, is confined to adult men and is much less common than it was years ago. Infections from barbers' instruments are now rare, and the organisms are usually acquired from animals.

1. **Subjective data.** Pruritus or pain occurs.

2. **Objective data**

a. The superficial type of infection looks like ringworm elsewhere (see objective data for tinea corporis).

b. The deeper type of infection is associated with marked inflammation, pustular folliculitis, and kerion formation. Loss of facial hair is common. The angle of the jaw is the most usual location.

C. **Tinea corporis,** or infection of the nonhairy skin, may be seen in any age group, but children are most susceptible. It occurs in all parts of the world, but is most prevalent in hot, humid climates and rural areas.

1. **Subjective data.** Tinea corporis may be either asymptomatic or mildly pruritic.

2. **Objective data.** The typical lesions start as erythematous macules or papules that spread outward and develop into annular and arciform lesions with sharp, scaling or vesicular, advancing borders and healing centers. Tinea corporis is most common on the exposed surfaces of the body, namely, the face, arms, and shoulders.

D. **Tinea cruris,** or ringworm of the groin ("jock itch"), is frequently found in obese men in the summertime. It is often associated with the simultaneous presence of tinea pedis. Heat, friction, and maceration predispose to this infection; it is most common in the tropics.

1. **Subjective data.** Symptoms include pruritus, which may be intense, and discomfort due to the inflamed intertriginous tissues rubbing together. Many eruptions are asymptomatic, however.

2. **Objective data (See color insert.).** The eruption affects both the groin and upper inner thigh symmetrically and often has a butterfly appearance with clearly defined, raised borders. Lesions often extend into the gluteal folds and onto the buttocks.

E. **Tinea of the hands (tinea manuum) and feet (tinea pedis).** Tinea pedis is the most common of all fungal diseases; 30–70% of the population at some time have had a fungal infection of the feet. Unlike other ringworm, tinea pedis is generally a disease of adult life. This infection, too, is found most often in tropical climates and in the summertime.

The causative fungi may be found in shoes, flooring, and socks and have been recovered from clothing more than 5 months after laundering. Occlusive footwear is a strong predisposing factor. Simple contact with infected scales is not enough for infection; concomitant trauma to the feet is necessary for infection to take place.

1. **Subjective data.** Pruritus is the most common symptom. Fissures may be painful and also are easy avenues for secondary local bacterial infection or lymphangitis. This is of particular importance in patients with diabetes, chronic lymphedema, and stasis syndromes.

2. **Objective data**

a. **Tinea pedis** may take several forms.

(1) Mild to severe interdigital scaling and maceration with fissures is the most common form.

(2) Widespread fine scaling in "moccasin-foot" distribution is very frequent. The scaling usually extends up onto the sides of the feet and lower heel, where it exhibits a characteristic clearly defined, fine polycyclic scaling border.

(3) Some fungi induce a vesicular or bullous eruption with large blisters.

b. **Tinea manuum** is usually seen as mild erythema with hyperkeratosis and scaling, mainly over the palmar surfaces. Hand infection is almost never found in the absence of foot involvement. Inflammatory lesions on the feet are often associated with a sterile vesicular "id" reaction on the hands, often misdiagnosed as a primary fungal infection. Unilateral involvement of either hands or feet is common and even helpful in making a clinical diagnosis.

F. Onychomycosis, or fungal infection of the nails, is seen in approximately 40% of patients with fungal infections in other locations. Fungi invade the nails by growing either into the ventral edge or extending from the distal lateral nail groove. The organisms become located in the soft keratin in the proximal nails; fungi carried to the distal nail may or may not be viable. Fingernails are less commonly involved than toenails.

1. **Subjective data.** The nails become brittle, friable, and thickened. Patients often complain that the nails not only are cosmetically embarrassing but catch and pull on clothing.

2. **Objective data.** Infection starts at the free margin or lateral borders of the nail as a white or yellow discoloration and progresses proximally. The nail may become thickened, distorted, and crumbly and may be lifted up by an accumulation of subungual keratin and debris. Destruction may be slight or very severe and leave only small remnants of keratinous material.

III. Assessment

A. Definitive diagnosis is made by the microscopic identification of hyphae and spores in scales or hair. In nails the presence of hyphae usually means dermatophyte infection; however, secondarily invading saprophytic fungi can also be seen at times. This procedure is discussed in detail on p. 214.

B. Infection may be confirmed, or in some instances identified in the absence of a positive scraping, by fungal culture. This technique is discussed on p. 215.

C. Examination of infected areas with long-wave ultraviolet light (Wood's lamp) may be used to make a diagnosis, screen large populations of children, or follow the course of therapy for tinea capitis caused by *Microsporum canis* or *M. audouini*. Scalp ringworm infection caused by many fungi does not fluoresce, however (see p. 215).

IV. Therapy

A. Prophylactic measures

1. Development of fungal infections is enhanced by heat, moisture, and maceration. If these environmental factors cannot be changed, chances for cure are less and those for relapse are excellent. Intertriginous or interdigital areas should be dried thoroughly after bathing and a simple talcum powder or antifungal powder (Tinactin) should be applied then and each morning.

2. Footwear should fit well and be nonocclusive (leather shoes or sandals are best; avoid plastic footwear or sneakers).

3. Patients with hyperhidrosis should wear absorbent cotton socks and avoid wool or synthetic fibers. Unless the hyperhidrosis can be controlled it may be impossible to clear concomitant fungal infection (see p. 286).

4. Clothing and towels should be changed frequently and be well laundered in hot water.

B. Local therapy. Infections of the body and groin, and superficial involve-

ment of the bearded area, palms, and soles, usually can be treated by topical measures alone (see also p. 258).

1. Acute, inflammatory lesions with blistering and oozing should be treated with intermittent (4–6 times a day) or continuous open wet compresses (see p. 313). Blisters should be decompressed but roofs left intact.

2. Clotrimazole (Lotrimin, Mycelex), miconazole (Monistat-Derm), haloprogin (Halotex), and tolnaftate (Tinactin) solution or cream applied 3id will cause involution of most superficial scaling lesions within 1–3 weeks. Treatment should be continued for at least 4 weeks in order to decrease the relapse rate. The first three are also effective against *C. albicans* infection. Overnight application of Keralyt gel for 1–2 weeks is effective for toe-web infection, presumably by removing the stratum corneum in which the fungi are growing.

3. Undecylenic acid and its salts (Desenex and others) have been confirmed as effective topical antifungal agents and should be used as mentioned in **B.2.** Most topical antifungal agents have a high initial cure rate (80–90%) but relapse or reinfection is very common.

4. Thick, hyperkeratotic involvement, as on the palms or soles, may require local therapy with medications containing keratolytic agents such as salicylic acid, which will cause softening and exfoliation of the skin.

   a. The most useful means of combining keratolytic and antifungal therapy is to apply Keralyt gel under occlusion overnight or for 2–3 hours in the evening, and to use an antifungal agent at other times. The use of Keralyt alone may be sufficient to rid the skin of fungal organisms.

   b. Verdefam solution, 3 and 5% sulfur and salicylic acid ointment, and half- or full-strength Whitfield's ointment are other keratolytic preparations that may be applied 2id or alternated with the preparations noted in **B.2.**

5. Interdigital tinea pedis in its more severe and macerated form is associated with an enormous overgrowth of aerobic bacteria. Thirty percent aluminum chloride hexahydrate applied 2id for 7–10 days will produce resolution of odor, itching, and maceration in most instances. Aluminum chloride dries the web space, making it less hospitable to bacteria and fungi, and also directly kills bacteria (see p. 253).

6. Topical treatment of the nails will rarely, if ever, result in total cure of onychomycosis.

   a. Forty percent urea ointment may be employed as a painless technique for avulsing symptomatic dystrophic nails. This ointment allows removal of the nail and also facilitates subsequent treatment with antifungal solutions. Compounding this formulation is complicated and it must be applied in a specific fashion (see South and Farber, 1980).

   b. Ten percent glutaraldehyde solutions buffered to pH 7.5 have been reported to be effective after application 2id for 1–4 months. Buffered glutaraldehyde has high bactericidal, sporicidal, fungicidal, and viricidal activity, but rapidly undergoes polymerization and loses activity after 2 weeks.

c. One percent 5-fluorouracil in propylene glycol solution has been reported to be useful for onychomycosis in a preliminary study (Bagatell, 1977).

d. Reduction of a thickened, crumbling nail mass with an emery board or electric rotary sandpaper drill will reduce complaints of a cosmetic nature or of mechanical difficulties.

e. Local application of clotrimazole (Lotrimin), miconazole (Monistat-Derm), haloprogin (Halotex), tolnaftate (Tinactin), or Verdefam solutions may be helpful occasionally.

f. Surgical avulsion of the toenails, concomitant with systemic griseofulvin therapy, is often the only treatment that will clear toenail onychomycosis.

C. Griseofulvin (see also p. 260), a fungistatic and fungicidal antibiotic derived from various species of *Penicillium,* is effective against all dermatophyte fungi but is of no value against bacteria, superficial fungal infections such as tinea versicolor, or yeast infections such as those caused by *C. albicans.*

1. Tinea pedis should be treated with ultramicrosized griseofulvin 0.25–0.33 gm every day for 3 months. This period reflects the data available on the time it takes for the stratum corneum of the soles and palms to completely shed and "restore" itself. For the plantar scaling type approximately 90% of patients will be "cured" at 3 months. After some recurrences within the next 3 months the final "cure" rate should be about 70%. Clotrimazole used alone would yield a final "cure" rate of 18% and there appears to be no advantage to using the two drugs simultaneously. For intertriginous tinea pedis combination griseofulvin and clotrimazole treatment would be expected to yield about a 90% 3-month "cure" with a final rate of 84% after 3 subsequent months without treatment. Griseofulvin alone is less effective, and clotrimazole alone least effective (final rate 20%) (Zaias et al., 1978).

2. Infection of nonhairy skin usually responds to the use of griseofulvin, 0.25–0.33 gm of ultramicrosized griseofulvin every day for 3–4 weeks, but it is needed only for extensive, recalcitrant, or recurrent lesions. Avoid terminating therapy until there is definite evidence of a cure, complete clearing of lesions, negative fungal scrapings, and a negative culture.

3. Tinea capitis due to *M. canis* or *M. audouini* will respond to 0.25–0.33 gm ultramicrosized griseofulvin every day for a period of 6–8 weeks. Alternatively, a single dose of 1.5–2.0 gm (which may be repeated, if necessary, in 3–4 weeks) will result in cure of most children so treated. Patients should be treated for 2 weeks beyond the time that Wood's light or KOH preparations are negative. *Trichophyton tonsurans,* now the most common cause of tinea capitis in the southern United States, requires griseofulvin administration for 6 weeks or longer. Approximately 2.5–3.3 mg/lb of body weight is the effective dose for children. In general, children weighing 30–50 lb may take up to 165 mg/day, and children weighing over 50 lb, up to 330 mg/day.

Therapy should be continued for at least 2 weeks after clinical and mycologic cure.

There is no further justification for cutting or shaving the hair, having the patient wear a skullcap, or irradiating the scalp. Local antifungal remedies add little to the results obtained from griseofulvin alone.

4. **Griseofulvin therapy of fungal disease of the nails** should be approached with the realization that prolonged administration may not lead to cure and that, even if it does, relapse is not uncommon. Fingernails respond more readily than toenails; in fact, infection of the first toenail responds hardly at all unless the nail is first removed.

   The starting dose of ultramicrosized griseofulvin should be 0.75–0.99 gm every day for the first month, with gradual lessening of the dose to 0.5–0.66 gm every day over the following several months. Duration of therapy for fingernails will be 6–9 months, for toenails 9–18 months. Local therapy adds little. Side effects at these higher antibiotic levels are most commonly headache or mild gastrointestinal discomfort. Photosensitivity may become a problem also.

5. Dogs and cats infected with ringworm fungi also can be treated with griseofulvin.

D. Ketoconazole (Nizoral), a new broad-spectrum oral imidazole antifungal agent, is an effective and safe treatment for recalcitrant and chronic dermatophytosis as well as other cutaneous and systemic fungal infections (see p. 261). This drug was approved for use by the FDA in 1981 and has great promise. With time, it may become the drug of choice for difficult dermatophyte infections. In a recent study of resistant dermatophyte infections, the cure rate for ketoconazole was 83% with a relatively low relapse rate, while that for griseofulvin was 32% with a relatively high relapse rate. One 200-mg tablet is taken once daily at the beginning of a meal. Patients who respond slowly may take 200 mg 2id. Initial improvement takes place in 5–7 days.

Tinea versicolor

I. **Definition and pathophysiology.** Tinea versicolor is a chronic, asymptomatic, superficial fungal infection caused by the organism *Pityrosporum furfur*. This organism represents the pathogenic filamentous form of the yeastlike *Pityrosporum orbiculare,* a normal skin resident. The eruption is found worldwide, is seen most commonly in young adults in temperate zones, and accounts for about 5% of all fungal infections. Although the fine scales are teeming with hyphae and spores, the organisms cannot readily be cultured. They are found only in the stratum corneum, never penetrate deeper, and cause no inflammatory response. Lymphocyte transformation studies demonstrate that while a majority of young adults are sensitized to *P. orbiculare* as well as to *C. albicans,* extracts of *P. orbiculare* are much less active antigenically than are those of *C. albicans.* This might explain the relative lack of inflammation in the lesions produced by *P. orbiculare* and the comparatively high incidence of chronic tinea versicolor.

Tinea versicolor develops either as a result of change in host resistance or because certain strains of *P. orbiculare* are capable of transforming into a more aggressive form. Factors predisposing to clinical infection include: (1)

pregnancy, (2) serious underlying diseases, (3) a genetic predisposition, (4) high plasma cortisol, as in patients taking corticosteroids, and (5) a warm and humid climate. Experimental tinea versicolor cannot be produced without occlusion. Tinea versicolor often infects people for years, because of inadequate treatment, reinfection, or an inherent predisposition to infection.

The decreased or increased pigmentation in affected areas has long been considered to be secondary to a "sun screening" effect of infected keratin. The infected areas may be darker than surrounding skin in wintertime, but they do not tan after sun exposure and in summer become lighter than surrounding areas. Although this "fungus filter" perhaps plays some part in the pathogenesis of the hypopigmentation, it appears that the pigmentary changes are related to fungus-induced effects on melanosome size and distribution as well as the release of dicarboxylic acids by *P. furfur*. In hypopigmented tinea versicolor, the fungus initiates the production of abnormally small, occasionally packed melanosomes that are not transferred to keratinocytes properly. Conversely, in hyperpigmented tinea versicolor, melanosomes are larger and singly distributed within keratinocytes in a fashion similar to that of normal black pigmentation.

II. **Subjective data.** The eruption is almost always asymptomatic and only of cosmetic significance.

III. **Objective data.** Lesions vary in color from white and pink to brown, but usually consist of tan, desquamating, round or perifollicular, coalescing macular patches found primarily on the trunk. Involved untreated areas may be lighter than surrounding skin in the summer and become relatively darker during the winter.

IV. **Assessment**

  A. Examination of scales under the microscope with potassium hydroxide (KOH) or Swartz-Medrik stain (SMS) will reveal numerous short, straight, and angular hyphae and clusters of thickwalled, round, and budding yeasts (see p. 214). A negative microscopic examination virtually excludes the diagnosis, in contrast to dermatophyte infections.

  B. The causative organism of tinea versicolor cannot be easily cultured on artificial media.

  C. Wood's light examination will intensify the pigmentary changes and allow the extent and margins of involvement to be seen more readily. Infected areas may show a gold-to-orange fluorescence.

V. **Therapy**

  A. Tinea versicolor may be treated with many therapeutic agents, all of which will be successful if used for an adequate length of time. The evening application of medication should follow a bath. In most cases the topical treatment should be applied to the entire torso from the neck to the waist, as lesions may be widespread as well as clinically inapparent. Most treatments will remove any evidence of active infection (scaling) within several days, but to ensure cure these regimens should be continued for several weeks. The pigmentary changes resolve much more slowly (months). In spite of seemingly adequate therapy, relapse or reinfection is common, but it always responds to retreatment. Tinea versicolor does not respond to griseofulvin.

B. The frequency of relapse has led some to recommend that therapy be continued for 2 consecutive nights each month for 1 year in order to ensure a cure.

C. Useful agents

1. **Selenium sulfide suspension** (Exsel, Selsun, Iosel) should be applied to the affected areas, allowed to dry, and then allowed to remain for 15 min for 7–14 consecutive days. As little as a 5–20-min application on alternate days for 2 weeks may be effective in some instances.

2. **Zinc pyrithione,** an antifungal and antibacterial agent incorporated into shampoos, is very effective against lipophilic yeasts such as *P. orbiculare* (see p. 295). Shampoos containing this chemical (Danex, DHS-Zinc, Head and Shoulders, Zincon) should be applied 5 min nightly for 14 days.

3. **25% sodium hyposulfite** should be applied to lesions 2id for several weeks. Tinver lotion (25% sodium thiosulfate, 1% salicylic acid, and 10% alcohol) is used in the same fashion.

4. **Keratolytic creams,** ointments, or lotions containing 3–6% salicylic acid (Keralyt gel; Sebulex shampoo; 3–6% sulfur and salicylic acid ointment; 6% salicylic acid cream; 3% salicylic acid in 70% alcohol) applied overnight for 1–2 weeks, or the use of salicylic acid soap, are also effective.

5. **Akrinol** cream contains the hexylresorcinol salt of 9-amino-acridine and should be applied 2id for 6 weeks to prevent relapse.

6. **Clotrimazole (Lotrimin), miconazole (Monistat-Derm), haloprogin (Halotex), or tolnaftate (Tinactin)** preparations will eradicate tinea versicolor, but they are more expensive and no more effective than any of the foregoing.

7. **Propylene glycol** 50% in water applied 2id for 2 weeks is an inexpensive and apparently effective treatment. A slight burning sensation may occur in a few patients after application of the solution.

8. **Retinoic acid cream (Retin–A cream)** applied 2id for 2 weeks will cure the tinea versicolor and may be accompanied by lightening of pigmentation in the areas to which it is applied. It may therefore be more useful in those particularly embarrassed by the hyperpigmentation of infected skin.

9. **Ketoconazole** (see p. 261) clears the majority of patients with tinea versicolor who have taken this drug orally, but equally good results are possible with topical therapy.

References

CANDIDIASIS

DeVillez, R. L., and Lewis, C. W.   Candidiasis seminar. *Cutis* 19:69–83, 1977.

Grayhill, J. R., Herndon, J. H., Kniker, W. T., and Levine, H. B.   Ketoconazole treatment of chronic mucocutaneous candidiasis. *Arch. Dermatol.* 116:1137–1141.

Kirkpatrick, C. H., and Alling, D. W.   Treatment of chronic oral candidiasis with clotrimazole troches: A controlled clinical trial. *N. Engl. J. Med.* 299:1201–1203, 1978.

Kirkpatrick, C. H., and Sohnle, P. G. Chronic Mucocutaneous Candiasis. In B. Safai and R. A. Good (eds.), *Immunodermatology*. New York: Plenum, 1981. Pp. 495–514.

Maibach, H. I., and Kligman, A. M. The biology of experimental human cutaneous moniliasis (*Candida albicans*). *Arch. Dermatol.* 85:233–257, 1962.

Petersen, E. A., Alling, D. W., and Kirkpatrick, D. H. Treatment of chronic mucocutaneous candidiasis with ketoconazole. *Ann. Intern. Med.* 93:791–795, 1980.

Ray, T. L., Hanson, A., Ray, L. F., and Wuepper, K. D. Purification of mannan from *Candida albicans* which activates serum complements. *J. Invest. Dermatol.* 73:269–274, 1979.

Rebora, A., Marples, R. R., and Kligman, A. M. Erosic interdigitalis blastomycetica. *Arch. Dermatol.* 108:66–68, 1973.

Rebora, A., Marples, R. R., and Kligman, A. M. Experimental infection with *Candida albicans*. *Arch. Dermatol.* 108:69–73, 1973.

Sohnle, P. G., and Collins-Lech, C. Relative antigenicity of *P. orbiculare* and *C. albicans*. *J. Invest. Dermatol.* 75:279–283, 1980.

Stone, O. J., and Mullins, F. J. Role of *Candida albicans* in chronic disease. *Arch. Dermatol.* 91:70–72, 1965.

Witten, V. H., and Katz, S. I. Nystatin. *Med. Clin. North Am.* 54:1329–1337, 1970.

DERMATOPHYTE INFECTIONS

Artis, W. M., Odle, B. M., and Jones, H. E. Griseofulvin-resistant dermatophytosis correlates with in vitro resistance. *Arch. Dermatol.* 117:16–19, 1981.

Baden, H. P. Fungal infections: Treatment with a keratolytic gel. *Cutis* 16:574–575, 1975.

Baer, R. L., and Rosenthal, S. A. The biology of fungous infections of the feet. *J. A. M. A.* 197:1017–1020, 1966.

Bagatell, F. K. Topical therapy for onychomycosis. *Arch. Dermatol.* 113:378, 1977.

Epstein, W. L., Shak, V., and Riegelman, S. Dermatopharmacology of griseofulvin. *Cutis* 15:271–275, 1975.

Fulton, J. E. Miconazole therapy for endemic fungal disease. *Arch. Dermatol.* 111:596–598, 1975.

Grant, L. V. A further look at the treatment of onychomycosis with topical glutaraldehyde. *J. Am. Podiatry Assoc.* 64:158–161, 1974.

Hildick-Smith, G., Blank, H., and Sarkany, I. *Fungal Diseases and Their Treatment*. Boston: Little, Brown, 1964.

Hunziker, N., and Brun, R. Lack of delayed reaction in presence of cell-mediated immunity in trichophyton hypersensitivity. *Arch. Dermatol.* 116:1266, 1980.

Jones, H. E., Reinhardt, J. H., and Rinaldi, M. G. Model dermatophytosis in naturally infected subjects. *Arch. Dermatol.* 110:369–374, 1974.

Jones, H. E., Simpson, J. G., and Artis, W. M. Oral ketoconazole: An effective and safe treatment for dermatophytosis. *Arch. Dermatol.* 117:129–134, 1981.

Leyden, J. J., and Kligman, A. M. Aluminum chloride in the treatment of symptomatic athlete's foot. *Arch. Dermatol.* 111:1004–1010, 1975.

Leyden, J. J., and Kligman, A. M. Interdigital athlete's foot: The interaction of dermatophytes and resident bacteria. *Arch. Dermatol.* 114:1466–1472, 1978.

Rebel, G., and Taplin, D. *Dermatophytes: Their Identification and Recognition* (2nd ed.). Coral Gables, Fla.: University of Miami Press, 1970.

Smith, E. B.   New topical agents for dermatophytes. *Cutis* 17:54–58, 1976.

South, D. A., and Farber, E. M.   Urea ointment in the nonsurgical avulsion of nail dystrophies: A reappraisal. *Cutis* 25:609–612, 1980.

Spiekermann, P. H., and Young, M. D.   Clinical evaluation of clotrimazole: A broad-spectrum antifungal agent. *Arch. Dermatol.* 112:350–352, 1976.

Tschen, E. H., Becker, L. E., Ulrich, J. A., Hoge, W. H., and Smith, E. B.   Comparison of over-the-counter agents for tinea pedis. *Cutis* 23:696–698, 1979.

Zaias, N.   Onychomycosis. *Arch. Dermatol.* 105:263–274, 1972.

Zaias, N., Battistini, F., Gomez-Urcuyo, F., Rojas, R. F., and Ricart, R.   Treatment of tinea pedis with griseofulvin and topical antifungal cream. *Cutis* 22:196–199, 1978.

TINEA VERSICOLOR

Allen, H. B., Charles, C. R., and Johnson, B. L.   Hyperpigmented tinea versicolor. *Arch. Dermatol.* 112:1110–1112, 1976.

Bamford, J. T. M.   Tinea versicolor treatment. *Arch. Dermatol.* 110:956, 1974.

Boardman, C. R., and Malkinson, F. D.   Tinea versicolor in steroid-treated patients: Incidence in patients with chronic ulcerative colitis and regional enteritis treated with corticotropin and corticosteroids. *Arch. Dermatol.* 85:44–52, 1962.

Burke, R. C.   Tinea versicolor: Susceptibility factors and experimental infection in human beings. *J. Invest. Dermatol.* 36:389–402, 1961.

Dorn, M., and Roehnert, K.   Dimorphism of *Pityrosporum orbiculare* in a defined culture medium. *J. Invest. Dermatol.* 69:244–248, 1977.

Faegemann, J.   Experimental tinea versicolor in rabbits and humans with *Pityrosporum orbiculare*. *J. Invest. Dermatol.* 72:326–329, 1979.

Faegemann, J.   Tinea versicolor and *Pityrosporum orbiculare:* Mycological investigations, experimental infections and epidemiological surveys. *Acta Derm. Venereol.* (Stockh.) [Suppl. 86], 1979.

Faegemann, J., and Bernander, S.   The activity in vitro of five different antimycotics against *Pityrosporum orbiculare*. *Acta Derm. Venereol.* (Stockh.) 59:521–524, 1979.

Faegemann, J., and Fredriksson, T.   An open trial of the effect of a zinc pyrithione shampoo in tinea versicolor. *Cutis* 25:667–669, 1980.

Faegemann, J., and Fredriksson, T.   Propylene glycol in the treatment of tinea versicolor. *Acta Derm. Venereol.* (Stockh.) 60:92–93, 1980.

McGinley, K. J., Lantis, L. R., and Marples, R. R.   Microbiology of tinea versicolor. *Arch. Dermatol.* 102:168–170, 1970.

Mills, O. H., Jr., and Kligman, A. M.   Tretinoin in tinea versicolor. *Arch. Dermatol.* 110:638, 1974.

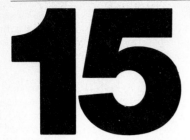

Herpes simplex

I. Definition and pathophysiology. Cutaneous herpes simplex infections take two distinct forms: (1) the painful and disabling primary infection, seen only in previously uninfected individuals without circulating antibody, and (2) the common, bothersome recurrent form of "cold sores" or "fever blisters." In the United States, 7% of the general population have two or more bouts of facial herpes yearly. By 4 years of age, approximately 50% of the population have antibodies to HSV. This percentage increases 60–70% by ages 10 to 14. Following primary infection effective immunity develops in some individuals, but 20–45% of the population will have recurrent disease. Twenty-three percent of the latter group have at least two episodes of recurrent facial herpes per year.

Herpes simplex (HSV) is a DNA virus, infects humans alone, and has an almost universal distribution. There are two types of herpesvirus: type 1, which is usually responsible for nongenital herpetic infections; and type 2, which is usually the agent involved in genital infections in both males and females. Type 2 herpesvirus exhibits biologic as well as morphologic differences from type 1. In addition to the potential threat to the fetus and neonate when the virus infects the reproductive tract during pregnancy, a possible etiologic role in cervical dysplasia and carcinoma has recently been documented. Women with genital herpes simplex infections appear to have 5–10 times greater likelihood of developing cervical carcinoma than do uninfected women and HSV-2 antigens have also been found associated with a high percentage of cases of atypical epithelial lesions of the vulva. It is unclear whether the findings are etiologically important or simply reflect infection by a ubiquitous agent.

Type 2 infection primarily involves persons beyond the age of puberty, is spread by sexual contact, and is one of the most common sexually transmitted diseases.

The majority of affected individuals probably have subclinical primary herpetic infections with type 1 or 2 virus or both; a few may subsequently excrete the virus in respiratory, vaginal, or other secretions and thus constitute a reservoir of infection. Virus excretion persists for 15–42 days after primary infections. Virus titer in recurrent facial-oral disease decreases dramatically by 2 days and most lesions are negative by 5 days. In women with recurrent genital herpes virus is present for a mean of 4.8 days, while 16% may continue to shed virus from lesions after 6 days. The primary infection, which has an incubation period of 3–12 days following exposure, runs a clinical course of 1–3 weeks; recurrent lesions heal more quickly (7–10 days). The risk of recurrence after first episodes of genital herpes is related to virus type and is more likely to occur in men than in women. Only 14% of HSV-1 infections recur, as compared to 60% of HSV-2 infections. Among patients with primary HSV-2 infections, the probability of recurrence is directly related to the presence and titer of antibodies to HSV-2 in convalescent phase serum.

After primary infection, the virus appears to remain latent in sensory ganglia. In patients with recurrent herpes, the virus is periodically reactivated and conducted to the epidermis via peripheral nerve fibers. It then replicates in the skin, producing the recurrent herpetic lesion. Trigger factors include emotional stress, physical trauma (including genital trauma for lesions in this area), sunburn (6 minimal erythema dose UVL radiation is sufficient), menses, fever, and systemic infections. Patients with atopic dermatitis risk the development of generalized lesions (eczema herpeticum) regardless of whether or not their eczema is active. Diseases or drugs that interfere with host response, particularly with the cell-mediated immune components, also predispose to widespread, slowly healing, and more destructive infections. Those with lymphoreticular malignancies or thymic defects and immunosuppressed transplant patients are most prone to severe HSV infections. In the compromised host, chronic cutaneous herpes simplex may develop. Lesions remain active for months, are usually periorificial, and can be destructive.

II. Subjective data

A. Primary symptomatic oral or genital infections

1. Infections on mucosal surfaces are preceded by a day or two of local tenderness.

2. The lesions are accompanied by severe and disabling pain and tender lymphadenopathy, often making it impossible for those with gingivostomatitis to eat or drink, or women with vulvovaginitis to walk or urinate.

3. High fever and purulent malodorous secretions accompany oral or vaginal infections.

4. Primary infection in men usually results in painful penile lesions, but it may also cause urethritis, with dysuria and discharge.

B. Recurrent lesions are preceded by several hours of a burning or tingling sensation in 80% of patients. They are uncomfortable, but much less so than the lesions of the primary infection. Virus is present in the lesion at the time of a prodrome.

III. Objective data (See color insert.)

A. Primary infection

1. **Gingivostomatitis** is the most frequent manifestation of primary infection.

   a. Vesicles, erosions, and maceration are seen over the entire buccal mucosa.

   b. Marked erythema and edema of the gingiva are typical.

   c. Submandibular adenopathy usually is present.

2. **Vulvovaginitis** is seen most frequently in girls and young women.

    a. It consists of widespread vesicles, erosions, and edema in the vulva, labia, and surrounding skin.

    b. These areas become very edematous, erythematous, and extremely tender.

    c. A profuse vaginal discharge is present and some women develop urinary retention.

    d. Bilateral, tender, inguinal adenopathy is usually present.

3. **Urethritis** in men is accompanied by a watery discharge and the occasional presence of vesicles around the urethral meatus.

4. **Inoculation herpes** is commonly found on the paronychial area ("herpetic whitlow") of nurses and physicians, particularly those involved with mouth care, and may also be found on previously traumatized or burned skin. The lesions are characterized by the sudden appearance of vesicles and are accompanied by extreme local pain, sometimes a sterile lymphangitis, and a systemic reaction. Herpetic whitlow is often misdiagnosed as a bacterial paronychia and mistreated with incision and drainage of lesions, with subsequent implantation of the virus into the incised tissue.

5. **Cervicitis** is often asymptomatic but nevertheless important to recognize in pregnant women because of the associated risk of fetal infection and spontaneous abortion. Pregnant women who acquire genital herpes during the first 20 weeks of pregnancy have an increased risk of abortions, whereas the infants of those who acquire infection after 20 weeks have an increased incidence of prematurity.

B. **Recurrent infection**

1. Multiple small vesicles, clustered together, appear at the site of premonitory symptoms.

    a. The vesicles may arise from normal skin or from an area that has a slight erythematous blush.

    b. Vesicles are initially clear, then become cloudy and purulent, dry and crust, and heal within 7–10 days.

    c. The mature lesion consists of grouped vesicles and/or pustules on an erythematous edematous base.

2. The presence of a yellow or golden crust on older lesions indicates bacterial superinfection.

3. Regional, often tender, adenopathy is almost always present. Lymphangitis and lymphadenitis may be seen, particularly with recurrent lesions of the hands.

4. The most common sites for lesions are on the face (lips, perioral area, cheeks, and nose) and neck. Next is the anogenital area, then the sacrum and buttocks. However, recurrent herpes can be seen anywhere on the skin. It is uncommon for recurrent lesions to be located inside the oral cavity except in the immunocompromised host.

IV. Assessment. Any doubt concerning the presence of a herpes simplex infection may be clarified by any of several diagnostic procedures:

A. Skin biopsy of a typical viral vesicle will reveal a characteristic picture: (1) an intraepidermal lesion in the mid-to-upper epidermis; (2) ballooning degeneration of cells; (3) acantholytic cells floating free; and (4) large, multinucleated viral giant cells. Intranuclear inclusions may be seen in the giant cells as well as in other infected epidermal cells.

B. A cytologic smear of the vesicle, for the purpose of looking for giant cells and inclusion bodies, is easily and quickly done (see p. 213). The smears are positive in about 75% of virus culture positive recurrent facial herpes, but in only approximately 40% of ulcerative genital lesions. It is important that the earliest vesicle be chosen for biopsy or cytologic smears. Lesions of herpes simplex, herpes zoster, and varicella will have an identical appearance on biopsy and tissue smear. Exfoliative cytology (Papanicolaou smear) is especially useful as a means of detecting asymptomatic cervical or vaginal infection in women.

C. The virus may be easily and rapidly grown from the vesicle fluid (24–48 hr).

D. Specific neutralizing antibody titers will rise after the first week of primary infection and peak at 2–3 weeks. Change in antibody titer cannot be used as a criterion for recurrent lesions.

E. If the appropriate facilities and reagents are available the following procedures may be carried out if indicated:

1. The virus may be easily identified under electron microscope.

2. The virus can be demonstrated in tissue specimens using immunofluorescent or immunoperoxidase techniques.

3. The virus may be typed by appropriate serologic tests.

V. Therapy

A. Prophylactic measures. There is no prophylactic therapy of proven value. The repeated use of vaccines (smallpox, polio, BCG, Lupidon G, influenza, yellow fever) has never been shown to reliably inhibit recurrent herpes simplex. Immune stimulants (levamisole, isoprinosine, interferon) are available for investigational use only and have not yet been shown to affect the course of recurrent herpes in the normal host. No immune defect is present in patients with recurring herpes infections. If a consistent trigger factor can be identified after careful questioning, specific measures may be taken to counteract these stimuli (i.e., use of sunscreens or avoidance of sun or other specific trauma). Genital herpes is a sexually transmitted disease, and primary infection can be prevented by avoiding sexual contact with an individual with active lesions. Pregnant women with active herpes vulvar lesions or in whom herpesvirus has been recovered by cervical or vaginal culture 4–6 weeks prior to delivery should have a cesarean section. Neonatal herpes, which may be acquired transplacentally or more often from direct inoculation in the birth canal, may be an overwhelming and fatal infection. If the virus is present in the canal at birth, the risk of infant involvement is 40% unless the infant is delivered abdominally before or within 4 hr of membrane rupture. If the fetus becomes infected at delivery it runs a 50% risk of mortality.

B. Active therapy

1. Primary infection

a. The primary infection is extremely painful, and adequate analgesia is important. If salicylates are inadequate, opiates may be needed for the first 7–10 days.

b. With first-episode primary genital herpes, 5% acyclovir (Zovirax) ointment applied within 6 days of onset 6 times daily for 7 days will decrease the duration of viral shedding and the time to complete crusting of lesions. Time to healing will not be shortened. Therapy does not prevent recurrences.

c. Acyclovir administered intravenously has been shown to decrease the duration of viral excretion and reduce healing times of severe initial episodes of genital herpes in healthy patients, and/or initial mucosal HEV-1 and HEV-2 infections in immunocompromised children and adults.

d. Cleansing mouthwashes (with benzalkonium chloride [Zephiran] 1:1000 or tetracycline suspension 250 mg/60 ml H_2O) both clean and soothe involved mucous membranes as well as decrease secondary bacterial superinfections.

e. Vulvovaginitis and genital lesions may be aided by sitz baths in tepid water with or without Aveeno colloidal oatmeal. Women unable to void may sometimes be able to do so while in a bath. If not, intermittent catheterization or a temporary indwelling Foley catheter is necessary.

f. This is one of the few instances in which topical anesthetics are justified (see p. 243). Dyclonine hydrochloride (Dyclone), Benadryl Elixir, or viscous Xylocaine may be used for oral lesions (see Aphthous Stomatitis, p. 20), and benzocaine aerosol (Americaine) or Quotane ointment may be beneficial symptomatically for the vulvar area. Application should be as frequent as is necessary to keep the patient comfortable. The benzocaine preparations may sensitize the skin and should not be used routinely.

2. Recurrent infection

a. There are no topical agents that have yet been shown to reliably shorten the healing time or lower the recurrence rate of cutaneous herpes simplex infections. Agents that have been shown to be ineffective, or that have not been clearly shown to be useful, include ethyl ether, chloroform, alcohol, idoxuridine (IDUR) (Stoxil, Herplex), adenine arabinoside (Vira-A), vitamins C, E, and B_{12}, lactobacillus, 2-deoxy-D-glucose, zinc, lysine, povidone-iodine, dye-light (photodynamic inactivation), silver sulfadiazine (Silvadene), nonoxynol-9 cream, and dimethyl sulfoxide (DMSO).

b. When lesions are vesicular apply cool compresses with tap water or Burow's solution (see p. 313) for 10 min 3–4 times a day.

    c. Apply topical antibacterials such as povidone-iodine ointment or bacitracin ointment to prevent bacterial superinfection.

    d. Some physicians believe that early and repeated application of a potent fluorinated steroid to the lesion will decrease its severity by inhibiting the inflammatory response. If this modality is used, it is essential to avoid the immediate periorbital area.

    e. Acyclovir, a new antiviral agent, has been shown to decrease virus titers in facial and genital herpes lesions treated topically, but time-to-healing was not shortened. IV acyclovir will decrease virus excretion, reduce pain, and promote rapid healing of recurrent HSV-1 and HSV-2 infections in *immunocompromised* children and adults. Further studies with this investigational drug are in progress.

3. Ocular infection. Patients with symptoms of corneal involvement (photophobia, pain) should be examined with a slit lamp. Herpes simplex keratitis is treated with trifluridine (Viroptic), IDUR (Herplex, Stoxil), or adenine arabinoside monophosphate (Vira-A, Ara-A); however, herpetic lesions of the lids and the immediate periorbital area, in the absence of ocular involvement, need not be treated with intraocular medication.

References

Bader, C., Crumpacker, C. S., Schnipper, L. E., Ransil, B., Clark, J. E., Arndt, K. A., and Freedberg, I. M.   The natural history of recurrent facial-oral infection with herpes simplex virus. *J. Infect. Dis.* 138:897–905, 1978.

Corey, L., Nahmias, A. J., Guinan, M. E., Benedetti, J. K., Critchlow, C. W., and Holmes, K. K.   A trial of acyclovir in genital herpes simplex virus infections. *N. Engl. J. Med.* 306:1313–1319, 1982.

Curry, S. S.   Cutaneous herpes simplex infections and their treatment. *Cutis* 26:41–58, 1980.

Douglas, R. G., and Couch, R. B.   A prospective study of chronic herpes simplex virus infection and recurrent herpes labialis in humans. *J. Immunol.* 104:289–295, 1970.

Guinan, M. E., MacCalman, W., Kern, E. R., Overall, J. C., Jr., and Spruance, S. L.   The course of untreated recurrent genital herpes simplex infection in 27 women. *N. Engl. J. Med.* 304:759–763, 1981.

Howard, W. R., Taylor, J. A., and Steck, W. D.   Lymphatic complications of manual herpes simplex infection. *Cutis* 23:580–583, 1979.

Juel-Jensen, B. E., and MacCullum, F. O.   *Herpes Simplex, Varicella and Zoster.* Philadelphia: Lippincott, 1972.

Kaufman, R. H., Dreesman, G. R., Burek, J., Korkonen, M. O., Matsun, D. O., Melnick, J. L., Powell, K. L., Purifoy, D. J. M., Courtney, R. J., and Adam, E.   Herpesvirus-induced antigens in squamous cell carcinoma in situ of the vulva. *N. Engl. J. Med.* 305:483–488, 1981.

Kibrick, S.   Herpes simplex infection at term: What to do with mother, newborn, and nursery personnel. *J.A.M.A.* 243:157–160, 1980.

Krueger, G. C., Spruance, S. L., and Overall, J. C., Jr.   Herpes simplex labialis: A review of pathogenesis, natural history, and therapy. *JCE Dermatol.* 19–37, 1978.

Logan, W. S., Tindall, J. P., and Elson, M. L.   Chronic cutaneous herpes simplex. *Arch. Dermatol.* 103:606–614, 1971.

Muller, S. A., Herrmann, E. D., and Winkelmann, R. K.   Herpes in hematologic malignancies. *Am. J. Med.* 52:102–114, 1972.

Nahmias, A. J., and Roizman, B.   Infection with herpes simplex viruses 1 and 2. *N. Engl. J. Med.* 289:667–674, 719–725, 781–789, 1973.

Raab, B., and Lorinez, A. L.   Genital herpes simplex—concepts and treatment. *J. Am. Acad. Dermatol.* 5:249–263, 1981.

Reeves, W. C., Corey, L., Adonus, H. G., Vouter, L. A., and Holmes, K. K.   Risk of recurrence after first episodes of genital herpes: Relation to HSV type and antibody response. *N. Engl. J. Med.* 305:315–319, 1981.

Rosato, F. E., Rosato, E. F., and Plottan, S. A.   Herpetic paronychia: An occupational hazard of medical personnel. *N. Engl. J. Med.* 283:804–805, 1970.

Schneidman, D., Barr, R., and Graham, J.   Chronic cutaneous herpes simplex. *J.A.M.A.* 241:592–594, 1979.

Wheeler, C. E., Jr.   Pathogenesis of recurrent herpes simplex infections. *J. Invest. Dermatol.* 65:341–346, 1975.

Wheeler, C. E., Jr., and Abele, D. C.   Eczema herpeticum, primary and recurrent. *Arch. Dermatol.* 93:162–173, 1966.

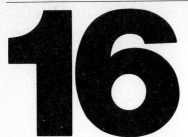

Herpes zoster and varicella

I. Definition and pathophysiology. Infection with the zoster-varicella virus will produce one of two clinical entities. Generalized, highly contagious, and usually benign chickenpox will develop in the nonimmune host, while localized and painful zoster (shingles) will develop in the partially immune host. Clinical manifestations reflect the interaction between this virus and the host immune mechanisms.

Chickenpox, usually acquired through droplets from a respiratory source, is seen primarily in the winter and spring, has an incubation period of 10–23 days, begins abruptly, and the lesions heal or even disappear within 7–10 days. Ninety percent of reported cases occur in children less than 10 years of age. Four percent of infections are subclinical. Almost every individual has been infected by young adulthood. The disease is communicable from 1 day prior to the appearance of the exanthem to 6 days after, and crusts are noninfectious. Signs, symptoms, and complications often become more severe with age; adolescents and adults may become severely ill, particularly when there is pulmonary involvement.

Zoster results from reactivation of latent virus residing in dorsal root or cranial nerve ganglion cells. It is seen sporadically with no seasonal variation; two-thirds of patients are over 40 years old. Lesions erupt for several days and usually are gone within 2–3 weeks in children and 3–4 weeks in adults. Zoster is a self-limited, localized disease which causes discomfort for several days but usually heals without complications. Lesions may be greater in number and persist for up to 7 months in the immunosuppressed. Postherpetic neuralgia, however, is seen with increasing frequency in those over 60 years of age and can be an extremely painful, chronic, and, at times, unremitting plague.

In patients with serious underlying conditions that alter immunologic competence, much more severe disease develops. In children with lymphoma or leukemia, varicella is a life-threatening infection; adults with such diseases often acquire zoster, which may then disseminate. Approximately 2–4% of zoster cases, in normal hosts, will disseminate. However, of all cases of disseminated zoster, about two-thirds of the patients will be found to have malignant disease, including about 40% with lymphoproliferative disorders. In Hodgkin's disease, dissemination may occur in 25% of cases with a mortality approaching 25%. In patients with any type of malignant disease, but particularly Hodgkin's disease, dermatomal zoster develops more frequently than in age-matched controls. The location of the dermatome affected is often related to a site of prior radiation therapy or to the presence of neoplastic lesions either centrally (lesions in or around the spinal column), causing neural irritation, or peripherally, as metastatic deposits. Immunosuppressive therapy for such diseases, or that used in transplantation programs, also predisposes to recurrence of zoster-varicella infection but not necessarily to dissemination.

II. Subjective data

A. Varicella

1. Varicella in children is preceded by little or no prodrome; there may be only 24 hr of malaise and fever. In adolescents and adults, fever and constitutional symptoms almost always precede the exanthem by 24–48 hr.

2. The appearance of cough, dyspnea, and chest pain within 2–5 days after the onset of the rash is indicative of severe pulmonary involvement.

3. Pruritus is the primary and most annoying feature of chickenpox, and the patient's scratching contributes to secondary bacterial infection and scarring.

B. Zoster. The appearance of zoster lesions is frequently preceded by a mild to severe preeruptive itch, tenderness, or pain; the last may be generalized over the entire nerve segment, localized to part of it, or referred. This pain may be confused with that of pleural or cardiac disease, cholecystitis or other abdominal catastrophe, renal or ureteral colic, sciatica, etc. Neurologic changes within the affected dermatome include hypesthesia, dyesthesia, or hyperesthesia. The interval between pain and eruption may be as long as 10 days, but averages 3–5 days. In some patients, particularly children, there are no sensory changes at all. The pain will usually subside within several weeks, but 73% of patients over 60 years of age have discomfort that persists over 8 weeks.

III. Objective data (See color insert.)

A. Chickenpox begins abruptly with the appearance of discrete, erythematous macules and papules located primarily over the thorax, scalp, and mucous membranes; the face and distal extremities remain less involved. Lesions progress rapidly from erythematous macules to 2- –3-mm clear, tense, fragile vesicles surrounded by an erythematous areola. As the lesions progress, they first become umbilicated and then within hours become cloudy and purulent, with crusts forming in 2–4 days. Varicella lesions appear in 3–5 distinct crops for up to a 5-day period, and lesions in **all** stages of development may be seen within one area (an important difference from smallpox). Crusts fall off in 1–3 weeks.

B. Zoster lesions appear first posteriorly and progress to the anterior and peripheral distribution of the nerve involved (see end-paper figures for dermatome charts). Only rarely will the eruption be bilateral. Erythematous macules, papules, and plaques are seen first, and in most instances grouped vesicles appear within 24 hr, although blisters never develop in some patients. Plaques may be scattered irregularly along a dermatomal segment or may become confluent. Mucous membranes within the dermatomes are also affected. The vesicles become purulent, crust, and fall off within 1–2 weeks. The presence of a few vesicles (10–25) outside the affected dermatome is usual and does not imply dissemination.

Zoster appears most often in thoracic and cervical segments. Lesions on the tip of the nose herald involvement of the nasociliary branch of the ophthalmic division of the trigeminal nerve, implying a strong possibility of concomitant keratoconjunctivitis. Paresis and permanent motor damage are more common than previously thought and are found mostly with involvement of the trigeminal and upper cervical and thoracic nerves.

C. Those predisposed to more severe disease may show hemorrhagic, bullous, and infarctive-gangrenous lesions, which will heal slowly with scarring.

IV. Assessment

A. Infection may be confirmed by a cytologic smear of the vesicle, by biopsy, or by serologic methods (see Herpes Simplex, p. 96).

B. Patients more at risk for severe varicella or those with disseminated zoster should be hospitalized and kept under strict precautions, in private rooms and away from seriously ill patients and those with lymphoproliferative disease or on immunosuppressive therapy. All patients with disseminated zoster or those severely ill with varicella should be investigated for underlying neoplastic or immunologic disease.

C. Approximately 50% of adults with varicella show nodular pulmonary infiltrates, but not all will manifest clinical respiratory disease. A chest x ray is indicated for evaluation.

V. Therapy

A. Varicella. Most patients with varicella require only symptomatic therapy.

1. Localized itching may be alleviated by application of a drying antipruritic lotion (calamine alone or with 0.25% menthol and/or 1.0% phenol). Lotion with phenol should not be given to pregnant women.

2. Antihistamines may help pruritus.

3. The patient should cut nails short and keep hands clean, and children should wear gloves, if necessary, to prevent excoriation.

4. Mouth and perineal lesions may be treated by rinses or compresses with hydrogen peroxide, saline, or other agents (see Herpes Simplex, p. 97).

5. Apply topical antibiotic ointments to locally infected lesions. If infection is widespread, it is most often due to Group A beta-hemolytic streptococcus or staphylococcus and systemic antibiotics should be used.

6. High-risk susceptible patients (those with lymphoma-leukemia or immunodeficiency, those on immunosuppressive drugs, the newborn child of a mother with varicella) under 15 years of age with close exposure to varicella or zoster should be passively immunized by use of varicella-zoster globulin (VZIG). This will effectively abort clinical infection if administered within 72 hr of exposure.

B. Zoster

1. Analgesics should be given as necessary. Opiates may be needed.

2. For the vesicular stages, one of the following may be effective:

a. Application of cool compresses with 1:20 Burow's solution.

b. Painting of lesions with equal parts of tincture of benzoin and flexible collodion, or with flexible collodion q12h.

c. Application of a drying shake lotion containing alcohol, menthol, and/or phenol.

d. Splinting the area with an occlusive dressing is often very useful in relieving pain. Lesions should be covered with cotton and then wrapped with an elastic bandage as for a fractured rib.

3. When lesions are crusted and/or secondarily infected, Burow's solution compresses should be applied (see p. 313) and systemic antibiotics used if appropriate.

4. Ocular involvement should be evaluated by an ophthalmologist. Herpes zoster keratoconjunctivitis is treated with topical ophthalmic corticosteroids. The distinction from herpes simplex keratitis is an important one. The treatment is different (see p. 98).

5. Acyclovir has been shown to improve the rate of healing of skin lesions and shorten the period of pain in acute herpes zoster after intravenous administration.

6. In patients 50–60 years of age it is possible to decrease the incidence of postherpetic neuralgia by the use of systemic corticosteroids (presumably by inhibiting perineural inflammation and fibrosis). Noss (1979) believes that systemic corticosteroids are the treatment of choice for herpes zoster accompanied by pain, in the trigeminal distribution, with facial paralysis, or with Ramsay Hunt syndrome. Eaglstein et al. (1970) administered prednisone or its equivalent at a dose of 60 mg every day for 1 week, 30 mg every day for the second week, and finally, 15 mg every day for the third week. Keczkes and Basheer (1980) dispensed prednisone 40 mg daily with gradual reduction over 4 weeks. Treatment should be started within the first 5–7 days of the eruption. The risk-benefit ratio must be determined for each patient. Systemic corticosteroids do not influence the healing time of the acute eruption and do not increase the risk of dissemination. They will decrease the severity of edema and often the pain, and are very useful in patients with severe facial swelling either with or without ocular involvement.

7. **Postherpetic neuralgia.** Already existing postherpetic pain is extremely difficult to alleviate. There are several approaches that have been suggested:

a. Chlorprothixene (Taractan) was effective in bringing relief to 29 of 30 patients in one study (Farber and Burks, 1974). Patients with severe neuralgia received 50–100 mg IM followed by 50 mg PO q6h for 7–10 days. Patients with moderate neuralgia took 50-mg tablets PO q6h for 4–10 days. Some improvement was noted within 72 hr. A later study reported pain relief in one of three patients at high doses, and prominent side effects (Nathan, 1978).

b. The use of a combination of a tricyclic antidepressant and a substituted phenothiazine medication may lead to almost complete relief of pain within 1–2 weeks after institution of therapy. Amitriptyline (Elavil) 75–100 mg every day should be used in combination with either perphenazine (Trilafon) 4 mg 3–4 times a day, fluphenazine hydrochloride (Permitil) 1 mg 3–4 times a day, or thioridazine (Mellaril) 25 mg 4id. It may be necessary to continue medication for months.

c. Beneficial results have been reported with the combined use of either carbamazepine (Tegretol) 600–800 mg/day or phenytoin sodium (Dilantin) 300–400 mg/day with 50–100 mg of nortriptyline (Aventyl, Pamelor) (Hatangdi et al., 1976); and with combined use of carbamazepine (Tegretol) up to 1000 mg/day and clomipramine up to 75 mg/day (Gerson et al., 1977).

d. Pain relief in patients with acute herpes zoster and in many patients with post–zoster neuralgia has been claimed to follow daily intralesional or subcutaneous injection of triamcinolone 0.2 mg/ml into the affected dermatome. Up to 30 ml of the drug diluted in saline or 60 mg of triamcinolone can be administered at each session.

e. Repeated cryosurgery to limited areas affected by postherpetic neuralgia has been reported to reduce sensitivity of trigger areas and produce long-term relief of pain (Suzuki, 1980).

f. Transcutaneous electrical stimulation has brought pain relief to a high percentage of patients treated in this fashion.

g. Neurosurgical intervention is occasionally necessary in patients with intractable pain.

References

Blank, H., Eaglstein, W. H., and Goldfaden, G. H.   Zoster: A recrudescence of VZ virus infection. *Postgrad. Med. J.* 46:653–658, 1970.

Brown, G. R.   Herpes zoster: Correlation of age, sex, distribution neuralgia and associated disorders. *South. Med. J.* 69:576–578, 1976.

Eaglstein, W. H., Katz, R., and Brown, J. A.   The effects of early corticosteroid therapy on the skin eruption and pain of herpes zoster. *J.A.M.A.* 211:1681–1683, 1970.

Epstein, E.   Treatment of zoster and postzoster neuralgia by the intralesional injection of Triamcinolone: A computer analysis of 199 cases. *Int. J. Dermatol.* 15:762–769, 1976.

Farber, G. A., and Burks, J. W.   Chlorprothixene therapy for herpes zoster neuralgia. *South. Med. J.* 67:808–812, 1974.

Gallagher, J. G., and Merigan, T. C.   Prolonged herpes zoster infection associated with immunosuppressive therapy. *Ann. Intern. Med.* 91:842–846, 1979.

Gershon, A. A., Stanberg, S., and Brunell, P. A.   Zoster immune globulin: A further assessment. *N. Engl. J. Med.* 209:243–245, 1979.

Gerson, G. R., Jones, B. B., and Luscombe, D. K.   Studies in the concomitant use of carbamazepine and clomipramine for the relief of post-herpetic neuralgia. *Postgrad. Med. J.* 53:104–109, 1977.

Gordon, J. E.   Chickenpox: An epidemiological review. *Am. J. Med. Sci.* 244:362–389, 1962.

Hatangdi, H. S., Boas, R. A., and Richards, E. G.   Postherpetic Neuralgia: Management with Antiepileptic and Tricyclic Drugs. In J. J. Bonica, et al. (eds.), *Advances in Pain Research and Therapy.* New York: Raven Press, 1976. Pp. 583–587.

Hope-Simpson, R. E.   The nature of herpes zoster: A long-term study and a new hypothesis. *Proc. R. Soc. Med.* 58:9–20, 1965.

Juel-Jensen, B. E., and MacCallum, F. O.   *Herpes Simplex, Varicella and Zoster.* Philadelphia: Lippincott, 1972.

Keczkes, K., and Basheer, A. M.   Do corticosteroids prevent post-herpetic zoster? *Br. J. Dermatol.* 102:551–555, 1980.

Luby, J. P.   Varicella-zoster virus. *J. Invest. Dermatol.* 61:212–222, 1973.

Mazur, M., and Dolin, R.   Herpes zoster at the N.I.H.:A 20-year experience. *Am. J. Med.* 65:738–743, 1978.

Miller, L. H., and Brunell, P. A.   Zoster, reinfection or activation of latent virus?: Observations on the antibody response. *Am. J. Med.* 49:480–483, 1970.

Nathan, P. W.   Chlorprothixine (Taractan) in postherpetic neuralgia and other severe chronic pain. *Pain* 5:367–371, 1978.

Nuss, D. D.   Herpes zoster: Treatment with high-dose prednisone. *Bull. Assn. Mil. Dermatol.* 5:13–15, 1979.

Peterslund, N. A., Ipsen, J., Schonheyden, H., Seyer-Hansen, K., Esmann, V., and Juhi, H.   Acyclovir in herpes zoster. *Lancet* 2:827–830, 1981.

Rogers, R. S., and Tindall, J. P.   Herpes zoster in children. *Arch. Dermatol.* 106:204–207, 1972.

Suzuki, H., Ogawa, S., Nakagawa, N., Kanayama, T., Tai, K., Saitoh, H., Ottshima, Y.   Cryocautery of sensitized skin areas for the relief of pain due to post-herpetic neuralgia. *Pain* 9:355–362, 1980.

Taub, A.   Relief of postherpetic neuralgia with psychotropic drugs. *J. Neurosurg.* 39:235–239, 1973.

Vonderheid, E. C., and Van Voorst Vander, P. C.   Herpes zoster-varicella in cutaneous T-cell lymphomas. *Arch. Dermatol.* 116:408–412, 1980.

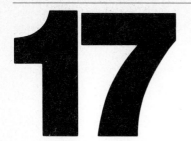

Hyperpigmentation and hypopigmentation

I. Definition and pathophysiology. Patients with pigmentary changes on their skin seek advice primarily for cosmetic reasons; they complain of having either too much or too little pigmentation, or they are unhappy with its distribution. Although pigment changes are usually asymptomatic and of no medical consequence, they may signify systemic disease.

A. Hyperpigmentation

1. **Melasma (chloasma)** is found most often on the facial areas of women who either are taking anovulatory drugs or are pregnant, and has been called "mask of pregnancy." However, it may also be found in men or women with no endocrinologic abnormalities. Its cause remains unknown, but sun is necessary for its development. It is present more frequently in dark Caucasians (e.g., Puerto Ricans and those of Mediterranean background).

2. **Freckles (ephelides),** like melasma, are present only on light-exposed skin, and the pigment is found only in the epidermis; neither are found on mucous membranes. Freckling is genetically determined, appears mostly by age 5–7, and is seen most in redheads, blondes, and other fair-skinned individuals. Paradoxically, there are fewer melanocytes in a freckle than in normal surrounding skin, but those that are present are large and able to form more melanin than usual. Freckles, like melasma, darken considerably in the summertime and may fade almost completely in the winter.

3. A **lentigo** is most often confused with a freckle. These hyperpigmented spots, which may appear at any age, are usually darker than freckles and are not induced by ultraviolet radiation. An increased number of melanocytes are present in the basal layer, and the epidermal rete ridges are elongated and clubbed. Lentigines are seen equally well in winter and summer and can be present on the palms, soles, and mucous membranes. The multiple lentigines ("leopard") syndrome is often associated with electrocardiographic changes. In the Peutz-Jeghers syndrome, lentigines on the lips and hands occur with small bowel polyposis. Such lentigines can be confused with the multiple, small, café-au-lait spots of neurofibromatosis. Solar ("senile") lentigines, commonly and incorrectly known as "liver spots," appear on the exposed surfaces of fair-skinned people long exposed to the sun, usually in association with other changes from sun damage, including wrinkling, dryness, and actinic keratoses.

4. **Postinflammatory hyperpigmentation** is common in more darkly pigmented persons and is more related to the nature of the insult than

to the degree of previous inflammation; it is severe following some conditions such as thermal burns and mild after others. There is an increase in epidermal melanin, but there may also be melanin granules present in dermal macrophages. Postinflammatory hyperpigmentation may persist for months to years.

B. Hypopigmentation

1. **Vitiligo** is a disorder in which areas of the skin are completely lacking melanin pigmentation. Pigment cells (melanocytes) cannot be detected in depigmented areas, even on inspection by electron microscopy. This is in contrast to albinism, in which melanocytes are present, but there is little or no pigmentation because of faulty or absent tyrosinase. The cause of vitiligo is unknown, but abnormal neurogenic stimuli, an enzymatic self-destruct mechanism, and an autoimmune mechanism have been postulated as pathogenetic factors. It appears to be inherited in some kinships and is found with increased frequency in patients with thyroid disease, Addison's disease, and pernicious anemia. In vitiligo patients there is also an increased incidence of halo nevi, diabetes mellitus, and alopecia areata. Lesions rarely repigment spontaneously.

2. **Postinflammatory** or **posttraumatic hypopigmentation** may be profound enough to mimic vitiligo, but frequently appears as slightly scaly, slightly lighter areas of skin (**pityriasis alba**). It is often seen following cutaneous diseases such as psoriasis and atopic dermatitis and in those instances may be related to the inability of altered epidermal cells to accept melanin granules rather than to the decreased production of pigment in melanocytes. Pityriasis alba is found most frequently on exposed areas (e.g., face) in children with atopic backgrounds. Postinflammatory hypopigmentation repigments slowly but in rare instances may be permanent, especially if scarring has occurred.

II. Subjective data.
There are no symptoms associated with melasma, freckles, lentigines, or postinflammatory changes. The depigmented areas of vitiligo sunburn easily.

III. Objective data

A. **Melasma** appears as large, tan macules with irregular borders in a reticulated pattern on the cheeks, upper lip, and forehead.

B. **Freckles** are small (usually 2–5 mm), pale to dark macules scattered irregularly on the face, shoulders, back, and other sun-exposed areas. There is usually a sharp line of demarcation between freckled and unexposed skin.

C. **Lentigines** may be the same size as freckles, or may be larger; they may be found anywhere on the cutaneous surface. **Solar ("senile") lentigines** are pale to dark brown macules found on the dorsum of the hand and on the face. They vary in color and size (from millimeters to centimeters in diameter) and may have indistinct borders.

D. **The lesions of vitiligo** are completely depigmented—pure white—except in the rare case of trichrome vitiligo, which has both depigmented and hypopigmented areas. They usually have sharp borders and are found symmetrically over bony prominences such as the wrists and around body orifices (lips, eyes, and anogenital areas). Injury to the skin of these patients may cause a temporary or permanent loss of pigment in that area. Scars, scratch marks, and bruises may thus heal with no pigment present. Hair growing from vitiliginous skin may or may not be white.

E. **Postinflammatory pigment changes** vary in size and are present only at the site of previous inflammation and trauma. The degree of hyper- or hypopigmentation may be mild or marked.

IV. **Assessment.** It is useful to examine pigmentary lesions under Wood's light (see also p. 215). When pigment is present in the epidermis the contrast between normal and hyperpigmented skin is enhanced. When pigment is present in the dermis, the contrast is not enhanced compared to ambient visible light.

Patients with generalized lentigines and those with vitiligo deserve a thorough history and physical examination to search for related systemic findings. Vitiligo patients, especially those in older age groups, need to be checked periodically for incipient or clinically apparent thyroid disease, particularly hypothyroidism. T_4 and TSH determinations provide adequate screening. Phenolic germicidal agents present in many household and industrial products may cause depigmentation indistinguishable from that of vitiligo.

V. Therapy

A. Treatment of hyperpigmentation

1. Lentigines and senile lentigines may be removed or their intensity of pigmentation diminished by light cryosurgical freezing (10–15 sec) with liquid nitrogen. Melanocytes are more sensitive to cold injury than keratinocytes and may be selectively damaged by this technique.

2. The intensity of pigmentation in melasma, freckles, and senile lentigines and the epidermal component of postinflammatory hyperpigmentation may be decreased by the conscientious application of 2–5% hydroquinone cream or lotion (Artra, Eldoquin, Eldoquin Forte, Melanex) 2–3 times a day for weeks to months (see p. 310). Hydroquinone is thought to act by inhibiting one or more steps in the tyrosine-tyrosinase pathway of melanin synthesis. It also affects the formation, melanization, and degradation of melanosomes and eventually causes necrosis of whole melanocytes. The hyperpigmented areas fade more rapidly and completely than surrounding normal skin; 80% of patients with melasma will note some improvement within an 8-week period.

   a. As the ability of the sun to darken these lesions is much greater than that of hydroquinone to "bleach" the pigment, **strict** avoidance of sunlight is imperative. Although sunscreens help, even visible light will cause some pigment darkening and, to be totally adequate, sun protection must therefore be opaque (Clinique Continuous Coverage, Reflecta, RVPaque, zinc oxide cream). Some hydroquinone products are available in an opaque base (Eldopaque, Eldopaque Forte) or with nonopaque sunscreens (Solaquin). Alternatively, a broad-spectrum sun protection factor (SPF) 15 sunscreen may be applied and the patient's makeup of choice put on over that.

Monobenzyl ether of hydroquinone (Benoquin) usually causes irreversible depigmentation and should be used only to eliminate residual areas of normally pigmented skin in patients with extensive vitiligo. It should not be used under any other circumstances.

b. A more effective method for decreasing skin pigment consists of concomitant use of 0.1% tretinoin and 0.05–2.0% hydroquinone. Twice daily application to hyperpigmented areas should induce considerable lessening of pigmentation within 6 weeks. Other approaches include use of 5.0% hydroquinone, 0.1% tretinoin, and 0.1% dexamethasone applied in one cream, or put on sequentially during the day. Peeling and redness usually precede hypopigmentation. Broad-spectrum SPF 15 sunscreen must be used at all times (e.g., Supershade 15, Total Eclipse), and women should apply a colored makeup of their choice *over* the sunscreen.

B. Treatment of vitiligo. There are four methods that may be useful:

1. Bleaching the surrounding skin in order to blur the margins of the lesion, or removing all remaining pigmentation in extensive cases.

Blurring of the margins of the lesion may be attempted with hydroquinone compounds (Artra, Eldoquin Forte, Melanex). Permanent removal of pigment requires the use of monobenzyl ether of hydroquinone (Benoquin) cream.

2. Complete avoidance of the sun, or conscientious use of broad-spectrum sunscreens, thus fading normal pigmentation in the fair-skinned individual and making the vitiligo less noticeable. Vitiligo patients should routinely use SPF 15 sunscreens effective against UVB (see p. 311) when outside to prevent sunburn in nonpigmented areas.

3. Attempting to repigment skin with the topical or systemic use of psoralen compounds.

As a general guide, if the vitiliginous skin is less than 6 sq cm (the size of a quarter or half-dollar), topical psoralens may be used; if a large portion of the body surface is involved, systemic psoralens and sunlight are indicated; if the area involved is extremely widespread, consider depigmentation with monobenzyl ether of hydroquinone.

Psoralen compounds, tricyclic furocoumarinlike molecules found naturally in a variety of plants throughout the world and also produced synthetically, radically increase the erythema response of skin to long-wave ultraviolet light (UVA) after either topical application or systemic administration. For this reason, therapy must be initiated gradually. There appears to be no toxicity associated with long-term trimethylpsoralen administration. Systemic treatment is begun with 0.6 mg/kg (40 mg for a 70-kg patient) of trioxsalen (Trisoralen) ingested with food 2 hr before 5 min per site (approximately 3 joule/sq cm of UVA) of noonday sun exposure. The best time for sun exposure is from 10:00 A.M. to 2:00 P.M., preferably 11:00 A.M. to 1:00 P.M. Exposure is increased by 5 min per day, until redness, beginning about 12–18 hr after sunning and becoming maximal at 48 hr, is achieved after each exposure. If repigmentation has not started after 20–30 treatments or 1½ hr exposure is reached (45 min to each side), increase trioxsalen to 0.9 mg/kg. If the desired results are still not seen after another 20–30 treatments, switch to 0.3 mg/kg of 8-methoxypsoralen (Oxsoralen) and indoor carefully monitored UVA light sources. A combination of 0.6 mg/kg of Trisoralen plus 0.3 mg/kg methoxsalen may be tried if either of the preceding fails. The beginning of repigmentation usually requires 30–50 treatments but this is variable. An alternative method for children or those who like to be outdoors utilizes longer exposures but specifies that the first treatment be late in the afternoon, i.e., 4:30 P.M., the second treatment at 4:00, the third at 3:30, etc. The danger of a severe burn is much greater with methoxsalen. Treatment should be 2–3 times weekly, never 2 days in a row. Patients should be instructed to wear plastic-lens sunglasses known to absorb UVA before and after exposure on treatment days (UVA passes through glass). On nontreatment days, sun exposure as tolerated is permitted for patients being treated with trioxsalen but not for those on methoxsalen. Cloudy weather does not interfere with treatment; ambient temperature also has no effect. Following treatment, a benzophenone containing sunscreen effective against UVA such as Total Eclipse, PreSun 15, Uval, Solbar, or Piz Buin Exclusiv Extrem Cream should be applied to all exposed skin; this will provide partial protection. Those who sunburn easily may benefit from using a UVB sunscreen such as Block Out or Pabanol all day, even during treatment. Prolonged exposure to sunlight beyond the treatment period is to be avoided for 8 hr after the medication has been ingested. Nontender, minimal pink coloration of the patches of vitiligo is acceptable, but if increasing redness develops, discontinue treatments until only faint pinkness remains.

Pigment reappears first as dots around hair follicles and then slowly spreads, becoming confluent. To be successful, therapy must continue for 9–18 months and often through several summers, beginning in early April and continuing through September. It is estimated that it takes about 150–300 exposures to bring about significant improvement. The age of the patient and duration of vitiligo do not affect the response rate. Lesions on the face and neck repigment more easily than those over bony prominences such as the dorsa of the hands, the elbows, and the knees. If treatment is discontinued before an area has completely filled in, the lesion is likely to gradually become white again. Psoralen therapy also increases the tolerance of vitiligo skin to sunlight, perhaps through thickening of the stratum corneum.

Topical 1% methoxsalen solution (Oxsoralen) should be used as follows:

a. Dilute to 0.1% solution with absolute alcohol.

b. Treatment should initially be administered once every 5 days and may be gradually increased to every 3 days.

c. Methoxsalen should be applied with a cotton swab, allowed to dry 1–2 min, and reapplied. The borders of the lesion should be protected with petrolatum and a sunscreen to prevent hyperpigmentation.

d. After a wait of 2 hr, the area should be exposed for 4 min to a black light source at 4 cm (1½ in.) or to 1 min of sunlight. A Wood's light, a small hand-held black light (e.g., UVL-21 or fluorescent UVA light source) may be used.

e. After treatment the area should be washed with soap and water and, if clothing does not cover the lesions, a benzophenone sunscreen or opaque sunscreen (see p. 311) should be applied. Benzophenone products have broad absorption and will protect from 250 to 360 nm; however, they provide only partial protection. Do not allow the treated area to be exposed to direct sunlight for 12 hr.

f. If erythema does not appear (first appearance in 24 hr with maximum at 48 hr), increase the exposure to black light during the next treatment by 2-min increments or exposure to sun by 30 sec until an adequate response is achieved. Never exceed 10 min sunlight exposure. Proceed cautiously, since even a small overexposure will result in blistering.

4. To hide the lesion with stains or cosmetics, use Covermark, an excellent cosmetic makeup; Dy-o-Derm, a stain that contains aniline dyes and dihydroxyacetone; or Vitadye, a cosmetic cover containing FD and C dyes and dihydroxyacetone. These latter agents do **not** provide protection against sunburn, and psoralen phototherapy can take place through such stains.

References

Arndt, K. A., and Fitzpatrick, T. B.   Topical use of hydroquinone as a depigmenting agent. *J.A.M.A.* 194:965–967, 1965.

Belliboni, N., and Yagima, M. E.   Epidemiology of pityriasis alba. *Ann. Brasileiros Dermatologica* 50:135–140, 1975.

Dawber, R. P. R.   Clinical associations of vitiligo. *Postgrad. Med. J.* 46:276–277, 1970.

Engasser, P. G., and Maibach, H. I.   Cosmetics and dermatology: Bleaching creams. *J. Am. Acad. Dermatol.* 5:143–147, 1981.

Epstein, J. H., and Farber, E. M.   Current status of oral PUVA therapy. *J. Am. Acad. Dermatol.* 1:106–117, 1979.

Fitzpatrick, T. B., Arndt, K. A., El Mofty, A. M., and Pathak, M. A.   Hydroquinone and psoralens in the therapy of hypermelanosis and vitiligo. *Arch. Dermatol.* 93:589–600, 1966.

Gano, S. E., and Garcia, P. L.   Topical tretinoin, hydroquinone and betamethasone valerate in the therapy of melasma. *Cutis* 23:239–241, 1979.

Gilchrest, B. A., Fitzpatrick, T. B., Anderson, R. C., and Parrish, J. A.   Localization of melanin pigmentation in the skin with Wood's lamp. *Br. J. Dermatol.* 96:245–248, 1977.

Gorlin, R. J., Anderson, R. C., and Blaw, M.   Multiple lentigines syndrome: Complex comprising multiple lentigines, electrocardiographic conduction abnormalities, ocular hypertelorism, pulmonary stenosis, abnormalities of genitalia, retardation of growth, sensorineural deafness and autosomal dominant hereditary pattern. *Am. J. Dis. Child* 117:652–662, 1969.

Jimbow, K., Obata, H., Pathak, M. A., and Fitzpatrick, T. B.   Mechanism of depigmentation by hydroquinone. *J. Invest. Dermatol.* 62:436–449, 1974.

Kahn, G.   Depigmentation caused by phenolic detergent germicides. *Arch. Dermatol.* 102:177–187, 1970.

Kligman, A. M., and Willis, I.   A new formula for depigmenting human skin. *Arch. Dermatol.* 111:40–48, 1975.

Lerner, A. B.   On the etiology of vitiligo and gray hair. *Am. J. Med.* 51:141–147, 1971.

Mehregan, A. H.   Lentigo senilis and its evolutions. *J. Invest. Dermatol.* 65:429–433, 1975.

Mosher, D. B., Parrish, J. A., and Fitzpatrick, T. B.   Monobenzylether of hydroquinone: A retrospective study of treatment of 18 vitiligo patients and a review of the literature. *Br. J. Dermatol.* 97:669–679, 1977.

Newcomer, V. D., Lindberg, M. C., and Sternberg, T. H.   A melanosis of the face (chloasma). *Arch. Dermatol.* 83:284–299, 1961.

Parrish, J. A., Fitzpatrick, T. B., Shea, C., and Pathak, M. A.   Photochemotherapy of vitiligo. *Arch. Dermatol.* 112:1531–1534, 1976.

Pathak, M. A., Fitzpatrick, T. B., and Parrish, J. A.   Treatment of melasma with hydroquinone. *J. Invest. Dermatol.* 76:324, 1981.

Pathak, M. A., Mosher, D. B., Fitzpatrick, T. B., and Parrish, J. A.   Relative effectiveness of three psoralens and sunlight in repigmentation of 365 vitiligo patients (abstract). *J. Invest. Dermatol.* 74:252, 1980.

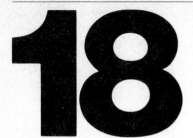

Infestations: pediculosis, scabies, and ticks

I. Definition and pathophysiology

A. Pediculosis. There are two species of blood-sucking lice specific for the human host: *Phthirus pubis* and *Pediculus humanus*. These wingless insects are obligate parasites and are host-specific for humans. The lice that inhabit the head or body are both types of *P. humanus*. They look similar to one another and will interbreed; however, they do have different physiologic feeding habits. The head louse is transmitted through shared clothing and brushes; the body louse, by bedding or clothing; and the pubic louse, from person to person and not infrequently on clothing, bedding, or towels. The chances of acquiring pediculosis pubis from one sexual exposure with an infected person is about 95%.

The adult *P. humanus* louse is 2–4 mm long, has 3 pairs of legs with delicate hooks at the tarsal extremities, and is gray white in appearance. The crab louse (*P. pubis*), which inhabits the genital region, is shorter (1–2 mm) and broader, and the first pair of legs is shorter than the clawlike second and third pair. The adult female louse has a lifespan of about 25 days and lays up to 10 eggs each day. As the lice feed, they inject their digestive juices and fecal material into the skin; it is this, plus the puncture wound itself, that causes pruritus. The ova (nits), which are oval, gray, and firmly attached to the hair, hatch in about 7–9 days and become mature in another week. Ova are laid very close to the scalp and hatch before the hair grows more than ¼ in. If no nits are found within ½ in. of the scalp and no lice are seen, treatment is not necessary because any nits more than ½ in. from the scalp are egg shells from a past infection.

B. Scabies is caused by infestation with the mite *Sarcoptes scabiei*. *S. scabiei* has four pairs of legs and transverse corrugations and bristles on its dorsal aspect. The 1.3×0.4 mm female mite, just visible to the human eye, excavates a burrow in the stratum corneum and travels as much as 5 mm every day for 1–2 months before dying. Each female lays a total of 10–38 eggs, which hatch in about 1 week, reach maturity in about 3 weeks, and start a new cycle. Fewer than 10% of deposited eggs produce adult mites. Most infected adults will harbor 10–12 adult mites.

Scabies is acquired principally through close personal contact, but may be transmitted through clothing, linens, or towels. The female can survive for at least several days away from human beings. The incubation period is usually less than 1 month but can be as long as 2 months. The severe pruritus is probably caused by an acquired sensitivity to the organism and is first noted 3–4 weeks after primary infestation, but sooner in subsequent infections. Immunofluorescent studies suggest a cutaneous vasculitislike pattern in dermal vessels, with the presence of IgM and C_3 conjugates. The delayed host response and these findings suggest a humoral component to the disease. Canine scabies (sarcoptic mange) causes crusting and hair loss over the ear margins, legs, and abdomen of dogs. This is highly communicable and may result in small epidemics in humans.

C. **Ticks** are large mites covered by a tough integument. These ectoparasites live by sucking blood from mammals, birds, and reptiles. They are found in trees, grass, bushes, or on animals (dogs, cattle); after attaching to human skin, the female tick feeds, becomes engorged after 7–14 days, and then drops off. Ticks are capable of transmitting several rickettsial (e.g., Rocky Mountain spotted fever), viral (e.g., encephalitis), and other (Lyme disease and erythema chronicum migrans) illnesses.

II. Subjective data

A. Extreme pruritus is the primary characteristic of pediculosis. In some sensitized patients, generalized pruritus, urticaria, and eczematous changes may develop.

B. Scabies is noted for severe itching, which becomes most marked shortly after the patient goes to bed. Early in the course only the sites of burrows are pruritic; later, the itching may become generalized.

C. Tick bites are painless; often they are discovered several days later when itching develops or the engorged tick is found. Occasionally symptoms of fever, headache, and abdominal pain may occur while the feeding tick remains attached. Children can very rarely develop a reversible flaccid paralysis that starts after the tick has been attached for several days.

III. Objective data

A. Pediculosis

1. **Scalp**

   a. Nits may be found most easily on the hairs on the occiput and above the ears.

   b. Adult lice are often impossible to find, and, in the average case, there will be fewer than 10 mature insects present.

   c. Secondary impetigo and furunculosis with associated cervical lymphadenopathy is a frequent complication.

2. **Body**

   a. Scratch marks, eczematous changes, urticaria, and persistent erythematous papules may be seen. Lesions frequently are most noticeable on the back.

   b. The lice will be found in the seams of clothing and only rarely on the skin. They can move as much as 3.5 cm in 2 hr.

3. **Pubic**

   a. Pubic and thigh hair can be infested by only a few or by uncountable numbers of nits.

   b. The yellow gray adults may be difficult to find.

    c. Small black dots present in infested areas represent either ingested blood in adult lice or their excreta.

    d. Body and axillary hair as well as the eyelashes and beard also should be examined for nits. Pubic lice can move 10 cm a day.

B. Scabies

  1. Multiple straight or S-shaped ridges or dotted lines, 5–20 mm long, that frequently resemble a black thread and end in a vesicle, represent the characteristic burrow, although this need not be present. Mites are also in papules and vesicles, the most common lesions.

  2. Sites of involvement are chiefly the interdigital webs of the hands, wrists, antecubital fossae, points of the elbows, nipples, umbilicus, lower abdomen, genitalia, and gluteal cleft. Lesions of the glans penis are characteristic in males. Infants and small children often have lesions on the palms, soles, head, and neck.

  3. Generalized urticarial papules, excoriations, and eczematous changes are secondary lesions caused by sensitization to the mite.

  4. Indurated erythematous nodules are more common than discrete burrows and are slow to resolve after treatment.

  5. Secondary bacterial infection with impetiginization and furunculosis is common.

  6. Canine scabies lesions are papules or vesicles without burrows seen on the trunk, arms, or abdomen.

C. Ticks. The engorged tick, often the size of a large pea, may resemble a vascular tumor or wart.

  1. Previously sensitized hosts may develop a localized urticarial response.

  2. The usual bite reaction shows small dermal nodules surmounted by necrotic centers.

  3. The site of a tick bite may also be marked by an eschar (a round crusted ulcer).

  4. Granulomatous response to tick bites causes lesions that resemble dermal fibromas (dermatofibroma, histiocytoma).

IV. Assessment

A. Unexplained pyoderma of the scalp, inflammatory cervical or occipital adenopathy, or itching with mild inflammation of the occipital scalp and nuchal area should be attributed to pediculosis until proved otherwise. It is necessary to be persistent in searching for nits. If suspicion is high, a therapeutic trial or reexamination in 2–3 days is indicated.

Unexplained pubic pruritus very frequently is a manifestation of pediculosis. In fastidious individuals few adult lice and nits will be found, and a careful search—ideally employing a hand lens—should be made, with special attention to the genital area.

B. The diagnosis of scabies is made by demonstrating the presence of the organisms, the eggs, or the oval, brown black fecal concretions called scybala, from a burrow or papule. A superficial epidermal shave biopsy is the best method. The best papules for examination are often small but very itchy. Raise the burrow or papule between the forefinger and thumb and use a No. 15 scalpel blade to "saw" off the top of the papule or entire burrow. This procedure is almost painless. Place material on a glass slide, cover with immersion oil, and examine under scanning power. Burrows or papules are found most often between the fingers, on the flexor aspect of the wrists, or on the ulnar aspect of the hands. It may sometimes be difficult to find either the burrow or the mite, and in that case the clinical picture of intense pruritus and papular and excoriated lesions will lead one to the correct diagnosis. It has been suggested that if topical tetracycline (Topicycline) is painted on a suspected area, let dry 3 min, and then washed and dried, scabetic burrows will then fluoresce when viewed under the Wood's light. The mite of canine scabies is easily demonstrated in scrapings from the dog, but rarely seen in preparations taken from human lesions.

V. Therapy

   A. Gamma benzene hexachloride (GBH), (Gamene, Kwell), a pesticide also known as lindane, is the treatment of choice for pediculosis and scabies (see p. 268). GBH is available as a shampoo for the treatment of pediculosis capitis and/or pubis, and in cream and lotion form for treating scabies and all forms of pediculosis. GBH also repels ticks and other arthropods and kills chiggers. Up to 10% of the topically applied drug may be absorbed percutaneously; alternative treatments should therefore be considered in infants, young children, and pregnant women. However, good toxicologic data about other treatment methods are lacking.

   GBH and benzyl benzoate kill the lice, but the dead organisms do not fall off hairs or body spontaneously. Most patients regard the continuing presence of dead organisms as evidence of continuing infestation and it is necessary to clearly instruct them otherwise. Application of a 1:1 solution of white vinegar and water followed by a shower, or combing the hair with a comb dipped directly into vinegar, may help dissolve the dead nits cemented to the hairs and wash off their remains. The only certain way to remove dead nits is with a fine-toothed comb or forceps.

    1. For pediculosis capitis or pubis, 1 oz of shampoo is worked into a lather and left on the scalp or genital area for 4 min. After thorough rinsing, the hair should be cleaned with a fine-toothed comb to remove nit shells. Retreatment is usually not necessary. Pediculocides have not been shown to be ovicidal, and since eggs attached to hair shafts require 7–10 days to hatch, a second application is needed after this interval only if living lice can be demonstrated or eggs are observed at the hair-skin junction. Combs and brushes should be soaked in 2% Lysol or a pediculocidal shampoo for about an hour or heated in water to about 65°C (149°F) for 5–10 min.

    2. For pediculosis corporis the patient need only wash with soap and water and apply topical antipruritic lotions. If lice get on the body, GBH should be used. Lice in clothing may be killed by being washed and/or dried by machine (hot cycle in each), or by boiling, followed by ironing the seams, dry-cleaning, or by applying dry heat at 140°F (60°C) for 20 min. Alternatively, they may be eliminated by dusting with 1% malathion powder or 10% DDT powder.

3. **Pediculosis pubis** should be treated with application of GBH cream or lotion to infested and adjacent areas for 8–12 hr. Alternatively, the shampoo can be used as described above. Clothing, linens, and towels should be washed in very hot water and/or dried for at least 20 min on the "hot" cycle, or dry-cleaned. Temperatures higher than 52°C (125°F) for 5–10 min kill both lice and their eggs. Alternatively, clothing and/or bedding may be sealed in a plastic bag for 30–35 days. This far surpasses the life span of lice and nits. Treatment may be repeated after 7 days if living lice are still present, or eggs are demonstrated at the hair-skin junction.

   a. Eyelash infestation with pediculosis pubis may be treated by applying:

      (1) Petrolatum applied thickly 2 times a day for 8 days with mechanical removal of nits; or

      (2) 0.025% Physostigmine ophthalmic ointment with a cotton-tipped applicator; or

      (3) Yellow oxide of mercury.

4. **Scabies** is treated by application of GBH cream or lotion to the entire body from the neck down, with particular attention to the interdigital webs, wrists, elbows, axillae, breasts, buttocks, and genitalia. Approximately 30–60 gm or 60–120 ml is required to cover the trunk and extremities of an average adult. Medication should be applied for 8–12 hr and then washed off. At that point, clothing should be thoroughly washed and/or dried by machine (hot cycle in each), or dry-cleaned and linens and towels changed; personal articles can be sealed in a plastic bag for 10 days. Transmission of scabies is unlikely after 24 hr of treatment. A second application 1 week later is necessary only if there is clear evidence of treatment failure.

B. Alternative treatments for scabies

1. Persistent itching in treated scabies patients may be due to either continued infestation, a slowly subsiding hypersensitivity response, or irritation from overuse of GBH.

   a. Lesions should again be examined for the presence of mites. If persistent infection is present, retreatment with GBH, or the alternative methods noted below should be used.

   b. Persistent pruritic nodules may remain in patients seemingly otherwise cured of scabies. These lesions are similar to prurigo (neurodermatitis) nodules and respond only to intralesional corticosteroid injection.

   c. If itching is related to sensitization, treatment with topical corticosteroids or with a short (7--10-day) tapering course of oral corticosteroids will bring relief.

2. **Crotamiton (10% N-ethyl-o-crotonotoluide; Eurax)** cream applied twice and left on during a 48-hr period is usually effective against scabies and has been said to act as an antipruritic agent (see p. 267). Although it is the usual alternate therapy, very little is known about its toxicity, and cure rates are probably lower than those with GBH.

3. **5–10% precipitated sulfur** in a water-washable base (or in pet-rolatum, which is messier), applied nightly for 3 nights, remains a reliable treatment. Patients may complain of the sulfur odor. This treatment is often chosen for infants and pregnant women, although sulfur, too, has produced toxicity and death in infants.

4. **20–25% benzyl benzoate** in an alcoholic vehicle or emulsion applied once daily for 48–72 hr may also be effective (see p. 267). It has neurotoxic side effects similar to those of GBH.

5. **10% thiabendazole** suspension applied twice daily for 5 days or 10-day courses of oral thiabendazole (25 mg/kg daily) have also been reported to be useful.

C. **Alternative treatments for pediculosis** are also available:

1. **Pyrethrins** (A-200 Pyrinate, RID), rapid-acting compounds derived from chrysanthemum plants, are the leading over-the-counter louse remedy. Medication is applied for 10 min and then rinsed off. It should not be used more than twice within a 24-hr period. This treatment is as effective as GBH for head and pubic lice.

2. **Copper oleate-tetrahydronaphthalene lotion (Cuprex)** applied for 15 min to infested areas may be used for the eradication of head and pubic lice.

3. **A 2–5% DDT emulsion, 10% DDT powder, 0.5% malathion lotion, or 1% malathion powder** are all effective against mature lice and larvae but not against nits. However, these preparations remain on the skin and clothing long enough for the nits to mature and be destroyed at that time. These agents are particularly effective in epidemics and in mass delousing.

4. **Trimethoprim/sulfamethoxazole (Bactrim, Septra)** PO once daily for 3 days, repeated in 10 days, seems effective in the treatment of pediculosis capitis. This therapy is not useful for treating scabies.

D. **Epidemiologic treatment.** Family, close friends, sexual contacts, and those sharing quarters of patients with pediculosis or scabies all should be considered for treatment to prevent reinfection or a small epidemic.

E. **Protection against tick infestation** is best accomplished by applying repellents to clothing. The most efficient agent is diethyltoluamide (deet) (see p. 302).

F. **Tick removal methods** are multiple and each has its advocates. The important consideration is that the organism not be crushed while being taken off the skin.

1. The easiest and most efficient method entails grasping the tick near its mouth with forceps and lifting it gently upward and forward. A needle or other sharply pointed object should be inserted between the tick and skin to help pry it out. If tick mouth parts break off in the skin they generally cause little damage. Tick removal within a few hours of attachment prevents transmission of disease.

2. There is little objective evidence that a tick may be induced to loosen its grasp by touching it with a hot object, such as a matchhead that has just been extinguished or a hot nail, or by applying a few drops of a solvent such as chloroform or gasoline.

References

Ackerman, A. B. Crabs: The resurgence of *Phthirus pubis*. *N. Engl. J. Med.* 278:950–951, 1968.

Baer, R. L. (ed.). The management of scabies and pediculosis: The proceedings of a symposium. *Cutis* [Suppl.] Sept., 1981.

Charlesworth, E. N., and Johnson, J. L. An epidemic of canine scabies in man. *Arch. Dermatol.* 110:572–574, 1974.

Falk, E. S. Serum immunoglobulin values in patients with scabies. *Br. J. Dermatol.* 102:57–61, 1980.

Felman, Y., and Nikitas, J. A. Scabies. *Cutis* 25:32–42, 1980.

Felman, Y., and Nikitas, J. A. Pediculosis pubis. *Cutis* 25:482–489, 1980.

Fernandez, H., Torres, A., and Ackerman, A. B. Pathologic findings in human scabies. *Arch. Dermatol.* 113:320–324, 1977.

Hoefling, K. K., and Schroeter, A. L. Dermatoimmunopathology of scabies. *J. Am. Acad. Dermatol.* 3:237–240, 1980.

Hubler, W. R., and Clabaugh, W. Epidemic Norwegian scabies. *Arch. Dermatol.* 112:179–181, 1976.

Marples, M. J. *The Ecology of the Human Skin.* Springfield, Ill.: Thomas, 1965.

Martin, W. E., and Wheeler, C. E., Jr. Diagnosis of human scabies by epidermal shave biopsy. *J. Am. Acad. Dermatol.* 1:335–337, 1979.

Mellanby, K. *Scabies* (2nd ed.). Hampton, England: Classey, 1943.

Newsom, J. H., Fiore, J. L., and Hachett, E. Treatment of infestation and phthirus pubis: Comparative effectiveness of synergized pyrethrins and gamma benzene hexachloride. *Sex. Trans. Dis.* 6:203–205, 1979.

Orkin, M., Epstein, E., and Maibach, H. I. Treatment of today's scabies and pediculosis. *J.A.M.A.* 236:1136–1139, 1976.

Orkin, M., Maibach, H. I., Parish, L. C., and Schwartzman, R. M. *Scabies and Pediculosis.* Philadelphia: Lippincott, 1977.

Pramanik, A. K., and Hansen, R. C. Transcutaneous gamma benzene hexachloride absorption and toxicity in infants and children. *Arch. Dermatol.* 115:1224–1225, 1979.

Rasmussen, J. E. The problem of lindane. *J. Am. Acad. Dermatol.* 5:507–516, 1981.

Schacter, B. Treatment of scabies and pediculosis with lindane preparations: An evaluation. *J. Am. Acad. Dermatol.* 5:517–527, 1981.

Smith, D. E., and Walsh, J. Treatment of pubic lice infestation: A comparison of two agents. *Cutis* 26:618–619, 1980.

19

Intertrigo

I. Definition and pathophysiology. Intertrigo is an inflammatory dermatosis involving body folds. It is most common in obese individuals during hot weather and is found principally in the inframammary, axillary, and inguinal folds, but it may also affect other similar areas (folds of the upper eyelids, neck creases, antecubital fossae, and umbilical, perineal, and interdigital areas). As a result of skin constantly rubbing on skin, the heat, moisture, and sweat retention lead to maceration, inflammation, and often secondary bacterial or *Candida albicans* infection.

Incontinence may contribute to intertrigo in several ways: excessive moisture, irritant chemicals present in urine and feces, and microbial contamination.

Other eruptions that localize in the body folds and must therefore be differentiated from simple intertrigo include seborrheic dermatitis, psoriasis, dermatophyte infections, erythrasma, and miliaria.

II. Subjective data. Mild or early involvement is associated with soreness or itching. The more intense the inflammation, the more severe the discomfort.

III. Objective data. Mild erythema is seen initially. This may then progress to more intense inflammation with erosions, oozing, exudation, and crusting. Finally, vegetative changes, overt purulence, and surrounding cellulitis may arise in these areas.

IV. Assessment

   A. Examine pustule contents or scales microscopically and by culture for evidence of bacterial, *Candida,* or dermatophyte infection.

   B. Initiate investigation for and treatment of associated medical conditions such as diabetes, obesity, and incontinence.

V. Therapy

   A. Environmental changes to promote drying and to aerate the body folds are essential.

   1. The living and working areas should be cool and dry. Air conditioning or fans will help. Have the patient disrobe for at least 30 min 2id and expose the involved folds to a fan or electric bulb to promote drying.

   2. Clothing should be light, nonconstricting, and absorbent, avoiding wool, nylon, and synthetic fibers. Bras should provide good support. Prolonged sitting and driving are obviously harmful.

   3. Wash, rinse, and dry intertriginous areas at least twice daily and liberally apply a talc-containing powder.

4. Occlusive, oily, or irritant ointments or cosmetics do more harm than good and should be avoided. In certain instances of incontinence, the benefit from a protective ointment may outweigh the potential harm. Lotions, sprays, powders, creams or gels may be useful.

5. Careful and prompt attention to soiling by incontinent patients is mandatory.

B. Specific measures

1. Apply cooling tap water or Burow's solution compresses or soaks 3–4 times a day to exudative areas.

2. Separate folds with absorbent material, e.g., cotton sheeting well dusted with drying powders. Cornstarch should not be used, as it will encourage bacterial and fungal overgrowth.

3. Initially, corticosteroid or steroid-antibiotic lotions, creams, or gels should be applied 2–3 times a day, but prolonged use should be avoided, since continued application of fluorinated steroids may lead to intertriginous striae and cutaneous atrophy. Hydrocortisone (1%), with or without iodochlorhydroxyquin (Vioform or Vioform-HC), will usually be effective and its use reduces concern about corticosteroid side effects.

4. Bland lotions (calamine) are soothing and drying.

5. Some physicians apply drying antiseptic dye preparations to these areas and instruct patients to use them once daily thereafter. One-half or full strength Castellani's paint (fuchsin, phenol, and resorcinol [see p. 264]) or 0.5–1.0% gentian violet solution may be used. These dyes are very effective but messy and may sting or burn on application.

6. Specific antimonilial treatment (see p. 80) may be helpful in cases where the organism has been demonstrated.

20

Keloids and hypertrophic scars

I. **Definition and pathophysiology.** Keloids and hypertrophic scars both represent an excessive connective tissue response to cutaneous injury. These fibroblastic lesions may differ only slightly in clinical and histologic appearance, but they represent quite different types of tissue growth and require somewhat different treatments.

The circumstances that increase the likelihood of developing keloids or hypertrophic scars are similar. Excessive or poorly aligned tension on a wound, the introduction of foreign material into the skin, and certain types of trauma, such as burns, are all provocative factors. Some areas of the body—presternal, shoulders, back, chin, ears, lower legs—are much more at risk. Most keloids appear within 1 year of local trauma. Black and deeply pigmented individuals are affected more frequently, and individuals 10–30 years old develop lesions much more commonly than do prepubescent children or older adults. The fibrous tissue that accumulates in hypertrophic scars and keloids is associated with increased cellularity and metabolic activity of fibroblasts. Myofibroblasts, cells with characteristics of both fibroblasts and smooth muscle cells, have recently been found to represent the principal cell in keloids. Relative amounts of type 3 collagen appear to be increased. The tumescence of these lesions is caused by an abundance of extracellular material. Collagenase activity in keloids has been found to be normal or increased; however, the collagen may be protected from degradation by proteoglycan and specific protease inhibitors. A familial predilection for keloid formation has been found, and both autosomal recessive and autosomal dominant inheritance patterns have been reported.

II. **Subjective data.** Keloids are usually asymptomatic, although some are pruritic and others may be quite painful and tender.

III. **Objective data (See color insert.)**

A. Hypertrophic scars appear as scars that are more elevated, wider, or thicker than expected. They correspond in size and shape to the inciting wound.

B. Keloids start as pink or red, firm, well-defined, telangiectatic, rubbery plaques that for several months may be difficult to distinguish from hypertrophic scars. Later, uncontrolled overgrowth causes extension beyond the site of the original wound, and the tumor becomes smoother, irregularly shaped, hyperpigmented, harder, and more symptomatic. The tendency to send out clawlike prolongations is typical of keloids.

IV. **Assessment.** Keloid formation is associated with other dermatologic diseases. These conditions, if present, should be investigated and treated aggressively. They include dissecting cellulitis of the scalp, acne vulgaris, acne conglobata, hydradenitis suppurativa, pilonidal cysts, foreign body reactions, and local infections with herpes or vaccinia virus.

V. Therapy

A. Hypertrophic scars usually require no treatment and often spontaneously resolve in 6–12 months. However, they will respond to intralesional corticosteroid injections as noted below, or they may be managed by careful reexcision, as they tend to recur much less readily than keloids.

B. Keloids

1. Prophylactic considerations are of paramount importance. Clearly, optional elective surgical procedures should be avoided in keloid-formers. When surgery is necessary for cosmetic reasons, early childhood is the best time. Scalpel surgery with strict aseptic technique and avoidance of wound tension is mandatory. Electrosurgery and chemosurgery should be avoided; cryosurgical procedures are usually not followed by keloid formation.

2. Intralesional corticosteroid injection by syringe or needleless jet injector often brings excellent results and is the treatment of choice. In skin fibroblast culture glucocorticoids specifically decrease collagen synthesis in comparison to total protein synthesis. In addition, glucocorticoids may enhance collagen breakdown in keloids.

   a. In this instance one strives to achieve with corticosteroids the effect we most often try to avoid: atrophy. Therefore, use of high concentrations of medication (triamcinolone, acetonide, or diacetate, 10, 25, or 40 mg/ml) injected undiluted at 4-week intervals is warranted. Multiple injections directly into the bulk of the mass over several months (to years) may be necessary.

   b. Initially it may be difficult to force much medication into the tough collagenous mass. As the lesion softens and flattens, injection is more easily accomplished. Freezing the keloid with liquid nitrogen by spray or cotton swab application prior to injection causes the lesion to become edematous and less dense during thawing and allows the corticosteroid to be injected more easily and accurately. In addition, the freezing itself may have a therapeutic effect.

   c. Injections at more frequent intervals may result in too marked a result, leading to a depressed atrophic lesion.

   d. Perilesional atrophy and perilymphatic atrophy around draining vessels may be seen but will resolve over the subsequent 3–12 months.

3. Small lesions (less than 5 cm) may respond to cryosurgery with liquid nitrogen or CO_2 repeated every 2–3 weeks.

4. Constant compression and pressure maintained for a minimum of 4–6 months is beneficial following excision of keloids or other surgical procedures. Many pressure devices have been described.

5. Application of 0.05% retinoic acid 2id for 3 months resulted in a favorable result in 77% of 28 intractable cases (DeLimpens, 1980).

6. Larger lesions or those in suitable areas may be reexcised or treated by radiation therapy, or both. When excising keloids it is desirable to dilute the local anesthetic 1:1 with a corticosteroid suspension and to reinject the healing wound with corticosteroids at 2–3 weekly intervals. Some also advocate postexcision x-ray therapy at 2-week intervals. Radiation therapy also is often beneficial, particularly with lesions of less than 6 months' duration.

References

Brent, B.   The role of pressure therapy in the management of earlobe keloids: Preliminary report of a controlled study. *Ann. Plast. Surg.* 1:579–581, 1978.

Ceilley, R. I., and Babin, R. W.   The combined use of cryosurgery and intralesional injections of suspensions of fluorinated adrenocorticosteroids for reducing keloids and hypertrophic scars. *J. Dermatol. Surg. Oncol.* 5:54–56, 1979.

DeLimpens, A. M. P. J.   The local treatment of hypertrophic scars and keloids with topical retinoic acid. *Br. J. Dermatol.* 103:319–323, 1980.

Editorial.   Keloids and x-rays. *Br. Med. J.* 3:592, 1974.

James, W. D., Bescenceney, C. D., and Odom, R. B.   The ultrastructure of a keloid. *J. Am. Acad. Dermatol.* 3:50–57, 1980.

Kiil, J.   Keloids treated with topical injections of triamcinolone acetonide (Kenalog): Immediate and long term results. *Scand. J. Plast. Reconstr. Surg.* 11:169–172, 1977.

Levy, D. S., Salter, M. M., and Roth, R. E.   Postoperative irradiation in the prevention of keloids. *Am. J. Roentgenol.* 127:509–510, 1976.

Lubritz, R. R.   Cryosurgery of benign lesions. *Cutis* 16:426–432, 1975.

Murray, J. C., Pollack, S. V., and Pinnell, S. R.   Keloids: A review. *J. Am. Acad. Dermatol.* 4:461–470, 1981.

Wilson, W. W.   Prophylaxis against postsurgical keloids: Results in patients. *South. Med. J.* 58:751–753, 1965.

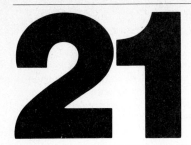

Keratoses

I. Definition and pathophysiology

A. Seborrheic keratoses are benign, noninvasive, hyperplastic epidermal lesions found most profusely on the face, shoulders, chest, and back. They are the most common skin tumor seen in the middle-aged and elderly population and are termed seborrheic only in relation to their greasy appearance and their location in areas that have many sebaceous glands. There is no known relationship to sebaceous gland function, seborrhea, or seborrheic dermatitis; their cause is unknown. In mature seborrheic keratoses, DNA synthesis is decreased while RNA and protein synthesis are increased. Concern about these lesions is primarily cosmetic; occasionally they cause anxiety because their dark color raises the question of melanoma.

B. Actinic (solar, senile) keratoses are premalignant lesions caused by the cumulative effects of solar radiation on the skin and are located solely on the exposed surfaces: face, ears, bald scalp, dorsa of the forearms, and hands. They may be seen in fair-skinned individuals in their twenties and thirties but are most common around age 50 and later. Lymphocytes and skin fibroblasts cultured from some actinic keratosis patients show a defect in DNA repair synthesis after ultraviolet irradiation. Also, autoradiographic labeling indices have been shown to average 5.4% in non-sun-exposed buttock skin, but were elevated to 11.2% in paralesional skin and 17.4% in actinic keratoses (Pearse and Marks, 1977). These findings suggest that actinic keratoses develop in epidermis that is itself abnormal, and that there may be a gradual progression of sun-damaged epidermis via the clinically obvious keratosis to skin cancer. Without treatment up to one-eighth of patients may have one or more lesions that will invade as squamous cell carcinoma; however, progression to very aggressive lesions accompanied by metastasis rarely occurs.

II. Subjective data

A. Seborrheic keratoses, particularly those in intertriginous areas, may itch intensely.

B. Actinic keratoses are usually asymptomatic.

III. Objective data (See color insert.)

A. Seborrheic keratoses start as small, multiple, flesh-colored, yellow or tan, waxy papules, and slowly grow to become dark brown or black, greasy, verrucous lesions with a distinct border. The rough scale may sometimes flake or be rubbed off but will always regrow. A variant of seborrheic keratoses termed **dermatosis papulosa nigra** is seen primarily on the cheeks in blacks as multiple small, dark, pedunculated papules.

B. Actinic keratoses first appear as flesh-colored to pink, flat or slightly raised, well-defined, scaly lesions. They feel rough or like sandpaper on palpation and usually arise from obviously sun-damaged skin (dry, wrinkled, atrophic, telangiectatic). Whereas parts of seborrheic keratoses can easily be scraped off with the fingernail or a tongue blade, this is not at all true of actinic lesions. A horny, keratotic, conical protuberance, termed a **cutaneous horn,** may develop from an actinic keratosis. (Cutaneous horns may also form on verrucous epidermal nevi, warts, seborrheic keratoses, and squamous cell carcinomas.)

IV. Assessment. Any doubts concerning the exact diagnosis of the keratosis may be resolved by pathologic examination of a 4-mm punch biopsy, shave biopsy, or curettage specimen. The base of all cutaneous horns should be submitted for histologic diagnosis. Shave biopsies or curettage specimens are often not sufficient for definitive histologic diagnosis.

V. Therapy

A. Seborrheic keratoses are benign lesions, and therapy should therefore be as simple, rapid, and cosmetically acceptable as possible. After treatment, a small area of hypopigmentation may be left at the site of the keratosis.

1. Simple curettage, with or without anesthesia, is the easiest method and leaves the best cosmetic result. Lesions lightly frozen with ethyl chloride, CO_2, or liquid nitrogen may sometimes be more easily scraped off. Monsel's solution (ferric subsulfate), ferric chloride, aluminum chloride, Gelfoam, Oxycel, weak acids (30% trichloroacetic), or pressure alone may be used for hemostasis. Light electrodesiccation will accomplish the same end but adds the possibility of inducing a small scar. Lesions should remain uncovered or have only a light, nonocclusive dressing.

2. Application of liquid nitrogen (15–20 sec) or dry ice will also result in removal of lesions without a subsequent cicatrix. Multiple areas can be treated easily without anesthesia by this method.

3. Excision or radiotherapy is unwarranted.

4. Lesions of dermatosis papulosa nigra may be treated by scissors excision, light electrosurgery, cryosurgery, or curettage; it is particularly important not to treat too aggressively so as to avoid posttreatment hypopigmentation.

B. Actinic keratoses

1. Prophylactic measures. Patients must first be told that these lesions are a result of damage from the sun and should be instructed to avoid further damage from solar radiation (see p. 311).

2. Single or isolated lesions may be treated by any of the following methods:

a. Cryotherapy with liquid nitrogen (20–30 sec) or dry ice application.

b. **Curettage and electrodesiccation** under local anesthesia. This is a simple and rapid procedure and the wound heals quickly; in addition, this method provides tissue for histologic diagnosis. Mild acids (30–50% trichloroacetic acid) or Monsel's solution (ferric subsulfate) may be used for hemostasis.

c. **Shave excision** (scalpel skimming) followed by electrosurgery or chemosurgery (acids).

d. **Excision and primary closure** is almost always a more extensive procedure than the lesion warrants.

3. **Multiple and/or extensive lesions** are best treated with application of topical 5-fluorouracil (5-FU). This has the advantage of easily treating large areas of involvement and also of eliminating subclinical keratoses. The primary disadvantage is the brisk inflammatory response that accompanies successful therapy. A small number of treated patients develop an allergic contact sensitivity to 5-FU. Medications should be used as follows:

a. **Sequential method**

(1) 5-FU is available as 1% (Fluoroplex), 2% (Efudex), and 5% (Efudex) solutions in propylene glycol, and 1% (Fluoroplex) and 5% (Efudex) creams (see p. 304). Alternatively, a 1% solution may be prepared by diluting a 10-ml ampule of 5-FU (Fluorouracil) with 40 ml of propylene glycol. At equivalent concentrations the solutions are more effective than creams. Higher concentrations induce a more severe inflammatory response but may be followed by slightly more complete involution of lesions and a lower recurrence rate. The higher concentration should always be used on areas other than the head and neck. On the face, the 1 or 2% solution or 1% cream often is sufficient.

(2) Medication should be applied twice daily with a nonmetal applicator, gloved hand, or fingers (followed by hand washing). Care should be taken to avoid the eyes, scrotum, and mucous membranes of the nose and mouth.

(3) The sequence of response is erythema, vesiculation, erosion, superficial ulceration, necrosis, and reepithelialization. Medication should be continued until the inflammatory response is at the ulceration and necrosis stage, which is usually 2–4 weeks. Patients may complain of intense burning and pain.

(4) At the point of ulceration, 5-FU may be stopped and a topical corticosteroid cream applied to hasten involution of the inflammation.

(5) Complete healing will be evident within 1–2 months. The cosmetic results are usually excellent. Residual postinflammatory hyperpigmentation occasionally follows this therapy.

(6) Patients should avoid excessive exposure to sunlight during 5-FU treatment or the intensity of the reaction may be increased.

b. Combined method (for face)

(1) Apply 1% 5-FU solution, and after 15 min apply 0.5% triamcinolone acetonide or other potent corticosteroid cream. Repeat nightly for 3 weeks.

(2) This method appears to be equally effective and may decrease or eliminate the brisk inflammation associated with the sequential method.

c. The effectiveness of the medication may be increased by applying both 5% 5-FU and 0.05% retinoic acid solution (tretinoin; Retin-A cream) together 2id until lesions exacerbate, and then continuing with 5-FU for another 2–3 weeks. The tretinoin may act to increase percutaneous penetration but may also possibly have a direct effect on keratoses. This is most useful for resistant areas such as the forearms or trunk.

d. 5-FU treatment should be repeated at yearly intervals in patients with severely sun-damaged skin.

4. Dermabrasion may also be effective for treatment of widespread facial actinic keratoses.

References

Arndt, K. A., and Freedberg, I. M.   Macromolecular metabolism in hyperplastic epidermal disease: A radio-autographic study. *Br. J. Dermatol.* 91:541–548, 1974.

Becker, S. W.   Seborrheic keratosis and verruca, with special reference to the melanotic variety. *Arch. Dermatol.* 63:358–372, 1951.

Breza, T., Taylor, R., and Eaglstein, W. H.   Noninflammatory destruction of actinic keratoses by fluorouracil. *Arch. Dermatol.* 112:1256–1258, 1976.

Dillaha, C. J., Jansen, G. T., Honeycutt, W. M., and Holt, G. A.   Further studies with topical 5-fluorouracil. *Arch. Dermatol.* 92:410–417, 1965.

Goette, D. K., and Odom, R. B.   Allergic contact dermatitis to topical fluorouracil. *Arch. Dermatol.* 113:1058–1061, 1977.

Graham, J. H.   Precancerous lesions of the skin. *Dermatol. Digest* March:16–22, 1970.

Lambert, B., Ringborg, U., and Swanbeck, G.   Ultraviolet-induced DNA repair synthesis in lymphocytes from patients with actinic keratoses. *J. Invest. Dermatol.* 67:594–598, 1976.

Leyden, J. J., and Kligman, A. M.   Studies on the allergenicity of 5-fluorouracil. *J. Dermatol. Surg. Oncol.* 3:518–519, 1977.

Pearse, D. D., and Marks, R.   Actinic keratoses and the epidermis on which they arise. *Br. J. Dermatol.* 96:45–50, 1977.

Pinkus, H.   Keratosis senilis: A biologic concept of its pathogenesis and diagnosis based on the study of normal epidermis and 1,730 seborrheic and senile keratoses. *Am. J. Clin. Pathol.* 29:193–207, 1958.

Pinkus, H.   Epithelial and fibroepithelial tumors. *Arch. Dermatol.* 91:24–37, 1965.

Robinson, T. A., and Kligman, A. M.   Treatment of solar keratoses of the extremities with retinoic and 5-fluorouracil. *Br. J. Dermatol.* 92:703–706, 1975.

Sanderson, K. A.   The structure of seborrheic keratoses. *Br. J. Dermatol.* 80:588–593, 1968.

Sbano, E., Andreassi, L., Feiniani, M., Valentino, A., and Baiocchi, R.   DNA repair after UV irradiation in skin fibroblasts from patients with actinic keratosis. *Arch. Dermatol. Res.* 262:55–61, 1978.

Spira, M., Freeman, R., Arfai, P., Gerow, F. J., and Hardy, S. B.   Clinical comparison of chemical peeling, dermabrasion and 5-FU for senile keratoses. *Plast. Reconstr. Surg.* 46:61–66, 1970.

Williams, A. C., and Klein, E.   Experiences with local chemotherapy and immunotherapy in premalignant and malignant skin lesions. *Cancer* 25:450–462, 1970.

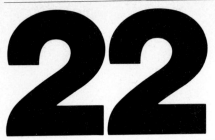

Milia

I. Definition and pathophysiology. Milia are asymptomatic, small, subepidermal, keratinous cysts found in individuals of all ages, most often on the face. Primary milia are noninflammatory collections of lamellated keratin most frequently found within the undifferentiated sebaceous cells that surround vellus hair follicles. Milia found in infants tend to disappear spontaneously in a few months, but lesions in adults are chronic. Most arise spontaneously, but others may be localized in areas of damaged skin associated with bullous disease (porphyria cutanea tarda, dermolytic bullous dermatosis) and in areas treated by dermabrasion. These secondary milia arise predominantly from eccrine duct epithelium.

II. Subjective data. Facial milia are of cosmetic significance only.

III. Objective data. Milia appear as tiny (1–2 mm), white, raised, round lesions covered by a thinned epidermis found primarily on the cheeks and eyelids. No orifice can be seen.

IV. Assessment. Inquire regarding previous inflammatory or blistering skin disease, trauma, or photosensitivity.

V. Therapy

    A. Milia are easily removed without anesthesia as follows:

        1. Gently incise the thin epidermis covering the milium with a No. 11 scalpel blade.

        2. Carefully sever and tease away any connection or adhesions between the cyst and the overlying skin.

        3. Apply mild pressure with a comedo extractor, curet, tongue blades, or the dull edge of the scalpel blade. The small keratin kernel should pop out as an intact ball.

    B. Light electrodesiccation with a fine needle is also an effective method.

References

Epstein, W., and Kligman, A. M. The pathogenesis of milia and benign tumors of the skin. *J. Invest. Dermatol.* 26:1–11, 1956.

Tsuji, T., Sugai, T., and Suzuki, S. The mode of growth of eccrine duct milia. *J. Invest. Dermatol.* 65:388–393, 1975.

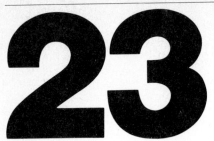

Molluscum contagiosum

I. Definition and pathophysiology. Molluscum contagiosum is a viral tumor limited to humans and monkeys and caused by a DNA-containing poxvirus. Although serial propagation of molluscum contagiosum virus (MCV) has been accomplished, there is no known animal model. The virus can be cultured on both human epidermis and amnion epithelium, and has been experimentally transmitted to human volunteers by injections of viral filtrate into the skin. MCV is a brick-shaped particle, approximately $300 \times 200 \times 100$ nm in size, which replicates in aggregates within the cytoplasm of infected cells. It may be seen in all cell layers of infected epidermis, but replication probably occurs in the more differentiated cell layers. Basal cell turnover and epidermal transit time are increased in MCV-infected epidermis. The disease is contracted from other people by direct contact, through fomites, and by autoinoculation. Children with atopic dermatitis may be more easily infected. Estimates of the incubation period range from 2 weeks to 2 months. Molluscum lesions formerly were found primarily in children on the face and trunk, but now they are also being seen very commonly in the pubic area and genitalia of sexually active young adults. Many lesions are self-limited in duration (6–9 months) but others will last for years.

II. Subjective data. Most lesions of molluscum are asymptomatic. Occasionally, large lesions become inflamed and look and feel like a furuncle. Chronic conjunctivitis or keratitis may accompany lesions located on or near the eyelids.

III. Objective data (See color insert.) Molluscum lesions are discrete, skin-colored or pearly white, raised, waxy-appearing, firm papules 1–5 mm in diameter, with a central punctate umbilication. They are found alone or in clusters on the face, trunk, lower abdomen, pubis, inner thighs, and penis. Mucosal lesions may be present.

IV. Assessment. Diagnosis may be confirmed by incising one of the papules, smearing the contents between two glass slides, staining (with Wright's, Giemsa's, or Gram's stain), and then viewing under low or high dry magnification. Molluscum bodies, which are cytoplasmic masses consisting of mature, immature, and incomplete virions and cellular debris, are ovoid, smooth-walled, and homogeneous, and are up to 25μ in diameter. The lesions most often confused with molluscum are warts.

V. Therapy. Molluscum can be successfully treated by any of the following methods:

A. Cryotherapy with liquid nitrogen (10–15 sec) or dry ice is generally the best treatment.

B. Removal of the lesion with a sharp curet. Anesthesia is often not necessary. Some recommend touching the base of the lesion with iodine or a mild acid (30% trichloroacetic acid).

C. Light electrodessication.

D. Application of a vesicant such as cantharidin (Cantharone) alone, or covered with Blenderm tape overnight. This method, though effective, may cause a severe inflammatory reaction. A keratolytic paint (Duofilm, Ti-Flex) may be used in the same fashion and will not cause as much inflammation.

References

Brown, S. T., and Weinberger, J.   Molluscum contagiosum: Sexually transmitted disease in 17 cases. *J. Amer. Venerol. Dis. Assoc.* 1:35–36, 1977.

Felman, Y. M., and Nikitas, J. A.   Genital molluscum contagiosum. *Cutis* 26:28–32, 1980.

Francis, R. D., and Bradford, H. B., Jr.   Some biological and physical properties of molluscum contagiosum virus propagated in tissue culture. *J. Virol.* 19:382–388, 1976.

Glickman, F. S., and Silvers, S. H.   Eczema and molluscum contagiosum. *J.A.M.A.* 223:1512, 1973.

Henao, M., and Freeman, R. A.   Inflammatory molluscum contagiosum: Clinicopathological study of seven cases. *Arch. Dermatol.* 90:479–482, 1964.

Leading article. Molluscum contagiosum. *Br. Med. J.* 1:459–460, 1968.

Mehregan, A. H.   Molluscum contagiosum: A clinicopathologic study. *Arch. Dermatol.* 84:123–127, 1961.

Pauly, C. R., Artic, W. M., and Jones, H. E.   Atopic dermatitis, impaired cellular immunity and molluscum contagiosum. *Arch. Dermatol.* 114:391–393, 1978.

Postlethwaite, R.   Molluscum contagiosum: A review. *Arch. Environ. Health* 21:432–452, 1970.

Shirodaria, P. V., Matthews, R. S., and Samuel, M.   Virus-specific and anticellular antibodies in molluscum contagiosum. *Br. J. Dermatol.* 101:133–140, 1979.

Steffen, C., and Markman, J.   Spontaneous disappearance of molluscum contagiosum: Report of a case. *Arch. Dermatol.* 116:923–924, 1980.

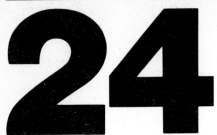

Pityriasis rosea

I. Definition and pathophysiology. Pityriasis rosea is a mild scaling eruption seen predominantly in adolescents and young adults during the spring and fall. It is self-limited in duration and thought to be viral in origin, although this is unproved. The lesions usually disappear within 6–8 weeks, and recurrences are uncommon.

II. Subjective data. Pityriasis rosea may be asymptomatic or, at times, intensely pruritic. The onset of the eruption is sometimes coincident with mild malaise and symptoms similar to a viral upper respiratory tract infection.

III. Objective data (See color insert.)

    A. The initial lesion is frequently a 2–6 cm, round, erythematous, scaling plaque, which may appear anywhere on the body. This "herald patch" is not present, or at least not noticed, in 20–30 percent of cases.

    B. Within several days to 2 weeks, small 1–2 cm pale, red, round to oval macular and papular lesions with a crinkly surface and a rim of fine scales appear in crops on the trunk and proximal extremities.

    C. The face, hands, and feet are usually spared except in children.

    D. The long axes of the lesions are oriented in the planes of cleavage running parallel to the ribs and classically are said to form a fir-tree-like pattern.

    E. Lesions may be few or almost confluent, slowly enlarging by peripheral extension, and can continue to appear for 7–10 days.

    F. Variants of pityriasis rosea at times seem to appear as commonly as the classic disease.

        1. In children the lesions are often papular.

        2. Vesicular and bullous lesions may be seen.

        3. Occasionally, eruptions may be limited to the shoulder or groin region.

        4. Urticarial, intensely inflammatory, and very symptomatic lesions are less common.

IV. Assessment

    A. The eruption is usually easily diagnosed by its morphology and distribution.

    B. A serologic test for syphilis should be drawn on all patients, since secondary syphilis may mimic pityriasis rosea almost exactly.

C. Other differential diagnostic considerations include tinea corporis, seborrheic dermatitis, acute psoriasis, and tinea versicolor.

D. Eight drugs have been incriminated in causing pityriasis rosea-like eruptions: (1) captopril, (2) arsenicals, (3) bismuth, (4) tripelennamine HCl, (5) methoxypromazine, (6) barbiturates, (7) clonidine, and (8) metronidazole.

E. Lesions that do not resolve in 8–14 weeks should suggest chronic parapsoriasis or pityriasis lichenoides et varioliformis acuta (PLEVA), and a punch biopsy is indicated.

V. Therapy

A. Most patients require no treatment.

B. Five consecutive daily doses of erythema-producing ultraviolet light (UVB) will decrease both the pruritus and extent of the eruption in 50% of those treated. Sunlight, too, appears to have a direct beneficial effect. There is some suggestion that those treated within the first week of rash will respond more readily.

C. Itching may also be somewhat alleviated with drying and antipruritic lotions, emollients, or antihistamines.

D. Topical corticosteroids or bursts of oral corticosteroids are of benefit only in more severe inflammatory variations. They are both ineffective and unwarranted in mild cases, and it is rarely necessary to use these medications.

References

Annotation. Pityriasis rosea. *Lancet* 1:33, 1968.

Arndt, K. A., Paul, B. S., Stern, R. S., and Parrish, J. A.   Treatment of pityriasis rosea with ultraviolet radiation. *Arch. Dermatol.* In press.

Björnberg, A., and Hellgren, L.   Pityriasis rosea: A statistical, clinical and laboratory investigation of 826 patients and matched healthy controls. *Acta Derm. Venereol.* (Stockh.) 42[Suppl. 50]:1–68, 1962.

Bunch, L. W., and Tilley, J. C.   Pityriasis rosea: A histologic and serologic study. *Arch. Dermatol.* 84:79–86, 1961.

Burch, P. R. J., and Rowell, N. R.   Pityriasis rosea: An autoaggressive disease? Statistical studies in relation to aetiology and pathogenesis. *Br. J. Dermatol.* 82:549–560, 1970.

Lipman, C. E.   Pityriasis rosea. *Br. J. Dermatol.* 79:533–539, 1967.

Merchant, M., and Hammond, R.   Controlled study of ultraviolet light for pityriasis rosea. *Cutis* 14:548–549, 1974.

Plemmons, J. A.   Pityriasis rosea: An old therapy revisited. *Cutis* 16:120–121, 1975.

Wilkin, J. K., and Kirkendall, W. M.   Pityriasis rosea-like rash from captopril. *Arch Dermatol.* 118:186–187, 1982.

25

Psoriasis

I. **Definition and pathophysiology.** Psoriasis is a chronic proliferative epidermal disease that affects 2–8 million people in the United States and 1–3% of the world's population. Its average age of onset is 7 years, but it may make its initial appearance late in life as well. The lesions, usually discrete scaling plaques, may become very extensive or even generalized. Histocompatibility antigens HLA-Cw6 and HLA-B13, B17, and Bw16 and Bw37 are present in a markedly higher frequency in psoriasis. When the latter two are both present, psoriasis tends to be more severe. The 5–10% of patients with an associated arthritis and those with pustular psoriasis are often HLA-B27 positive and 13,17-negative. The finding of these genetic markers implies that the HL-A chromosomal region includes loci that are part of the genotype resulting in susceptibility to psoriasis. There is a familial pattern in 30% of cases, and the inheritance is most consistent with a dominant mode. However, there is considerable genetic heterogenicity and it seems likely that in any family two or more genes may be involved.

The pathogenesis of psoriasis remains unclear, but important abnormalities identified include alterations in cyclic nucleotides, prostaglandins, and polyamines. Immunologic abnormalities have been demonstrated as well, and include antibodies to stratum corneum, deposition of IgG and complement on cells in dermis, and cellular immune defects. The time necessary for a psoriatic epidermal cell to travel from the basal cell layer of the epidermis to the surface and be cast off is 3–4 days, in marked contrast to the normal 26–28 days. There is controversy about the mechanism underlying the rapidly increased epidermal transit time. There is some evidence to suggest a shortened cell cycle time (37 rather than 163 hr) but an alternative explanation holds that in psoriatic skin a higher proportion of cells enters the active cell cycle from the resting state (G_0). In any event, the six- to ninefold transit time increase does not allow the normal events of cell maturation and keratinization to take place. This is reflected clinically by profuse scaling; histologically by a greatly thickened epidermis with increased mitotic activity, and by the presence of immature nucleated cells in the horny layer; under the electron microscope by reduced production of the intracellular filaments and granules seen with normal keratinization; and biochemically by increased synthesis and degradation of nucleoproteins. Beneath the plaques of proliferative epithelium lies an extremely vascular dermis.

The course of psoriasis is prolonged but unpredictable. In most patients the disease remains localized. In some, however, its severity is incompatible with a productive and happy life. Spontaneous clearing is quite rare, but unexplained exacerbation or improvement is common. Stress and anxiety frequently precede flare-ups of the disease.

II. Subjective data

A. Most lesions are asymptomatic.

B. Pruritus may be noted in 20% of patients.

C. Those with generalized disease may demonstrate all the signs and symptoms of an exfoliative dermatitis (loss of thermoregulation with findings of warm skin, a feeling of chilliness and shivering, increased protein catabolism, and cardiovascular stress).

D. Monoarticular or polyarticular pain, tenderness, and morning stiffness, especially in the small joints of the hands and feet, are the early manifestations of psoriatic arthritis. Intense pain in larger joints and the cervical and/or lumbosacral spine also may be present.

III. Objective data (See color insert.)

A. The psoriatic lesion is an erythematous, sharply circumscribed plaque covered by loosely adherent, silvery scales. Acute lesions tend to be small and guttate (drop-shaped).

B. Inapparent scaling can be made noticeable by scratching the surface of a psoriatic lesion.

C. Any body area may be involved, but lesions tend to occur most often on the elbows and knees, scalp, genitalia, and in the upper gluteal fold.

D. Lesions of active psoriasis often appear in areas of epidermal injury (Koebner reaction). Scratch marks, surgical wounds, or a sunburn may heal with psoriatic lesions in their place.

E. The nails may show punctate pitting or profuse collections of subungual keratotic material, clinically reflecting psoriatic involvement of the nail matrix or nail bed, respectively. A yellow brown subungual discoloration ("oil spot") is characteristic. Patients with distal interphalangeal joint involvement or arthritis mutilans usually have adjacent nail involvement.

F. Exfoliative psoriasis is indistinguishable clinically from other exfoliative dermatoses (see Assessment, **B.**). It may occur spontaneously, follow a systemic illness or drug reaction, or occur as a reaction to some drugs or to steroid withdrawal.

G. In acute psoriatic arthritis, one or several joints are erythematous and swollen—the distal phalanx classically has a "sausage" appearance. Long-standing or rapidly progressive disease may lead to severe bone destruction. Almost 50–55% of patients with psoriatic arthritis have asymmetric oligoarticular arthritis, 25% have a symmetric arthritis, and another 25% have spondyloarthritis with or without peripheral arthritis; 5% of patients show a destructive polyarthritis. The majority of patients with asymmetric arthritis have a mild or moderately progressive course, but about 50% with symmetric arthritis suffer with progressive, slowly destructive arthritis.

IV. Assessment

A. The medical history may reveal a cause for the onset or exacerbation of psoriatic lesions. For example, acute psoriasis or a flare-up in chronic lesions may follow streptococcal pharyngitis by 7–10 days. Psoriasis may be precipitated or exacerbated in patients ingesting lithium carbonate.

B. Other causes of exfoliative dermatitis (exfoliative erythroderma) include generalized eczematous dermatitis (e.g., atopic, contact, allergic), drug reactions, lymphoma, leukemia, and several rather uncommon skin diseases; 8–10% of cases are idiopathic.

C. Biopsy of lesions will reveal a psoriasiform epidermal thickening, but the histologic picture often is not diagnostic.

D. Hyperuricemia is proportional to the amount of cutaneous involvement and is related to the increased nucleic acid degradation associated with accelerated epidermopoiesis. It rarely causes symptoms or requires therapy.

E. Patients with psoriatic arthritis will typically have an elevated erythrocyte sedimentation rate and by definition will have negative tests for rheumatoid factor. X-ray films of the hands may show characteristic subcortical cystic changes with relative sparing of the articular cartilage.

V. Therapy

A. It is important to emphasize that psoriasis is a treatable disease. Optimism and encouragement are justified and make it easier for the patient to conscientiously apply sometimes awkward and messy dressings. All agents that are effective are toxic to epidermal cells, although mechanisms vary. Pharmacologic data concerning the mode of action of most of these topical medications are limited.

B. **Treatment for mild to moderate cutaneous involvement** (for scalp care and for nail care, see p. 147)

1. **Repeated exposure to sunlight or middle-wavelength, sunburn spectrum, ultraviolet light (UVB)** from artificial sources to the point of mild erythema will induce flattening or clearing of many lesions. A standardized 3 times weekly UVB protocol will induce complete clearing in an average of 23 treatments (Adrian et al., 1981). UVB phototherapy is probably the most rapid and effective method of inducing remission in mild to severe disease. UVB inhibits epidermal mitosis and presumably acts by this mechanism.

2. **Potent fluorinated corticosteroids** applied 2–3 times a day to local lesions are quite useful, especially in reducing scaling and thickness. Overnight or 24-hr occlusive therapy with these medications or with flurandrenolide tape (Cordran Tape) will initiate involution in most lesions. Corticosteroids exert their beneficial effects in this setting as mitotic inhibitors.

   Patients should apply corticosteroid (from potency group 1–4, p. 274) to lesions without occlusion during the day; in the evening, apply medication to plaques immediately after bath or shower, and occlude with plastic wrap or suit for 4 hr or overnight (see p. 274 for occlusion techniques). As lesions subside, decrease the use of occlusion and increase the use of a bland emollient (e.g., Eucerin).

3. **Injection of intralesional corticosteroids** beneath isolated chronic plaques will cause involution within 7–10 days (triamcinolone acetonide, diluted to 2.5-5.0 mg/ml).

4. **Coal tar therapy** (see also p. 307) may be combined with or alternated with topical corticosteroids: tars such as Estar or T/Derm, which are

nearly colorless, or 1–5% crude coal tar ointment, which is very messy but may be more effective, is applied overnight. This may be followed by exposure to ultraviolet light (UVL) or sunlight. Tars sensitize the skin to long-wave UVL (UVA) and also appear to have a direct beneficial effect on psoriasis. Recent data have shown that tars offer no advantage over lubricants such as petrolatum used along with an **aggressive** UVB treatment protocol (LeVine et al., 1980). However, they do inhibit DNA synthesis directly and have an atrophogenic effect on skin. When used along with less aggressive UVL treatment, it has been suggested that tars have a "light-sparing" effect.

As directed in the instructions for corticosteroids, but on alternate nights, the patient should apply a tar formulation overnight and be exposed to UVL the following morning; or apply corticosteroid cream with or without occlusion during the day, tar overnight, and UVL exposure in the morning. The latter regimen is the protocol sometimes used to treat hospitalized psoriatics.

5. **Other topical agents**

   a. **Keralyt gel** (6% salicylic acid, 60% propylene glycol, 20% ethyl alcohol) applied under occlusion to hydrated skin overnight is the most effective way to remove thick, adherent scaling. It is sometimes useful to start therapy by alternating the use of Keralyt overnight and corticosteroid during the day, and then to stop using the keratolytic gel as the psoriasis improves and the lesions become flat and less hyperkeratotic.

   b. **Salicylic acid,** 2–10%, in other formations might also help remove scales and crusts and may be used along with corticosteroid or anthralin therapy (see p. 145). Formulations commonly used include 3–10% salicylic acid cream, 3–6% sulfur and salicylic acid ointment, and 3% sulfur, 3% salicylic acid, 4% cetyl alcohol-coal tar distillate (Pragmatar) cream.

   c. **Mercury compounds** are very allergenic and not commonly used, but they can be effective topical agents. Long-term use has been reported to cause renal tubular damage. Ammoniated mercury cream (5%) may be used alone but is often combined with other agents as follows and used 2–3 times a day:

      (1) Tar solution 2–10%.

      Salicylic acid 1–5%.

      Ammoniated Hg 5–10%. This cream may be compounded at various concentrations with or without the tar or salicylic acid. Higher concentrations may be irritating.

      (2) Tar distillate 5%.

      Ammoniated Hg 5%.

      Methanamine sulfosalicylate 2%, available as Unguentum Bossi.

C. **Treatment for more severe or widespread involvement**. The management of severe or extensive psoriasis is a problem that can be best handled by a dermatologist.

1. **The anthralin (dithranol) paste method** is very effective for widespread lesions consisting primarily of thick plaques (see p. 303). Its disadvantages are that anthralin may be a primary irritant, it stains clothing and skin, and it is difficult to apply. Anthralin paste can be used on an outpatient or inpatient basis and will clear up the lesions on most patients within 2–3 weeks. The patient should use anthralin as follows:

   a. Bathe at bedtime in a coal tar bath (Balnetar, liquor carbonis detergens, Polytar, Zetar) and scrub scales off.

   b. Liberally apply 0.1% or 0.2% anthralin with 0.2% salicylic acid and 5.0% hard paraffin in zinc oxide paste (Anthra-Derm, Lasan Unguent; see Farber and Harris, 1970, for details) to lesions with a tongue blade or gloved fingers. The anthralin concentration may be gradually increased to 0.4% or greater. A new anthralin product in a vanishing cream, Drithocreme, has recently become available in 0.1%-, 0.25%-, and 0.5%-concentrations, and is used similarly.

   c. Cover paste with powder and gauze dressing or stockinette, or simply wear old pajamas, and leave on 8–12 hr.

   d. Remove paste or cream in the morning. A bath or mineral oil will aid removal.

   e. A low-strength corticosteroid cream (fluocinolone 0.01%, triamcinolone 0.025%) may be used during the day.

   f. UVL treatment may be used but does not add appreciably to the final result.

   g. Use old sheets and bed clothing, since anthralin will stain them a violet color. Treat intertriginous areas cautiously with a 1:10 dilution of the paste and with sheeting separating body folds. Anthralin stain may be removed from the skin with 3–6% salicylic acid cream or ointment, which may also be used to rim lesions to limit the paste margins.

   h. Two alternative methods for effective use of anthralin have been described. The first utilizes nonirritating and nonstaining lower strengths of 0.01–0.05% (Brody and Johanssen, 1977; Montes et al., 1979), and the other recommends using high concentrations (1.0%) for short periods of 1 hr daily (Schaefer et al., 1980).

2. **Aggressive UVB phototherapy** is the most rapid and most effective single agent regimen for clearing psoriasis. It may be used by specific protocols 3 times a week (Adrian et al., 1981), 5 times a week (LeVine and Parrish, 1980), or daily (LeVine et al., 1979). The latter will clear most patients in 18 treatments. All protocols involve application of lubricants to psoriatic plaques prior to phototherapy. In our departmental teaching hospitals these treatments have supplanted the tar and UVL therapy described next.

3. **Tar and UVL therapy (Goeckerman regimen)** is best an inpatient treatment, since tars are messy to apply and potent ultraviolet hotquartz or fluorescent lights are needed. Tars and middle-wavelength ultraviolet light (UVB) act as separate antipsoriatic agents.

a. Apply tar (Estar, T/Derm), a heavy layer of 1–5% crude coal tar in Aquaphor or petrolatum with 1% polysorbate 80 (Tween 20), or other tar preparation in the evening. If these are too irritating or drying, use 10% liquor carbonis detergens in hydrophilic ointment or Nivea oil.

b. In the morning, remove the tar by rubbing with a towel and cotton-seed or mineral oil and then bathing. If a tar layer is present, UVL will not reach the skin.

c. Expose the skin to minimal erythema doses of UVL—an amount that will produce slight redness 12 hr later. This is equivalent to 20–30 min of sunlight; exposure time for artificial light sources is usually determined by experience and may be 30 sec or many minutes. Whenever possible careful radiometry of light sources should be performed on a regular basis so that accurate cumulative and individual treatment doses can be recorded. Production of a mild phototoxic effect (sunburn) is probably necessary for an effective response. Gradually increase the duration of light exposure daily.

d. Bathe and remove scales with a stiff brush. Too vigorous brushing, however, may cause a Koebner reaction.

e. After bathing, liberally rub tar onto involved areas. Alternatively, steroids with occlusion may be used during the day, being applied after UVL exposure, with tars applied only overnight. Using the latter method, lesions will flatten more quickly, but there will be no overall difference in the time necessary for total clearing or length of remission.

f. After a 2- –3-week in-hospital stay, most patients will clear and prolonged clinical remission of psoriasis will occur.

4. **Photochemotherapy** (see also p. 220) will bring about marked improvement when used for widespread, severe psoriasis. A photoactive drug (a psoralen) is administered orally, followed 2 hr later by exposure to long-wave UVL (UVA). Psoralens form photoadducts with DNA in the presence of UVA and in this way probably reduce the increased epidermal turnover characteristic of psoriasis. Repeated PUVA (psoralen plus ultraviolet-A) exposure causes disappearance of lesions in almost all patients with 10–20 treatments over 4–8 weeks. Psoriasis often recurs weeks to months after PUVA ceases, and twice-monthly treatment is necessary to keep most patients free of their disease. Scalp, body folds, and other areas not exposed to UVA respond poorly to the therapy. Outdoor use of PUVA is also possible, although more hazardous (Robertson et al., 1978; Basler, 1979; Parrish et al., 1977).

5. **Combined therapies** appear to be most effective of all in clearing recalcitrant widespread and severe psoriasis. These include PUVA-UVB (Momtaz and Parrish, 1981), methotrexate-PUVA (Morison et al., 1982), and methotrexate-UVB (Paul et al., in press). The latter, for example, combines thrice weekly UVB treatments with once weekly methotrexate administration for 8 weeks. This regimen cleared all of 26 cases of disabling psoriasis in one-half the number of UVB treatments (12) required without methotrexate, and utilized relatively low

amounts of each agent, thereby reducing cumulative methotrexate and UVL toxicity.

6. **Retinoids,** synthetic derivatives of vitamin A and its metabolite vitamin A acid, have a direct effect on the growth and differentiation of keratinizing and nonkeratinizing epithelium. The aromatic drug etretinate (Ro 10-9359), not yet approved for use in the United States, is the most useful, especially in pustular and erythrodermic psoriasis. However, only about 50% of patients respond, and side effects are frequent and troublesome. The greatest usefulness of retinoids will be their combined use with PUVA, UVB phototherapy, or topical agents such as corticosteroids.

7. Some psoriatics undergoing hemodialysis or peritoneal dialysis for renal failure have experienced improvement in their skin disease. This has been further evaluated and the value of dialysis in the treatment of psoriasis is questionable, at best, at this time.

D. Scalp care

1. **Mild involvement** may be treated by the patient with a tar shampoo (10% liquor carbonis detergens in tincture of green soap, Pentrax, Polytar, Sebutone, T-gel, Zetar) and steroid lotion or solution 2id (Synalar, Valisone, Halog).

2. **More severe involvement** should be treated as follows:

   a. If scaling is thick, it is necessary to first remove the scales and then apply something to inhibit their reformation. This is best accomplished by having the patient apply a keratolytic gel (Keralyt gel) to a hydrated scalp and then cover it with an occlusive plastic shower cap for several hours or overnight. This will effectively loosen the scales, after which a steroid lotion or solution (Halog, Synalar, Valisone) should be applied under a shower cap for the rest of the night, or without occlusion during the day.

   b. Alternatively, chronic thick plaques may also be treated by the patient as follows:

      (1) Apply anthralin (Lasan Unguent) or 3% sulfur, 3% salicylic acid, 4% tar distillate (Pragmatar) cream, or phenol/saline lotion (P&S liquid) or, in severe cases, 20% oil of cade, 10% sulfur, 5% salicylic acid ("20-10-5" ointment) in hydrophilic ointment to the scalp, leaving on overnight.

      (2) Use tar shampoo (e.g., T/Gel) in the morning.

      (3) Reapply the preparation as for overnight during the day until scaling is decreased. At that point, substitute a steroid lotion or solution.

   c. Intralesional corticosteroid injections will clear isolated plaques (see **V.B.3,** p. 143).

E. Nail care.
There is no consistently effective therapy for psoriatic involvement of the nails. The nails will often improve coincidentally with remission of cutaneous lesions and will almost always improve after systemic antimetabolite therapy.

1. Removal of subungual debris and application of corticosteroids under occlusion may offer some benefit.

2. Injection of small amounts of triamcinolone acetonide (about 0.3 mg; or 0.1 ml at 3 mg/ml) into the nail bed at 2- -3-week intervals will result in cure or improvement in about 75% of treated nails, but it is painful and time-consuming. Onycholytic nails respond least well. There will be about a 50% recurrence rate when treatment is stopped.

3. Forty percent urea ointment may be useful in removing hypertrophic or dystrophic psoriatic nails. Subsequent topical therapy to the denuded nail bed and proximal nail fold may result in regrowth of "normal" nails in one-half of those treated (South and Farber, 1980).

4. 1% 5-fluorouracil solution (Fluoroplex) applied twice daily to nail margins has been reported to decrease the severity of involvement by 75% in two-thirds of patients within 3–6 months.

F. **Psoriatic arthritis** may respond to a variety of pharmacologic agents. In general when the disease is mild to moderate, it should be treated with either aspirin or a nonsteroidal anti-inflammatory drug; if unresponsive or more severe, with hydroxychloroquin; and if relentless, disabling, or destructive to joints, with gold or immunosuppressive agents. Splinting and local heat should also be used.

1. **Aspirin** must be taken to near toxicity in order to be effective.

2. **Nonsteroidal anti-inflammatory agents** are very effective in early psoriatic arthritis and there is some opinion that they may be more useful than aspirin. Indomethacin is given in doses of 75–100 mg/day, although amounts up to 150 mg/day may be required. It is essential that these drugs be administered in amounts sufficient to exert their anti-inflammatory effects. Ibuprofen (Motrin) dosage should be 2400 mg/day, or naproxen (Naprosyn) 500–750 mg/day. Other similar agents include fenoprofen (Nalfon), tolmetin (Tolectin), sulindac (Clinoril), and zomepirac (Zomax). All of these medications are gastrointestinal irritants and are contraindicated in patients with ulcer disease. They all also affect platelets in a manner similar to aspirin and if given to patients already on anticoagulants may result in bleeding and clotting problems. There is no clear evidence that any one of the nonsalicylate nonsteroidal anti-inflammatory agents is more effective than any other in controlling the inflammation of psoriatic arthritis.

3. **Hydroxychloroquin (Plaquenil)** has recently been shown to induce a beneficial response in 75% of 100 patients with psoriatic arthritis. The use of this antimalarial drug was **not** accompanied by an exacerbation in psoriasis (Schur et al., 1979), contrary to previous beliefs.

4. **Gold or folic acid antagonists,** particularly methotrexate, are very useful in intractable cases unresponsive to the more conventional therapies. 6-Mercaptopurine may be more effective against the arthritis component but is less useful for the cutaneous lesions. Gold or immunosuppressive drugs may put psoriatic arthritis into remission.

5. Spondylitis associated with psoriatic arthritis is treated with the same medications as spondylitis of other causes. The nonsteroidal anti-inflammatory drugs described above are the initial agents of choice and the disease usually responds well.

6. Distal arthritis limited to the DIP (distal interphalangeal) joints and present with adjacent nail involvement remains notoriously recalcitrant to most therapies.

G. **Acute psoriasis** should be treated gently with just emollients or topical steroids. Avoid tars, salicylic acid, and aggressive UVL therapy, since they may be irritating and lead to a more widespread eruption and chronic course.

H. **Antimetabolite therapy** with agents that inhibit DNA synthesis (hydroxyurea, methotrexate) is reserved for those patients unresponsive to other approaches and for whom the disease is an economic and social disaster. These agents have potentially serious side effects and should never be considered unless topical therapy has proved ineffectual.

References

Adrian, R. M., Parrish, J. A., Momtaz, T. K., and Karlin, M. J.   Outpatient phototherapy of psoriasis. *Arch. Dermatol.* 117:623–626, 1981.

Basler, R. S. W.   Psoralen and sunlight for psoriasis in the Southwest. *Cutis* 24:386–388, 1979.

Blecker, J. J.   Intradermal triamcinolone acetonide treatment of psoriatic nail dystrophy with Port-O-Jet. *Br. J. Dermatol.* 92:479, 1975.

Brody, I., and Johansson, A.   A topical treatment program for psoriasis with low strength anthralin concentrations. *J. Cutan. Pathol.* 4:233–243, 1977.

Cram, D. L.   Psoriasis: Current advances in etiology and treatment. *J. Am. Acad. Dermatol.* 4:1–14, 1981.

Current status of oral PUVA therapy for psoriasis. *J. Am. Acad. Dermatol.* 1:106–117, 1979.

Dorwart, B. B., Gall, E. P., Schumacher, H. R., and Krauss, R. E.   Crysotherapy in psoriatic arthritis: Efficacy and toxicity compared to rheumatoid arthritis. *Arth. Rheumatol.* 21:513–515, 1978.

Eisen, A., and Seegmiller, J.   Uric acid metabolism in psoriasis. *J. Clin. Invest.* 40:1486–1494, 1961.

Farber, E. M., and Harris, D. R.   Hospital treatment of psoriasis: A modified anthralin program. *Arch. Dermatol.* 101:381–389, 1970.

Lazarus, G., and Gilgor, R.   Psoriasis, polymorphonuclear leukocytes and lithium carbonate. *Arch. Dermatol.* 115:1183–1184, 1979.

LeVine, M. J., White, H. A. D., and Parrish, J. A.   Components of the Goeckerman regimen. *J. Invest. Dermatol.* 73:170–173, 1979.

LeVine, M. J., and Parrish, J. A.   Outpatient phototherapy of psoriasis. *Arch. Dermatol.* 116:552–554, 1980.

Lomholt, G.   *Psoriasis: Prevalence, Spontaneous Course and Genetics.* Copenhagen: GEC Gad, 1953.

Marisco, A. R., Eaglstein, W. H., and Weinstein, G. D.   Ultraviolet light and tar in the Goeckerman treatment of psoriasis. *Arch. Dermatol.* 112:1249–1250, 1976.

Methotrexate therapy for psoriasis: Guideline revisions. *Arch. Dermatol.* 108:35, 1973.

Momtaz, T. K., and Parrish, J. A.   Combined UVB and PUVA in the treatment of psoriasis. *J. Invest. Dermatol.* 76:303, 1981.

Montes, L., Welborn, W., and Brody, I.   Low strength anthralin in psoriasis. *J. Cutan. Pathol.* 6:445–456, 1979.

Morison, W. L., Momtaz, T. K., Parrish, J. A., and Fitzpatrick, T. B.   Combined methotrexate-PUVA therapy in the treatment of psoriasis. *J. Am. Acad. Dermatol.* 6:46–51, 1982.

Pariser, H., and Murray, P. F.   Intralesional injections of triamcinolone: Effects of different concentrations on psoriatic lesions. *Arch. Dermatol.* 87:183–187, 1963.

Parrish, J. A., et al.   Photochemotherapy of psoriasis using methoxsalen and sunlight: A controlled study. *Arch. Dermatol.* 113:1529–1532, 1977.

Paul, B., Stern, R. S., Arndt, K. A., and Parrish, J. A.   Combined methotrexate-UVB treatment of psoriasis. *J. Am. Acad. Derm.* In press.

Peachey, R. D., Pye, R. J., and Harman, R. P. M.   The treatment of psoriatic nail dystrophy with intradermal steroid injections. *Br. J. Dermatol.* 95:75–78, 1976.

Peck, G. L.   Retinoids in dermatology. *Arch. Dermatol.* 116:283–284, 1980.

Robertson, D., McCarty, J., and Jarratt, M.   Treatment of psoriasis with 8-methoxypsoralen and sunlight. *South. Med. J.* 71:1345–1349, 1978.

Schaefer, H., Farber, E., Goldberg, L., and Schalla, W.   Limited application period for dithranol in psoriasis: Preliminary report on penetration and clinical efficacy. *Br. J. Dermatol.* 102:571–573, 1980.

Schur, P. H., Kammer, G. M., and Soter, N. A.   Clinical, immunologic and genetic study of 100 patients with psoriatic arthritis. *Arth. Rheum.* 22:656, 1979.

South, D. A., and Farber, D. A.   Urea ointment in the nonsurgical avulsion of nail dystrophies: A reappraisal. *Cutis* 25:609–612, 1980.

Tannenbaum, L., Parrish, J. A., Pathak, M. A., Anderson, R. R., and Fitzpatrick, T. B.   Tar phototoxicity and phototherapy for psoriasis. *Arch. Dermatol.* 111:467–470, 1975.

Thiers, B.   Psoriasis. *J. Am. Acad. Dermatol.* 3:101–104, 1980.

Weinstein, G. D., and Frost, P.   Abnormal cell proliferation of psoriasis. *J. Invest. Dermatol.* 50:254–259, 1968.

Whyte, H. J., and Baughman, R. D.   Acute guttate psoriasis and streptococcal infection. *Arch. Dermatol.* 89:350–356, 1964.

Wolff, K., Fitzpatrick, T. B., Parrish, H. A., Gschnait, F., Gilchrest, B., Honigsmann, H., Pathak, M. A., and Tannenbaum, L.   Photochemotherapy for psoriasis with orally administered methoxsalen. *Arch. Dermatol.* 112:943–950, 1976.

Zaias, N.   Psoriasis of the nail: A clinical-pathologic study. *Arch. Dermatol.* 99:567–579, 1969.

26

Rosacea and periorificial (perioral) dermatitis

I. Definition and pathophysiology

A. Rosacea is a chronic disorder of unknown etiology that affects the central face and neck. It is characterized by two clinical components: a vascular change consisting of intermittent or persistent erythema and flushing, and an acneform eruption with papules, pustules, cysts, and sebaceous hyperplasia. There is no correlation between the sebum excretion rate and the severity of rosacea. Onset is most often between ages 30–50. Although women are affected 3 times as frequently, the disease may become more severe in men; it is much more common in light-skinned, fair-complexioned individuals.

Ocular changes (blepharitis, conjunctivitis, and keratitis) and sebaceous hyperplasia of the nose (rhinophyma) may be associated with rosacea. Differential diagnostic considerations include: (1) acne vulgaris, which is characterized by a wider distribution of lesions and the presence of comedones; (2) periorificial dermatitis; (3) seborrheic dermatitis; (4) the malignant carcinoid syndrome; (5) lupus erythematosus; and (6) photodermatoses.

B. Periorificial dermatitis is a distinct clinical entity that can be easily confused with rosacea, seborrheic dermatitis, or acne. It primarily affects young women, is usually found around the mouth but occasionally around the nose or eyes, and is of unknown cause. As with rosacea, prolonged use of fluorinated topical corticosteroids can cause an eruption with similar features and can perpetuate preexisting disease.

II. Subjective data

A. The facial lesions of rosacea and periorificial dermatitis often cause justifiable concern about personal appearance.

B. Rosacea papules and cysts can be painful; periorificial dermatitis papules may itch or cause a burning sensation.

C. Patients with rosacea may complain of feelings of facial heat and congestion.

III. Objective data

A. Rosacea (See color insert.)

    1. Recurrent erythema, located in the middle third of the face (midforehead, nose, malar areas, and chin), may later lead to a persistent flush and telangiectasia.

2. Acneform papules, pustules, and cysts may be present; comedones are not.

3. Rhinophyma, which predominantly affects men, is associated with follicular dilatation, irregular thickening of the skin, and hypertrophic soft masses centered about the tip of the nose.

B. Periorificial dermatitis

1. Discrete 1--3-mm erythematous or flesh-colored papules and pustules are seen singly, in clusters, or in plaques around the mouth, sparing the vermilion border. Lesions may occasionally occur around the nose and on the malar areas below and lateral to the eyes. The glabella may be affected as well.

2. There is often a persistent erythema of the nasolabial folds that may extend around the mouth onto the chin.

3. Long-standing lesions show a flatter, more confluent eruption, with superimposed dry scaling.

IV. Therapy

A. Rosacea

1. **Precipitating factors.** Patients who flush easily should avoid hot food and drinks and activities that induce this change. These may include teas, coffee, sunlight, extremes of heat and cold, and emotional stress. It has been demonstrated that the flushing caused by coffee, for example, is induced by a temperature of 60°C, but not by cold coffee or caffeine alone. If flushing is not caused by these factors, there is no evidence that avoidance will result in improvement of the disease. Vasodilator drugs which affect peripheral blood vessels will also exacerbate rosacea flushing.

2. **Systemic antibiotics**

   a. The most effective treatment for rosacea is the administration of tetracycline. Therapy should be initiated at 250 mg 4id until symptoms subside, after which the dosage can be slowly decreased or discontinued. Occasionally it is necessary to use larger doses (1.5–2.0 gm every day) for short periods of time in order to induce remission. Long-term administration usually is needed. Tetracycline is most effective in decreasing the acneform component and clearing the keratitis but will also diminish erythema.

   After discontinuing tetracycline therapy 25% of patients can be expected to relapse within a few days; about 60% will have a relapse within 6 months. Keratitis seems always to recur quickly and requires continual treatment.

   b. If tetracycline is ineffective, erythromycin or minocycline should be tried.

   c. Metronidazole (Flagyl) 200 mg 2id has been shown to be as effective as oxytetracycline for papulopustular rosacea.

   d. Ampicillin (250 mg 2–3id) also has been shown to be useful.

   e. Low doses of clonidine (Catapres), an alpha-adrenergic agonist, may prove effective in erythematotelangiectatic rosacea.

f. Some patients with severe rosacea will respond to oral isotretinoin (see p. 237).

3. **Topical therapy** for the acneform lesions is similar to that for acne vulgaris.

   a. Topical tetracycline lotion (Topicycline) applied twice daily is frequently useful in papulopustular rosacea. If ineffective or contraindicated, topical erythromycin or clindamycin lotions should be tried as in the treatment of acne vulgaris (see p. 240).

   b. Preparations containing benzoyl peroxide, sulfur in concentrations of up to 15%, or both (Sulfoxyl) can be useful (see p. 239).

   c. Ultraviolet light (UVL) therapy is of no benefit.

   d. Topical corticosteroids are occasionally used to decrease erythema and inflammation. The high-potency fluorinated steroid preparations should never be used, since they might induce more widespread and irreversible telangiectasia. 1% hydrocortisone cream is acceptable.

4. Large telangiectatic vessels may be destroyed by argon laser surgery or by electrosurgery, using the epilating needle (see p. 205).

5. Surgical reduction of the soft tissue enlargement in rhinophyma may be accomplished by a surgical shave, dermabrasion, or electrosurgery.

B. Periorificial dermatitis

1. **Systemic antibiotics** used as described for rosacea are the only reliable therapy. Periorificial dermatitis usually clears within 3–8 weeks, and it is then often possible to taper off tetracycline. Some patients need longer-term maintenance therapy.

2. **Topical therapy** with antibiotics previously described may be helpful. Fluorinated corticosteroids must be assiduously avoided. Hydrocortisone 1% or other nonfluorinated corticosteroid cream may be of symptomatic benefit but will not cure the eruption.

References

ROSACEA

Arndt, K. A. Argon laser therapy of small vascular lesions. *Arch. Dermatol.* 118:220–224, 1982.

Goldsmith, A. J. B. The ocular manifestations of rosacea. *Br. J. Dermatol.* 65:448–457, 1953.

Knight, A. G., and Vickers, C. F. H. A follow-up of tetracycline-treated rosacea: With special reference to rosacea keratitis. *Br. J. Dermatol.* 93:577–580, 1975.

Leydin, J. J., Thew, M., and Kligman, A. M. Steroid rosacea. *Arch. Dermatol.* 110:619–622, 1974.

Marks, R. Concepts in the pathogenesis of rosacea. *Br. J. Dermatol.* 80:170–171, 1968.

Marks, R. Rosacea. *Weekly Update: Dermatology* 617:2–7, 1979.

Marks, R., and Ellis, J. Comparative effectiveness of tetracycline and ampicillin in rosacea: A controlled trial. *Lancet* 2:1049–1052, 1971.

Nunzi, E., Rebora, A., Hamerlinck, F., Corman, R. F. Immunopathological studies on rosacea. *Br. J. Dermatol.* 103:543–551, 1980.

Pye, R. J., Meyrick, G., and Burton, J. L. Skin surface composition in rosacea. *Br. J. Dermatol.* 94:161–164, 1976.

Saihan, E. M., and Burton, J. L. A double-blind trial of metronidazole versus oxytetracycline therapy for rosacea. *Br. J. Dermatol.* 102:443–445, 1980.

Wilkin, J. K. Vasodilator rosacea. *Arch. Dermatol.* 116:598, 1980.

Wilkin, J. K. Oral thermal-induced flushing in erythematotelangiectatic rosacea. *J. Invest. Dermatol.* 76:15–18, 1981.

PERIORIFICIAL DERMATITIS

Bendyl, B. J. Perioral dermatitis: Etiology and treatment. *Cutis* 17:903–908, 1976.

Cochran, R. E. I., and Thomson, J. Perioral dermatitis: A reappraisal. *Clin. Exper. Dermatol.* 4:75–80, 1979.

Cotterill, J. A. Perioral dermatitis. *Br. J. Dermatol.* 101:259–262, 1979.

MacDonald, A., and Feiwal, M. Perioral dermatitis: Aetiology and treatment with tetracycline. *Br. J. Dermatol.* 87:315–319, 1972.

Sneddon, I. B. Perioral dermatitis. *Br. J. Dermatol.* 87:430–434, 1972.

Wilkinson, D. S. What is perioral dermatitis? *Inter. J. Dermatol.* 20:485–487, 1981.

Wilkinson, D. S., Kirton, V., and Wilkinson, J. D. Perioral dermatitis: A 12-year review. *Br. J. Dermatol.* 101:245–257, 1979.

27

Seborrheic dermatitis and dandruff

I. Definition and pathophysiology. Seborrheic dermatitis and dandruff each may cause a scaling on the scalp that is often associated with itching. There are, however, distinctions that can be found between the two disorders. Dandruff is noninflammatory, increased scaling on the scalp that represents the more active end of the spectrum of physiologic desquamation. On a normal scalp approximately 487,000 cells/sq cm can be found after a detergent scrub; scalps affected with dandruff and seborrheic dermatitis liberate up to 800,000 cells/sq cm. Although it has long been thought that microorganisms caused or contributed to the production of dandruff, it is now clear that no organism or combination of organisms is in any way responsible. Neither is seborrhea a causative factor: dandruff subjects produce no more sebum on their scalps than do controls.

Seborrheic dermatitis is an inflammatory, erythematous, and scaling eruption that occurs primarily in "seborrheic" areas, i.e., those with a high number and activity of sebaceous glands such as the scalp, face, and trunk. Although seborrheic dermatitis occurs in neonatal and postpubertal life—times during which sebaceous glands are most active—no direct relationship between the amount or composition of sebum and the presence of dermatitis has been documented. Reducing sebum excretion affects neither dandruff nor seborrheic dermatitis. This disease is one of accelerated epidermal growth resulting in retention of nuclei in stratum corneum cells that have not had sufficient time to completely mature. On a normal scalp there are approximately 3700 nucleated cells/sq cm; on scalps with dandruff there are 25,000, and on those with seborrheic dermatitis the count is 76,000. It has been postulated that prolonged retention of sebum on the skin may in some way act as an irritant or alter epidermal function following its percutaneous reentry. A constitutional predisposition to seborrheic dermatitis seems to exist, and emotional or physical stress also may be important. There is both increased sebum output and an increased incidence of seborrheic dermatitis in Parkinson's disease and some other neurologic conditions.

II. Subjective data. The lesions of seborrheic dermatitis and dandruff are often asymptomatic, but pruritus is not uncommon and may at times be intense.

III. Objective data

    A. Dandruff appears simply as noninflammatory, diffuse scaling on the scalp only.

    B. With seborrheic dermatitis, there is erythema, greasy scaling, and at times exudation; involved areas may have better-defined borders. Mild erythema and fine, dry scaling may also be found on the eyebrows, eyelids, nasolabial and postauricular folds, moustache, beard, and presternal areas. Inframammary folds, the groin, gluteal crease, and umbilicus are also affected. Lesions may become thick, semiconfluent, yellow, and greasy. Secondary impetiginization and folliculitis may occur.

C. Seborrheic marginal blepharitis, which consists of erythema and scaling of eyelid margins and cilia, is often associated with mild granular conjunctivitis. Seborrheic dermatitis in other sites is often not present.

IV. Therapy

A. Agents effective in eliminating the scaling of dandruff and seborrheic dermatitis appear to act by varying mechanisms. Selenium sulfide (see p. 294) and tars (see p. 307) inhibit mitotic activity. Zinc pyrithione (see p. 295) is directly cytotoxic and salicylic acid (see p. 306) disrupts the bonds that cause stratum corneum cells to stick together. There are no studies comparing efficacy of antiseborrheic shampoos. The following agents are listed in rough approximation of usefulness:

1. The most effective antiseborrheic shampoos contain 2½% **selenium sulfide** (Exsel, Iosel, Selsun). They should be applied 2–3 times weekly for 5–10 min each time.

2. Preparations containing 1–2% **zinc pyrithione** (Danex, DHS-Zinc, Head and Shoulders, Zincon) work almost as well.

3. **Salicylic acid-sulfur shampoos** (Ionil, Sebulex, TiSeb, Vanseb) are less effective but show definite activity.

4. **Tar** shampoos (DHS-T, Ionil T, Pentrax, Sebutone, T/Gel, TiSeb-T, Zetar) inhibit epidermal proliferation through cytostatic effects, after an initial burst of transient hyperplasia.

5. **Chloroxine** (Capitrol) shampoo contains a synthetic antibacterial compound similar to the hydroxyquinoline compounds used in dermatology for many years. Comparative efficacy studies with this shampoo appear to be unavailable.

6. Any nonmedicinal shampoo, particularly those containing **surfactants and detergents,** will remove scales and lead to subjective clinical improvement and decreased desquamation for about 4 days. These agents should be used every 2 days to control dandruff.

B. If the lesions are extensive or very inflammatory, also have the patient apply either a topical corticosteroid solution, lotion, or spray. (Valisone or Diprosone lotion is generally most effective; Synalar solution and other corticosteroid lotions are also useful.) Alternatively, a sodium sulfacetamide lotion (Sebizon) 2–3 times a day may be used.

C. Thick crusts may be more easily removed by overnight applications of a keratolytic gel (Keralyt gel), with or without plastic cap occlusion; 3% sulfur, 3% salicylic acid, 4% cetyl alcohol-coal tar distillate (Pragmatar) cream; Baker's P&S liquid; "20-10-5" ointment (see Psoriasis, p. 147); or a 30-min compress with warm mineral oil, prior to shampooing.

D. Seborrheic dermatitis lesions on other areas respond rapidly to a corticosteroid cream such as 1% hydrocortisone applied 1–3 times a day. Aerosols or lotions are easier to apply to hairy areas. Prolonged application of high-potency fluorinated corticosteroids may lead to disfiguring telangiectasia and atrophy. Other useful topical agents for glabrous skin include sulfur-containing medications such as 10% sulfacetamide lotion (Sebizon); 3% sulfur, 3% salicylic acid, 4% cetyl alcohol-coal tar distillate (Pragmatar) cream; or formulations such as precipitated sulfur 3–10%, salicylic acid 1–5%, and tar 2% in an ointment base or 1–3% sulfur in calamine lotion.

E. Seborrheic blepharitis is treated 1–3 times a day with either sulfacetamide (Sebizon) alone or with a 10% sulfacetamide/0.2% prednisolone/0.12% phenylephrine suspension (Blephamide, Sulfapred, Vasocidin) or similar preparations (Cetapred, Metimyd, Optimyd). It is essential to monitor intraocular tension concurrent with intermittent or chronic steroid therapy in or around the eye.

References

Frost, P., and Horwitz, S. N. *Principles of Cosmetics for the Dermatologist.* St. Louis: Mosby, 1982.

Kligman, A. M., Marples, R. R., Lantis, L. R., and McGinley, K. J. Appraisal of antidandruff formation. *J. Soc. Cosmet. Chem.* 25:73–91, 1974.

Leyden, J. J., McGinley, K. J., Kligman, A. M. Role of microorganisms in dandruff. *Arch. Dermatol.* 112:333–338, 1976.

Lowe, N. L., Breeding, J. H., and Wortzman, M. S. New coal tar extract and coal tar shampoos: Evaluation by epidermal DNA synthesis suppression assay. *Arch Dermatol.* 118:487–489, 1982.

Marks, R., Bhogal, B., and Wilson, L. The effect of betamethasone valerate on seborrheic dermatitis of the scalp. *Acta Derm. Venereol.* (Stockh.) 54:373–375, 1974.

McGinley, K. J., Leyden, J. J., Marples, R. R., and Kligman, A. M. Quantitative microbiology of the scalp in non-dandruff, dandruff, and seborrheic dermatitis. *J. Invest. Dermatol.* 64:401–405, 1975.

Parrish, J. A., and Arndt, K. A. Seborrheic dermatitis of the beard. *Br. J. Dermatol.* 87:241–244, 1972.

Priestly, G. C., and Brown, J. C. Acute toxicity of zinc pyrithione to human skin cells in vitro. *Acta Dermatol. Venereol.* (Stockh.) 60:145–148, 1980.

Priestly, G. C., and Savin, J. A. The microbiology of dandruff. *Br. J. Dermatol.* 94:469–471, 1976.

Veien, N. K., Pilgaard, C. E., and Gade, M. Seborrheic dermatitis of the scalp treated with a tar/zinc pyrithione shampoo. *Clin. Exper. Dermatol.* 5:53–56, 1980.

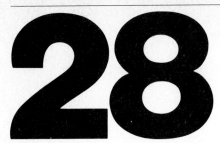

Sexually transmitted disorders (STDs)

Syphilis, gonorrhea, chancroid, lymphogranuloma venereum, and granuloma inguinale have long been considered the five venereal diseases. However, it is now quite apparent that there are numerous disorders that can be transmitted through close personal contact, and the expanded list included herein more truly reflects the actual sexually transmitted and sexually acquired diseases.

In the United States there were an estimated 1.6–2.0 million cases of gonorrhea, and an estimated 80,000–85,000 cases of primary and secondary syphilis in 1979. The rates per 100,000 population reported by state health departments were: gonorrhea 459; primary and secondary syphilis 11.4; chancroid 0.4; lymphogranuloma venereum 0.1; and granuloma inguinale 0.0. Rates per 1000 patient visits to STD clinics for other STDs were nongonococcal urethritis (NGU) 256; trichomoniasis 128; pediculosis pubis 37/24 (male/female); genital warts 33/36; genital herpes 29/18; and scabies 11/5. Entities will be discussed in this section in order of the incidence of new cases per 100,000 population found in hospital clinics in England. Our experience seeing patients in ambulatory venereal disease and dermatology clinics would probably differ in order of incidence but the diseases are the same. Note that four of the five least common disorders are the "classic" venereal diseases. This does not diminish their importance as infectious diseases of general concern, but it does point out that the spectrum of this type of communicable disorder is broad and the number of people affected by more common sexually transmitted disorders is high. Although some of these conditions are uncommon or do not have dermatologic findings, they all enter into the differential diagnosis and consideration of therapy and hence all will be discussed.

Nongonococcal urethritis (NGU)
(Incidence 208/100,000)

I. **Definition and pathophysiology.** NGU is an inflammation of the urethra not caused by *Neisseria gonorrhoeae*. A small proportion of cases is associated with trichomoniasis or candidiasis, but in about 90% of cases a pathogen cannot be identified by routine methods. *Chlamydia trachomatis,* an obligate intracellular bacterium that is cultured like a virus, can be isolated from almost half of the etiologically diagnosed cases if appropriate culture and antibody tests are available. Of the 15 immunotypes of *C. trachomatis,* types D through K are usually associated with genital and perinatal infection. The mycoplasma *Ureaplasma urealyticum* causes another 10–30% of cases. The cause of the remaining *Chlamydia*-negative NGU is not clear. Postgonococcal urethritis represents simultaneously acquired gonorrhea and NGU; this explains its high incidence when gonorrhea is treated with drugs other than tetracycline.

II. Subjective data. Patients with NGU have variable symptoms; dysuria, when present, is usually not severe.

III. Objective data. The urethral discharge in NGU is usually scant and is white or clear in appearance.

IV. Assessment. The diagnosis is established by the clinical presentation and a Gram's stain of urethral discharge that shows polymorphonuclear leukocytes but no organisms. Specifically there are no gonococci or *Candida albicans* on Gram's stain; no *Candida* on KOH smear or SMS (Swartz-Medrik stain); no trichomonas on saline wet mount; no bacteria on methylene blue and/or Gram's stain of a spun-down midstream urine. There will be no growth for these agents in the appropriate media: Thayer-Martin (gonococcus), Feinberg-Wittington or Bushby (*Trichomonas*), Sabouraud's (*Candida*), and phenyl ethyl alcohol/MacConkey (urinary tract bacteria).

V. Therapy

A. Tetracycline 500 mg 4id for at least 7 days or **doxycycline** 100 mg 2id for at least 7 days. The majority of patients will be cured on initial treatment but there is a 40% relapse rate in *Chlamydia*-negative NGU within 6 weeks. Steady sexual partners should be treated.

B. Erythromycin 500 mg 4id for at least 7 days is an alternative treatment particularly useful for tetracycline-resistant *U. urealyticum.*

C. Patients with multiple recurrences should be referred to a urologist to rule out structural abnormalities.

Gonorrhea
(Incidence 124/100,000)

I. Definition and pathophysiology. Infection with *N. gonorrhoeae* occurs most often as an anterior urethritis in men and as an asymptomatic or minimally symptomatic endocervical colonization in women. Transmission of the gonococcus is almost wholly by sexual practices and their variations, except for conjunctivitis in infants and at times vulvovaginitis in prepubescent girls. Gonorrhea is diagnosed more in the male and at least half of all reported cases are 25 years of age or younger. The majority of the 2–3 million Americans infected each year reside in urban areas.

Neisseria are gram-negative, nonmotile, non–spore-forming cocci that tend to grow in pairs with the adjacent sides flattened. Humans are the only natural host of *Neisseria*. *N. gonorrhoeae* is differentiated from nonpathogenic *Neisseria* through growth on selective antibiotic-containing media (Thayer-Martin agar) and from the meningococcus by sugar fermentation patterns on appropriate media.

Pathogenic gonococci have tiny proteinaceous surface projections called pili, which cause the organisms to stick to each other as well as to mucosal cells. The gonococcus enters the body by penetrating through columnar epithelial cells of the genitourinary tract and produces an acute inflammatory response.

II. Subjective data

A. Males

1. After an incubation period of 2–5 days 80–90% of men have the sudden onset of uncomfortable sensations along the urethra followed by frequent, painful urination.

2. After a variable period of time (10–14 days or longer) infection may spread to the posterior urethra, prostate, seminal vesicles, and epididymis, causing pain and a feeling of fullness in the perineum or scrotum.

B. Females

1. Seventy to eighty percent of infected women have gonococci present in the endocervical canal or urethra with no symptoms or with nonspecific symptoms such as vaginal discharge, urinary frequency, or dysuria.

2. Pelvic inflammatory disease (salpingitis, parametritis, and localized peritonitis) causes fever, nausea, vomiting, and abdominal pain and may follow an acute infection or occur months later.

III. Objective data

A. Males. A profuse mucopurulent discharge is present.

B. Females

1. A mild discharge may be seen.

2. Patients with pelvic inflammatory disease have acute abdominal pain and fever that simulates appendicitis or other acute surgical conditions.

IV. Assessment

A. Diagnosis

1. In men, the finding of intracellular gram-negative diplococci within polymorphonuclear leukocytes in a Gram-stained smear of a urethral exudate allows the presumptive diagnosis of gonococcal urethritis to be made with at least 99% accuracy. A urethral culture should be obtained from men suspected of asymptomatic urethral colonization, or for confirmation of adequate treatment.

2. In women, a smear will show about 5% false-positives and 50% false-negatives and is therefore of no diagnostic use. Cervical culture on Thayer-Martin media will detect 80–85% of those infected, and the addition of a culture of the anus will increase the yield to over 90%.

B. Extragenital infections and complications

1. **Pharyngeal infections,** usually asymptomatic, are present in about 20% of patients with anogenital gonorrhea who practice fellatio.

2. **Anal infections** in men are usually the result of anal intercourse among homosexuals. Fifty percent of women with gonorrhea will also have anal infection presumably because of contiguity but not neces-

sarily from intercourse. Anal infection is almost always asymptomatic.

3. **Disseminated infection (gonococcemia, arthritis-dermatitis syndrome)** appears initially as a triad of fever, migratory polyarthralgias and tenosynovitis, and characteristic skin lesions with subsequent development of stationary large-joint septic arthritis. Women are more commonly affected, and pregnancy and menstruation appear to predispose to dissemination.

   a. The cutaneous lesions are countable in number and are usually located distally over joints.

   b. They start as minute erythematous papules resembling mosquito bites, then progress to become pustules or, later, hemorrhagic infarcts. They are often tender.

4. **Other much less common complications** include meningitis, endocarditis, and pericarditis.

V. Therapy

A. **Uncomplicated infection in adults.** There are several possible regimens, each with advantages and disadvantages. Coexisting chlamydial infection may be present in up to 45% of gonorrhea patients.

   1. **Tetracycline** 500 mg PO 4id for 7 days. **Doxycycline** 100 mg PO 2id for 7 days may be substituted. This regimen is effective against coexisting chlamydial infections but requires patient compliance and is ineffective against anorectal infections in men.

   2. **Amoxicillin,** 3.0 gm, or **ampicillin,** 3.5 gm, either with **probenecid** 1.0 gm PO. This is an effective oral single-dose treatment but is ineffective against chlamydial or anorectal and pharyngeal infections.

   3. **Procaine penicillin** 4.8 million units IM at 2 sites with 1.0 gm **probenecid** PO. This is a parenteral, single-dose therapy but has the disadvantage of injections, procaine or penicillin reactions, and lack of effectiveness against *Chlamydia.*

   4. **Amoxicillin/ampicillin** as above **2,** followed by tetracycline as above **1.** This combines a single-dose therapy with one effective against chlamydial infections. However, this regimen has not yet been evaluated.

   5. Comments: Single-dose treatment is preferred in patients unlikely to complete multiple-dose regimens. IM procaine penicillin is preferred in homosexual men with anorectal infections or spectinomycin in penicillin-allergic patients. High failure rates have been reported in patients with pharyngeal infection treated with ampicillin or spectinomycin, and tetracycline or procaine penicillin is preferred. Penicillin-allergic patients (other than homosexual men) should be treated with tetracycline or doxycycline. If intolerant of those drugs, use spectinomycin 2.0 gm IM in 1 injection. Patients with incubating syphilis are likely to be cured by all the regimens described except spectinomycin, and all should have a serologic test for syphilis at the time of diagnosis. Treatment of choice during pregnancy is ampicillin or amoxicillin or, if allergy exists, IM spectinomycin. Erythromycin can be added to treat coexistent chlamydial infection.

B. Pelvic inflammatory disease (ambulatory patients)

1. Either cefitoxin 2.0 gm IM, **or** amoxicillin 3.0 gm PO, **or** ampicillin 3.5 gm PO, **or** procaine penicillin 4.8 million units IM at 2 sites; each along with probenecid 1.0 gm PO, **followed by** doxycycline 100 mg PO 2id for 10–14 days. Tetracycline 500 mg 4id can be used but is less active against some anaerobes and requires greater patient compliance.

   a. A cephalosporin plus a tetracycline is effective against gonorrhea, including penicillinase-producing organisms, and *Chlamydia*. Penicillinase-producing *N. gonorrhoeae* will not be adequately treated by the combination of either amoxicillin, ampicillin, or procaine penicillin plus doxycycline.

C. Disseminated infection

1. **Crystalline penicillin G** 10 million units IV for at least 3 days or until improvement, followed by ampicillin 500 mg PO 4id to complete 7 days, or

2. **Ampicillin or amoxicillin** plus probenecid as for anogenital infection, then 500 mg 4id to complete at least 7 days, or

3. **Tetracycline** 500 mg PO 4id for at least 7 days, or

4. **Cefoxitin** 1.0 gm or cefotaxime 500 mg 4id IV for at least 7 days, or

5. **Erythromycin** 500 mg PO 4id for at least 7 days.

6. **Hospitalization** is usually indicated, especially for patients who appear to have septic arthritis or other complications, have an uncertain diagnosis, or are unreliable.

D. Treatment failure. All patients with a positive follow-up culture after initial treatment for anogenital or urethral infection with penicillin, ampicillin, or tetracycline should receive 2 gm of spectinomycin IM. Failure is usually due to reinfection but could be from infection from penicillinase-producing *Neisseria gonorrhoeae* (PPNG). PPNG isolates resistant to spectinomycin may be treated with cefoxitin 2.0 mg IM with probenecid 1.0 gm PO, or cefotaxime 1.0 gm IM in a single dose without probenecid. PPNG pharyngeal infection should be treated with 9 tablets of trimethoprime sulfamethoxazole (80 mg/400 mg) taken as a single dose for 5 days. Consult the latest CDC recommendations periodically.

E. Epidemiologic treatment

1. Those known to have been recently exposed to gonorrhea should be examined and treated with the same treatment as those known to have the disease.

2. Acceptable regimens for prophylaxis or neonatal gonococcal and chlamydial ophthalmia include either tetracycline or erythromycin ointment or drops. 1% silver nitrate solution is effective against gonococcal ophthalmia but will not prevent chlamydial ophthalmia.

Candida albicans infection
(Incidence 83/100,000)

Candida albicans organisms may cause eruption by direct infection or through an irritant action. See p. 79 for more discussion.

Warts and condyloma acuminata
(Incidence 50/100,000)

These slow-growing viral lesions may be found on any area of the anogenital region, and they have clearly been shown to be sexually transmitted. See p. 191 for more discussion.

Trichomoniasis
(Incidence 43/100,000)

I. **Definition and pathophysiology.** The protozoan flagellate *Trichomonas vaginalis* may infect as many as 10–20% of sexually active males and females; in women it causes an infection of the vagina and urethra that may extend to involve the adjacent skin. Transmission is by sexual intercourse as well as from contaminated material or instrumentation. Organisms can be cultured from the urethra in 80% of infected women and about 70% of their male sexual partners.

II. **Subjective data**

   A. When symptoms are present, vulvar pruritus is the predominant problem.

   B. Dysuria and dyspareunia may be complaints.

   C. Men can have mild urethral pruritus associated with dysuria and frequency.

III. **Objective data**

   A. The vaginal discharge is characteristically cream-colored, frothy, and purulent.

   B. Signs of secondary irritant inflammation—edema, erythema, and excoriation of external genitalia—are often seen.

IV. **Assessment**

   A. Diagnosis is made by visualizing motile $10 \mu \times 20 \mu$ trichomonads on a wet mount.

   1. Mix a drop of discharge with a drop of saline on a slide, apply cover slip, view at 100–400× magnification with the condenser down.

   2. Wet mount will be positive in only 75–80% of patients from whom trichomonads can be cultured.

   3. Other suggestive features include vaginal secretions with a pH greater than 4.7 and a predominance of leukocytes.

   B. Organisms may be cultured on Feinberg-Wittington or other media.

V. **Therapy**

   A. Metronidazole (Flagyl) 2 gm PO in a single dose for the patient and for partner(s). Intravaginal metronidazole and other intravaginal medications are ineffective and should not be used.

   B. Recurrent discharge may represent relapse or reinfection with *Tri-*

chomonas, but because metronidazole therapy alters the normal vaginal flora, *C. albicans* vaginitis must be considered. If single-dose treatment fails, then treat with metronidazole 250 mg PO 3id for 7 days.

C. Metronidazole should not be used during pregnancy. Acidifying douches may give adequate relief of symptoms.

1. Clotrimazole, 100 mg intravaginally at bedtime for 7 days, may improve symptoms and effect some cures.

Herpes simplex
(Incidence 17/100,000)

Approximately 90% of genital herpes infections are with the type 2 virus. Some authorities in the United States claim that this is the third most common sexually transmittable disease. See p. 93 for more discussion.

Pediculosis pubis
(Incidence 13/100,000)

Scabies
(Incidence 4.8/100,000)

Both of these disorders present as moderate to severe pruritus in the pubic area and often elsewhere. See p. 115 for more discussion.

Syphilis
(Incidence 3.7/100,000; primary and secondary only)

I. **Definition and pathophysiology.** Syphilis is caused by a delicate spirilliform organism *Treponema pallidum,* characterized by thinness, motility, and the closeness and regularity of its 6–14 corkscrewlike spirals. These spirochetes, 6–15 μ long and 0.25 μ thick, pass through intact mucous membranes or abraded skin and are disseminated by the bloodstream throughout the body within hours. Approximately 3 weeks later (10–40 days) the primary lesion appears at the site of infection. This chancre persists 1–5 weeks and then spontaneously disappears. It is followed about 6 weeks later (2 weeks–6 months, average 9 weeks after inoculation) by the signs and symptoms of secondary syphilis, which also disappear without therapy within a month. If primary and secondary syphilis is left untreated, the clinical disease will disappear and serologic tests will revert to nonreactive in about 33% of patients. Thirty-three percent will continue to have positive serologic tests for syphilis but enjoy good health, and 33% will later develop signs of late syphilis. (Late [tertiary] syphilis is now not commonly seen.) Of the latter, about 25% can be expected to die primarily as a result of the disease; 80% of these deaths are related to cardiovascular problems.

II. **Subjective data**

A. The lesions of primary syphilis are either painless or much less discomforting than would be expected. Extragenital lesions may hurt.

B. Secondary syphilis is usually asymptomatic; specifically, the lesions rarely itch. Patients often note a flulike syndrome with headache, malaise, sore throat, and arthralgias.

III. Objective data (See color insert.)

A. **The primary chancre** is usually a single, firm erosion or ulcer covered with a crust. Occasionally, multiple chancres are present.

Bilateral nontender inguinal adenopathy may be palpated.

B. **The secondary rash** consists of generalized, faint, red brown macules and papules.

   1. The palms and soles are characteristically involved.

   2. Lesions on mucous membranes appear as raised white "mucous patches."

   3. Other findings may include generalized lymphadenopathy, patchy hair loss, and smooth-surfaced yet warty intertriginous plaques termed *condyloma lata.*

IV. Assessment

A. Definitive diagnosis is made by viewing the causative spirochete by dark-field microscopy in specimens collected from primary and secondary lesions.

T. pallidum is not stained by ordinary reagents and is so narrow that it cannot be visualized under the normal light microscope.

B. Invasion of the human host by this spirochete leads to production of multiple antibodies of two basic types, reflected in the two kinds of serologic tests for syphilis (STS).

   1. The nonspecific, nontreponemal antibodies (reagins), directed against a lipoidal antigen that results from interaction of host and parasite, are measured by floculation tests (VDRL [Venereal Disease Research Laboratories] and RPR [rapid plasma reagin]).

   These tests are sensitive, easy to perform, and are the screening tests of choice.

   2. The specific treponemal tests measure antibody directed against the treponemal organism.

      a. The fluorescent treponemal-antibody tests (FTA), the reference test at present, employ the Nichol-strain treponemes on the slide as antigen to which the patient's serum is added.

      b. This test is needed to confirm the presence or absence of true treponemal infection in those with a positive nontreponemal test but no history or knowledge of syphilis or other treponemal disease.

V. Therapy

A. **Early syphilis: primary, secondary, latent syphilis of less than 1 year's duration**

   1. **Benzathine penicillin G,** 2.4 million units IM once. Penicillin-allergic patients should take tetracycline 500 mg 4id for 15 days. Confirmed penicillin-allergic patients who cannot take tetracycline may be treated with erythromycin 500 mg 4id for 15 days.

B. **Syphilis of more than 1 year's duration, cardiovascular, late benign syphilis**

1. **Benzathine penicillin G,** 2.4 million units IM weekly for 3 weeks.

    Penicillin-allergic patients should take tetracycline 2 gm daily for 30 days. Confirmed penicillin-allergic patients intolerant of tetracycline may take erythromycin 2 gm daily for 30 days. There are no data to document efficacy of tetracycline or erythromycin treatment.

2. **Cerebrospinal examination** is mandatory for patients with possible neurosyphilis and is suggested for all other patients in this group to rule out asymptomatic neurosyphilis.

    a. Symptomatic or asymptomatic neurosyphilis may be treated with either:

    (1) Aqueous penicillin G 12–24 million units IV for at least 10 days, followed by benzathine penicillin G 2.4 million units IM weekly for 3 weeks, or

    (2) Procaine penicillin G, 2.4 million units daily, plus probenecid 2 gm daily both for 10 days, followed by benzathine penicillin G, 2.4 million units IM weekly for 3 weeks, or

    (3) Benzathine penicillin G, 2.4 million units IM weekly for 3 weeks.

C. Pregnant patients should be treated with penicillin, or, if allergic to penicillin, with erythromycin stearate, ethylsuccinate, or base.

D. Retreatment. The STS generally returns to normal within 6–12 months after treatment of primary syphilis or 12–18 months after treatment of secondary syphilis. Retreatment (same treatment as for syphilis of more than 1 year's duration) should be considered if:

1. Clinical disease continues or recurs.

2. The quantitative STS titer measured at 3-month intervals does not decrease at least fourfold (2 tube dilutions) within 1 year.

3. The quantitative STS titer increases fourfold (2 tube dilutions), representing either relapse or reinfection.

E. Penicillin, ampicillin, and tetracycline treatment of gonorrhea is curative for *incubating* syphilis.

Molluscum contagiosum
(Incidence 2.0/100,000)

Many adult patients with molluscum have lesions in the anogenital region. See p. 137 for more discussion.

Chancroid
(Incidence 0.11/100,000)

I. Definition and pathophysiology. Chancroid, seen 20 times more commonly in men than in women, is an autoinoculable, localized, sexually transmitted disease caused by coccobacillus *Hemophilis ducreyi*. The incubation period is only 24–72 hr; some lesions may heal within a few days.

II. **Subjective data.** Severe pain from both the genital lesion and lymph node is typical and helps differentiate the disease from syphilis. A foul odor may suggest chancroid even prior to evaluation.

III. **Objective data**

   A. The primary lesions consist of single or multiple (in about 50% of cases), round to oval, deep ulcers with irregular outlines, sharply defined but ragged and undetermined borders, and a purulent base. The lesion is soft to palpation and is surrounded by an erythematous halo.

   B. Balanitis, phimosis, and paraphimosis are frequent.

   C. Inguinal lymphadenitis, present in about 33–50% of cases, develops 1–3 weeks after the primary lesion, is most often unilateral, and resembles an abscess (bubo). Suppuration, breakdown, and sinus tract formation can occur.

IV. **Assessment**

   A. Diagnosis is suggested by viewing this small organism on Wright's, Giemsa's, or Gram's stain under the microscope. Tissue should be taken from under the undermined borders or from material aspirated from an unruptured lymph node.

   1. *H. ducreyi* is a short, gram-negative rod with rounded ends, usually found outside the cells and in bands in parallel rows ("school of fish").

   2. Under the best of conditions smears are positive in less than 50% of cases.

   B. The diagnosis is best made by isolation of the organism on appropriate (and newly described) selective culture media.

   C. Up to 15% of these patients may also be simultaneously infected with syphilis and have a "mixed chancre."

V. **Therapy**

   A. **Erythromycin** 2 gm daily, or

   B. **Trimethoprim/sulfamethoxazole,** DS (160/800 mg), PO 2id.

   C. Duration of therapy should be for 10 days or until ulcers and lymph nodes have healed.

   D. Fluctuant nodes should be aspirated through healthy skin, but **not** incised, drained, or excised.

Lymphogranuloma venereum
(Incidence 0.06/100,000)

I. **Definition and pathophysiology.** Lymphogranuloma venereum is a systemic disease caused by the obligate intracellular parasite *Chlamydia trachomatis* immunotypes L_1, L_2, and L_3. A 7- –12-day incubation period is followed by an evanescent primary lesion, then inflammatory lymphangitis and serious late sequelae.

II. **Subjective data**

   A. The primary lesion is painless.

   B. The inguinal adenitis is tender and is accompanied by malaise, arthralgia, and fever.

III. Objective data

A. The primary lesion, seen 1–3 weeks after inoculation but most often going unnoticed, may be a transient papule, vesicle, or rarely, an ulceration.

B. Inguinal adenitis, present 2–3 weeks after the primary lesion and 3–6 weeks after inoculation, is unilateral in 66% of cases, initially discrete and movable, and later firm, oval, and elongated. Overlying skin is adherent, edematous, and violaceous in color and may form grooves between the matted nodes; suppuration may occur.

C. The presence of LGV immunotypes of *C. trachomatis* in the rectum is associated with severe acute proctitis that mimics Crohn's disease of the rectum. The non-LGV immunotypes cause a mild proctitis with or without symptoms.

D. Erythema nodosum is seen in 2–10% of cases.

E. Late changes of chronic disease may include proctitis, rectal stricture, perirectal abscesses and fistulae, and severe genital swelling. Malignant transformation occurs in about 2% of cases.

IV. Assessment

A. The complement fixation test becomes positive within 1 month after onset of infection in 80–90% of patients. If only convalescent serum is available, a titer of 1:16 or greater suggests LGV.

B. The organism can be cultured only with special media; this is not a clinically useful procedure.

C. The Frei test, a 72-hr intradermal reaction performed with specific antigen grown on chick yolk sacs, becomes positive 2–3 weeks after the onset of adenopathy. This reagent, however, is no longer available.

D. The differential diagnosis includes pyogenic lymphadenitis, syphilis, chancroid, granuloma inguinale, and metastatic tumor.

V. Therapy

A. **Tetracycline** 500 mg PO 4id for 2–3 weeks.

B. Alternative (but not well-evaluated) regimens include:

   1. **Doxycycline** 100 mg PO 2id for at least 2 weeks.

   2. **Erythromycin** 500 mg PO 4id for at least 2 weeks.

   3. **Sulfamethoxazole** 1.0 gm PO 2id for at least 2 weeks. Other sulfonamides may be used in equivalent dosage.

C. **Aspiration,** but not incision, of suppurating adenitis should be performed before spontaneous breakdown of tissue.

Granuloma inguinale
(Incidence 0.03/100,000)

I. Definition and pathophysiology. This mildly contagious, chronic, granulomatous disease involves the skin and lymphatics in the anogenital area and is usually considered a sexually transmittable disease. The organism, *Calymmatobacterium (Donovania) granulomatis*, is related to the *Klebsiella* species. The incubation period is probably 3–6 weeks.

II. Subjective data. Lesions cause no discomfort but are usually malodorous.

III. Objective data

A. The insidious onset of tissue breakdown leads to an irregular ulcer with a soft, beefy red, friable, exuberant growth base.

B. Inguinal swellings are not lymphoadenitis but represent subcutaneous perilymphatic granulomatous lesions that may eventually break through the skin, causing sinus formation.

IV. Assessment. Diagnosis is confirmed by finding the organisms (Donovan bodies) in the lesions.

A. Remove a piece of the lesion with a scalpel or punch.

B. Smear undersurface of tissue onto slides, or crush between two slides.

C. Fix with alcohol, stain with Wright's or Giemsa's stain.

D. Donovan bodies will be found within mononuclear cells; they appear as straight or slightly curved rods with more deeply staining poles, thus creating a "safety pin" appearance. The organism is gram-negative and stains red with Giemsa's and blue or purple with Wright's stain. The capsule appears pink on Wright's stain.

V. Therapy

A. **Tetracycline** 500 mg PO 4id for 3 weeks, or

B. **Sulfisoxazole** 4 gm PO followed by 500 mg PO 4id for 3 weeks. Cotrimoxazole is also effective.

C. Fluctuating gland masses indicate a need for aspiration.

Other diseases

Other infections that may be sexually transmitted include those caused by cytomegalovirus, hepatitis B virus, and *Corynebacterium (Hemophilus) vaginalis*.

References

Abrams, A. J.   Lymphogranuloma venereum. *J. A. M. A.* 205:199–202, 1968.

Corey, L., and Holmes, K. K.   Sexual transmission of hepatitis in homosexual men: Incidence and mechanism. *N. Engl. J. Med.* 302:435–438, 1980.

Felman, Y., and Nikitas, J. A.   Syphilis serology today. *Arch. Dermatol.* 116:84–89, 1980.

Holmes, K. K.   Gonococcal infection: Clinical, epidemiologic and laboratory perspectives. *Adv. Intern. Med.* 19:259–285, 1974.

Holmes, K. K., Handsfield, H. H., Wang, S. P., Wentworth, B. B., Turck, M., Anderson, J. B., and Alexander, E. R.   Etiology of nongonococcal urethritis. *N. Engl. J. Med.* 292:1199–1205, 1975.

Jacobs, N. F., Jr., and Kraus, S. J.   Gonococcal and nongonococcal urethritis in men: Clinical and laboratory differentiation. *Ann. Intern. Med.* 82:7–12, 1975.

King, A., and Nicol, C.   Venereal Diseases (4th ed.). Baltimore: Williams & Wilkins, 1980.

Kraus, S. J., Werman, B. S., Biddle, J. W., Sottnek, F. O., and Ewing, E. P. Pseudogranuloma inguinale caused by *Haemophilus ducreyi*. *Arch. Dermatol.* 118: 494–497, 1982.

Kuberski, T.   Granuloma inguinale (Donovahosis). *Sex. Trans. Dis.* 7:29–36, 1980.

Quinn, T. C., Goodell, S. C., Mkrtichiam, P. A.-C., Schuffler, M. D., Wang, S. P., Stavin, W. E., and Holmes, K. K.   *Chlamydia Trachomatis* proctitis. *N. Engl. J. Med.* 305:195–200, 1981.

Sexually transmitted diseases: Extract from the Annual Report of the Chief Medical Officer of the Department of Health and Social Security for the year 1978. *Br. J. Vener. Dis.* 56:178–181, 1980.

Sexually transmitted diseases treatment guidelines 1982: Morbidity and mortality. Weekly report 31, 25 (August 20, 1982). Atlanta, Ga.: U.S. Dept. Health and Human Services, CDC, 1982.

Sparling, P. F.   Diagnosis and treatment of syphilis. *N. Engl. J. Med.* 284:642–653, 1971.

U. S. Dept. Health and Human Services. STD Fact Sheet: Basic Statistics on the Sexually Transmitted Disease Problem in the United States. Atlanta, Ga.: Centers for Disease Control, JJS Publ. No. (CDC) 81–8195, 1981.

Taylor-Robinson, D., and McCormack, W. M.   The genital mycoplasmas. *N. Engl. J. Med.* 302:1003–1010, 1063–1067, 1980.

29

Skin tags

I. **Definition and pathophysiology.** Skin tags (acrochordons) are small papillomas found commonly on the sides of the neck, axillae, upper trunk, and eyelids of the middle-aged and elderly. Obesity, pregnancy, menopause, and endocrine disorders such as acromegaly predispose to these benign epithelial hyperplastic lesions.

II. **Subjective data.** Skin tags are cosmetically bothersome but asymptomatic. Occasionally, a lesion will twist on its stalk and become painful, erythematous, and necrotic.

III. **Objective data.** The lesions are single or multiple, 1–3 mm in diameter, soft, flesh-colored or hyperpigmented papillomas, which are usually pedunculated.

IV. **Assessment.** Treatment of obesity or an underlying endocrinologic abnormality will decrease the likelihood of new lesion formation. Lesions may be confused with seborrheic keratoses, dermal nevi, or warts.

V. **Therapy.** Treatment is easily accomplished with any of the following methods:

A. Grasp the tag with forceps and sever the base with a sharp scissors or a scalpel blade. Hemostasis may be secured by pressure, Monsel's solution (ferric subsulfate solution), mild acids (30% trichloroacetic acid), or an electrosurgical spark. The lesion may be anesthetized with ethyl chloride or refrigerant spray prior to excision, but this is rarely necessary. Never use electrosurgical apparatus around flammable ethyl chloride spray.

B. Touch each lesion with a light electrosurgical spark or remove it with the cutting current. Administration of local anesthesia is usually unnecessary and causes as much pain as the treatment itself. Multiple lesions may be treated at one time.

Reference

Pinkus, H.   Epithelial and fibroepithelial tumors. *Arch. Dermatol.* 91:24–37, 1965.

30

**Sun reactions
and sun protection**

I. **Definition and pathophysiology.** The sun radiates a broad spectrum of energy that may be categorized in terms of the wavelength of the electromagnetic waves. That radiation reaching the earth's surface may be broadly subdivided into: (1) infrared (range 700 nm–100 μ), felt as heat or a sensation of warmth; (2) visible (range 400–700 nm), the energy that stimulates the retina, and (3) ultraviolet (range 290–400 nm), wavelengths shorter than visible beginning next to the violet end of the color spectrum (see also p. 218).

The ultraviolet spectrum is subdivided into three bands. UVA radiation (320–400 nm, long wavelength) can cause immediate pigment darkening of preformed melanin, may play an additive role in assisting UVB (see below) in causing sunburn or aging, and in the presence of some drugs (psoralens, antibiotics such as Declomycin, sulfonamides, phenothiazides, chlorothiazides, sulfonylureas, and others) may induce severe phototoxicity (sunburn and blistering). UVB radiation (280–320 nm, middle wavelength) causes erythema and sunburn, stimulates melanocytes to make melanosomes and to make them more rapidly and thereby causes a tan. After chronic exposure it induces the changes of aging and carcinogenesis. UVC radiation (range 200–280 nm) from sunlight is absorbed by the ozone layer in the atmosphere and does not reach the earth's surface. This radiation kills bacteria, can cause mild conjunctivitis or sunburn, and is used in operating-room germicidal lamps.

Sunburn is usually the result of excessive exposure to UVB ultraviolet light but may be a response to excessive UVC from artificial light sources or UVA in the presence of a topical or systemic photosensitizing agent. It is seen most commonly after exposure to the sun but may also follow exposure to sunlamps or occupational light sources (welding arcs [250–700 nm], photoengraving [250–700 nm], bactericidal or cold quartz lamps [254 nm]). UVB is not screened out by thin clouds on overcast days but is fully absorbed by window glass and is partially absorbed in the smoke and smog around large cities. Much UVL reaches the skin through reflection from snow, sand, or sidewalks; hats and umbrellas provide only moderate protection.

Tolerance to sunlight is based on the amount of melanin in the skin and an individual's genetic capacity to produce melanin following exposure to the sun, i.e., suntan. Based on response to the first 30-min exposure to summer sun and the tan that develops in persons with white skin, sun-reaction skin types can be classified as follows: skin type 1 always burns easily, never tans; skin type 2 usually burns easily, tans minimally; skin type 3 burns moderately, tans gradually; skin type 4 burns minimally, tans readily; skin type 5 are heavily pigmented individuals such as darker Mediterraneans, Mongolians, and Indians, and skin type 6 are blacks. Types 1 and 2 persons often have light skin color and blue eyes, may have red scalp hair and may or may not have freckling. However, some persons with darker hair and blue or green eyes have type 1 and 2 sun reactions. People with type 1 and 2 will exceed their sunburn threshold tolerance in 10–20 min of noontime temperate summer sunlight. Four to eight times the minimal erythema dose (MED) will produce a moderate to severe burn. A number of genetic (e.g., xeroderma pigmentosum), metabolic (e.g., pellagra and porphyria cutanea tarda), neoplastic (e.g., actinic keratosis, basal cell carcinoma), connective tissue (e.g., lupus erythematosus), immunologic (e.g., solar urticaria, drug photoallergy), and idiopathic (e.g., hydroa aestivale, polymorphous light eruption) diseases may be caused or exacerbated by light exposure. These will not be further discussed in this chapter.

II. Subjective data

A. A mild sunburn will be tender to the touch and cause a hot, taut, drawn feeling.

B. Severe burns are accompanied by intense pain, inability to tolerate contact with clothing and sheets, and constitutional symptoms, including nausea, tachycardia, chills, and fever.

III. Objective data

A. The earliest sign of a burn is a pink to scarlet hue of the skin and mild edema. The more severe the burn, the earlier it will be evident. Sun exposure will cause immediate erythema, which then fades. A delayed erythema appears in 2–4 hr, becomes maximum in 14–20 hr, and lasts 24–72 hr.

B. This may progress to a vivid erythema, intense edema, and blistering.

C. Peeling follows as a consequence of increased epidermal turnover during the repair response, usually a week or more after the burn.

D. Hyperpigmentation is seen as a result of UVB-induced new pigment formation and protects against further sunburn. This is evident as immediate pigment darkening of preformed melanin (2–24 hr) and delayed tanning, reflective of new pigment formation (4–7 days).

E. UVA reactions follow a slower time course; erythema becomes evident as late as 48 hr, and the reaction may become more severe for several days (see p. 221).

F. UVC reactions are seldom severe; overexposure to short-wave ultraviolet light rarely leads to blistering but can lead to conjunctivitis and keratitis.

IV. Assessment.
The patient's history will usually be adequate to explain the clinical picture. It is important to be certain that there are no predisposing or underlying causes (drug administration, topical application of photosensitizers, or systemic illnesses such as lupus or porphyria).

V. Therapy

A. Preventive measures. Sun-protective topical medications are available as sunscreens, which contain chemical substances such as paraaminobenzoic acid (PABA), PABA esters such as glyceryl PABA and padimate O, benzophenones, cinnamates, salicylates and anthranilates (see p. 311) that absorb UVL; or sunshades, which contain opaque materials such as titanium dioxide, talc, or zinc oxide that reflect the light.

1. **Sun protection factors (SPF).** The SPF value is the ratio of the time required to produce erythema through a sunscreen product to the time required to produce the same degree of erythema without the sunscreen. The SPF usually ranges from 2 (minimal protection) to 15 (super protection).

2. **Sunscreen indications.** Individuals with skin types 1 and 2 should apply sunscreens daily, with type 3 for protracted sun exposure, and for types 4–6 none is necessary. Patients with conditions that react adversely to light (e.g., systemic lupus erythematosus, solar urticaria, porphyrias) also need constant protection.

3. **Sunscreen UVL absorption.** Most sunscreens have their peak absorption in the UVB range between 290 and 320 nm. Of the commonly used sunscreen agents, only the benzophenones and anthranilates have substantial absorption in the UVA range, from 320–400 nm. The action spectrum for most photosensitivity reactions is in the UVA range.

4. **Method of use.** The term substantivity refers to a product's ability to remain effective under the stress of prolonged exercise, sweating, and swimming. PABA esters may be more effective than PABA in ethanol, and cream-based vehicles may in some cases be more resistant to removal than those in alcohol bases. Whatever product is used should be applied 1–2 hr before exposure and reapplied generously several times during exposure particularly after swimming or sweating.

5. **Adverse effects.** PABA may stain clothing yellow especially after exposure to the sun. Contact dermatitis occasionally develops from use of PABA, PABA esters, benzophenones, and cinnamates; glyceryl PABA is the most common cause. Patients allergic to benzocaine, procaine, paraphenylenediamine, and sulfonamides may have allergic reactions to PABA.

6. Some sunscreens for various skin types:

   a. Skin types 1 and 2 persons need maximal protection from SPF 15 sunscreens such as Total Eclipse, Super Shade 15, PreSun 15 (PABA esters plus benzophenones), Pabanol (PABA in alcohol), and TiSol (no PABA or PABA esters).

   b. Skin type 3 individuals may use products such as Sundown, PreSun, Block Out, Uval (no PABA or PABA esters).

7. **Lipstick sunscreens** include RVPaba, SunStick, and PreSun #15 Lip Protection. The first two give best protection in the UVB range; the latter has broader-spectrum UVL absorptive capacities.

B. **A mild sunburn** should be treated as follows:

   1. Apply cool tap water or Burow's solution compresses 20 min 3–4 times a day or more frequently.

   2. A topical corticosteroid spray, lotion, cream, or gel may reduce inflammation and pain.

   3. Use emollients (Eucerin, Lubriderm, Nivea, petrolatum) to soothe and relieve dryness.

4. Most proprietary over the counter (OTC) burn remedies contain local anesthetics (benzocaine, dibucaine, or lidocaine), antiseptics, emollients, and fragrant materials. There is little need for any of these ingredients in the care of a sunburn, and only 20% benzocaine (Americaine) has been demonstrated to be at all effective. The vehicles of "anesthetic" sprays, creams, and lotions may be cooling and the ointments lubricating, thus lessening the symptoms, but this must be weighed against the hazard of becoming sensitized, especially to benzocaine. As burns are intrinsically self-healing, it is mandatory that the therapy be less noxious than the disease.

C. Severe sunburn

1. Instruct patients to call immediately if they are overexposed to sunlamps or to sunlight, since it is easier and more effective to abort severe inflammation than to treat an already established reaction. A short course of systemic corticosteroids may reduce a potentially severe sunburn; prednisone 40–60 mg or its equivalent should be given daily for 3 days, then discontinued. Some recent studies have been unable to confirm that prednisone suppresses sunburn, but the clinical impression still remains that it may often be useful.

2. Topical care of established severe sunburns entails almost continuous cool compresses, topical steroids and emollients, a cradle for bed linens, analgesics as needed, and careful surveillance for bacterial superinfection.

3. Some fair-skinned individuals may increase their tolerance of UVL through systemic administration of psoralen compounds. These drugs will increase the capacity of the skin to produce melanin after sun exposure and also will result in retention of melanin granules in a thickened stratum corneum. Two hours prior to sun exposure, trioxsalen (Trisoralen) 30 mg should be taken, and exposure during the first week should be gradually increased (see p. 110 for more detailed treatment description). Use of medication without subsequent exposure to light will be ineffective.

References

Dalili, H., and Adriani, J. The efficacy of local anesthetics in blocking the sensations of itch, burning and pain in normal and "sunburned" skin. *Clin. Pharmacol. Ther.* 12:913–920, 1971.

Eaglstein, W. H., Taplin, D., Mertz, P., and Smiles, K. A. An all-day test for the evaluation of a topical sunscreen. *J. Am. Acad. Dermatol.* 2:513–520, 1980.

Epstein, J. H. Adverse Cutaneous Reactions to the Sun. In F. D. Malkinson and R. W. Pearson (eds.), *Year Book of Dermatology.* Chicago: Year Book, 1971. Pp. 5–35.

Fitzpatrick, T. B., Parrish, J. A., Haynes, H. A., and Gonzalez, E. Comparison of two sunscreens with different SPFs under natural conditions in Florida sunlight. *Dermatol. Capsule Comment* 3(5):1–3, 1981.

Greenwald, J. S., Parrish, J. A., Jaenicke, K. F., and Anderson, R. R. Failure of systemically administered corticosteroids to suppress UVB-induced delayed erythema. *J. Am. Acad. Dermatol.* 5:197–202, 1981.

Harber, L. C., and Bickers, D. R. *Photosensitivity Diseases.* Philadelphia: Saunders, 1981.

Kligman, L. H., Akin, F. J., and Kligman, A. M. Sunscreens prevent ultraviolet carcinogenesis. *J. Am. Acad. Dermatol.* 3:30–35, 1980.

Leading article. Unhealthy tan. *Br. Med. J.* 2:494–495, 1970.

Macleod, T. M., and Frain-Bell, W. A study of physical light screening agents. *Br. J. Dermatol.* 92:149–156, 1975.

Parrish, J. A., White, H. A. D., and Pathak, M. A. Photomedicine. In T. B. Fitzpatrick, et al. (eds.), *Dermatology in General Medicine* (2nd ed.). New York: McGraw-Hill, 1979. Pp. 942–994.

Sayre, R. M., Marlowe, E., Agin, P. P., LeVee, G. J., and Rosenberg, E. W. Performance of six sunscreen formulations on human skin: A comparison. *Arch. Dermatol.* 115:46–49, 1979.

Sunscreens. *Med. Lett. Drugs Ther.* 21:46–48, 1979.

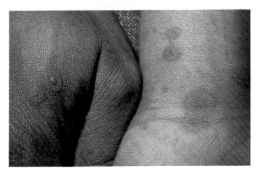

1. Erythema multiforme—
iris (target) lesions

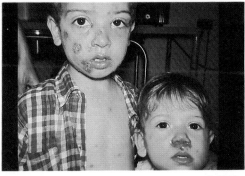

2. Strawberry nevus

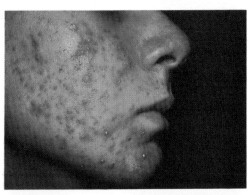

3. Acne—papules, pustules,
and scarring

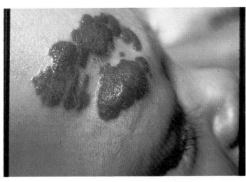

4. Impetigo

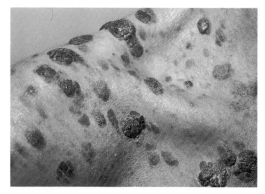

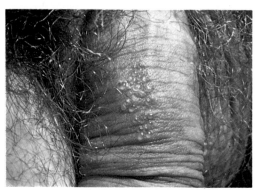

5. Seborrheic keratoses

6. Herpes simplex

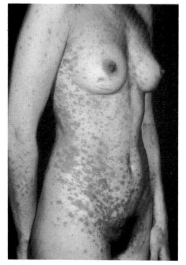

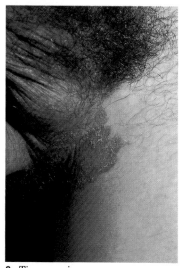

7. Pityriasis rosea

8. Tinea cruris

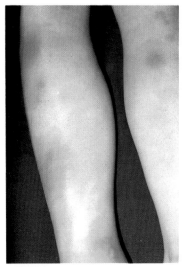

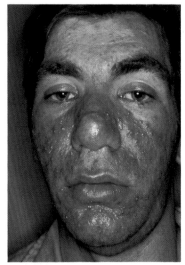

9. Erythema nodosum

10. Rosacea

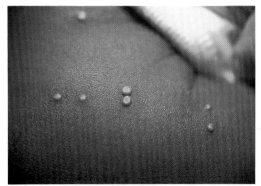

11. Molluscum
contagiosum

12. Psoriasis

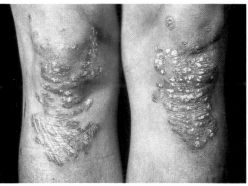

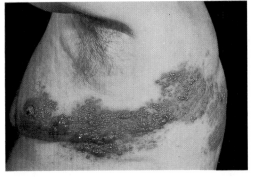

13. Herpes zoster

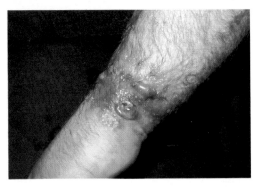

14. Contact dermatitis to leather (watchband)

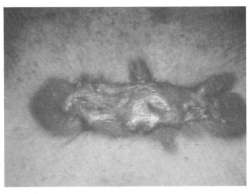

15. Keloid

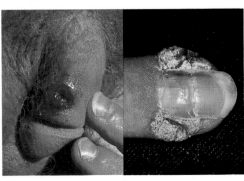

16. Primary syphilis—chancre

17. Periungual warts

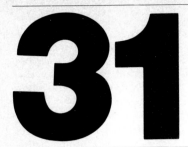

Urticaria

I. Definition and pathophysiology. Urticaria (hives) affects 20% of the population at some time during their lives. The same reaction taking place in submucosa or deeper dermis and subcutaneous tissue is termed **angioedema.** The injection of histamine or a histamine-releasing chemical into the skin, or release of histamine from mast cells following antigen-antibody reactions results in vasodilatation, increased vascular permeability, and extravasation of protein and fluids. Urticaria seems to be mediated principally by histamine, but the precise role of other mast-cell-related mediators such as slow-reacting substance of anaphylaxis, eosinophil chemotactic factor of anaphylaxis, platelet-activating factor, kinins, as well as prostaglandins remains to be elucidated.

Acute urticaria is most often mediated by B-lymphocyte-produced IgE and is seen in patients with anaphylaxis, serum sickness, or atopy, or as a reaction to insect bites, foods, infection, or drugs. Urticaria of more than 6 weeks' duration, termed **chronic urticaria,** may have a multiplicity of trigger factors; the exact cause remains in doubt in 80–90% of cases. Immunologic cases of chronic urticaria include reactions to drugs, or less frequently, to foods and food additives, inhalants, parasitic infestations, or Hymenoptera venom. The mean duration of urticaria alone is 6 months, angioedema alone 1 year, and urticaria with angioedema about 5 years (see Champion et al., 1969).

Hives may also accompany infections, collagen vascular disease, and malignant tumors. Hives with arthralgias or arthritis may be an early sign of anicteric hepatitis or a manifestation of an underlying necrotizing vasculitis. Stress and anxiety are often thought to be important etiologic factors. Urticaria induced by cold or ultraviolet light is uncommon.

There are two common types of physical urticaria. **Cholinergic urticaria** (generalized heat urticaria) is induced by acetylcholine, not histamine, and is triggered by heat, exercise, change in temperature, or emotions. The lesions are usually smaller than those of allergic urticaria and are more evanescent. **Dermatographic lesions** are hives induced by trauma (scratching) or pressure (standing, tight clothing or shoes). Types of **IgE-dependent physical urticarias** include cholinergic urticaria, dermatographism, acquired cold-induced urticaria, and sometimes, solar urticaria. Although everyone will respond to cutaneous trauma with a triple response of Lewis (erythema, flare, wheal), in dermatographism the response is excessive, even to stimuli of low intensity.

Nonimmunologic urticaria is found in as many as 5–8% of patients receiving radiocontrast media, and in those exposed to drugs such as opiates, antibiotics (notably polymyxin B), and curare, which directly release histamine from mast cells and basophils. Approximately 1% of individuals experience urticaria or anaphylactic reactions to aspirin and related nonsteroidal anti-inflammatory agents, and aspirin intolerance in patients with chronic urticaria ranges from 20–50%. Aspirin-intolerant patients also react to indomethacin. Up to 15–20% of such patients react to the ubiquitous azo dyes, notably tartrazine, and some manifest responses to benzoate preservatives. These agents may cause urticaria by altering arachidonic acid metabolism.

Hereditary angioedema is a dominantly inherited disorder in which a normal serum inhibitor of the activated first component of complement is either deficient or absent. These patients suffer recurrent episodes of cutaneous angioedema as well as attacks of laryngeal edema and gastrointestinal involvement, thought to be mediated by the complement cascade.

II. **Subjective data.** Intense pruritus is the typical symptom of urticaria. Stinging and prickling sensations are also described.

III. **Objective data**

A. Urticarial wheals are raised, erythematous, and edematous plaques with sharply defined, serpiginous, or polycyclic borders surrounded by an erythematous halo. Intensely edematous lesions will have a blanched center. Their diameters may range from millimeters to several centimeters. Individual lesions last up to 8–12 hr; those staying in one location for more than 24 hr cannot be considered true urticaria but must be regarded as a more fixed eruption such as erythema multiforme or urticarial vasculitis (urticaria perstans). The continuous spectrum of urticarialike lesions, ranging from the evanescent wheal of true urticaria to the relatively fixed edema of erythema multiforme, makes precise diagnosis difficult at times.

B. The lesions of cholinergic urticaria are small, 1- -3-mm, punctate, papular wheals surrounded by a large macular erythematous flare. They disappear spontaneously in 30–60 min.

IV. **Assessment.** A detailed and perceptive history and thorough physical examination frequently will reveal the cause and type of urticaria. If this is not rewarding, then other types of investigation, though usually unproductive, must nevertheless be pursued in patients with chronic urticaria. Pertinent tests would include CBC, differential, ESR, urinalysis, liver function tests, T4, and also complement levels (C3 and CH50) if there is suspicion of collagen-vascular disease, or necrotizing vasculitis. Total eosinophil counts may implicate an allergic cause such as drugs or atopy. Analysis of serum for cryoproteins or hepatitis-associated antigens and antibodies may permit specific diagnosis. Assessment of complement components C1, C4, C1INH may prove diagnostic for forms of C1INH deficiency. Occasionally a brief trial of a rigid elimination diet is warranted, and examination of fresh stool for ova and parasites is undertaken. Biopsy of chronic urticaria lesions is indicated and will occasionally show perivascular inflammatory changes suggestive of lupus erythematosus or vasculitis. Skin testing is rarely of value. Dermatographism can be evaluated by firmly stroking the skin with a tongue blade or similar blunt surface.

V. **Therapy**

A. **Anaphylactic and acute urticarial reactions:** therapy outlined on p. 32.

B. **Chronic urticaria**

1. Identification and treatment or removal of the trigger factor is the most important and the only effective long-term therapy.

    a. Avoidance of aspirin or food additives has been claimed to improve 50% of patients with chronic idiopathic urticaria.

2. Local measures

    a. Cool or ice water compresses or tepid baths with Aveeno colloidal oatmeal may eliminate itching.

    b. Antipruritic lotions or emulsions may help: 0.25% menthol ± 1% phenol in calamine lotion or Eucerin (see p. 289 for other preparations).

3. Systemic measures

    a. Antihistamine therapy with H1 antagonists is the therapy of choice (see p. 246 for types of antihistamines, method of action, and how to choose the appropriate agent). Hydroxyzine (Atarax, Vistaril) is often the best drug for chronic urticaria. It may be used alone or with other antihistamines, and dosage should be pushed to the limit of tolerance or to subsidence of symptoms. If hydroxyzine is ineffective, chlorpheniramine maleate (Chlor-Trimeton) or cyproheptadine hydrochloride (Periactin) should be used next, either alone or in combination. There is conflicting evidence concerning the effect of combining H1- and H2-antihistamines in the treatment of chronic idiopathic urticaria.

    b. If lesions are more acute or severe, or if angioedema is present, inject 0.3–0.5 ml epinephrine (1:1000) subcutaneously or IM q1–2h.

    c. Use of the H1-antihistamine chlorpheniramine, 4 mg PO 4id, plus the H2-antihistamine cimetidine, 400 mg PO 4id, has been shown to be more effective than placebo or either drug given alone for symptomatic dermatographism. Chlorpheniramine given alone produces no significant benefit, while cimetidine given alone produces marked exacerbation in itching. Combined H1- and H2-antagonist therapy is also helpful in acquired cold urticaria.

    d. It is rarely necessary or justified to use systemic corticosteroids. However, in some instances, when all diagnostic and therapeutic methods have been exhausted, a 2-week course of corticosteroids (starting at 40–60 mg prednisone or equivalent) will temporarily suppress the disease. Occasionally, after this treatment, the urticaria will not recur.

References

Braverman, I. M.   Urticaria as a sign of internal disease. *Postgrad. Med.* 41:450–454, 1967.

Champion, R. H.   Drug therapy of urticaria. *Br. Med. J.* 4:730–732, 1973.

Champion, R. H., Roberts, S. O. B., Carpenter, R. E., and Roger, J. H.   Urticaria and angioedema: A review of 554 patients. *Br. J. Dermatol.* 81:588–597, 1969.

Commens, C. A., and Greaves, M. W.   Cimetidine in chronic idiopathic urticaria: A randomized double-blind study. *Br. J. Dermatol.* 99:675–679, 1978.

Davies, M. G., and Greaves, M. W.   The current status of histamine receptors in human skin: Therapeutic implications. *Br. J. Dermatol.* 104:601–606, 1981.

Jacobson, K. W., Branch, L. B., and Nelson, H. S.   Laboratory tests in chronic urticaria. *J. A. M. A.* 243:1644–1646, 1980.

Kaur, S., Greaves, M., and Eftekhari, N.   Factitious urticaria (dermatographism): Treatment by cimetidine and chlorpheniramine in a randomized double-blind study. *Br. J. Dermatol.* 104:185–190, 1981.

Monroe, E. W., and Jones, H. E.   Urticaria. *Arch. Dermatol.* 113:80–90, 1977.

Moore-Robinson, M., and Warin, R. P.   Some clinical aspects of cholinergic urticaria. *Br. J. Dermatol.* 80:794–799, 1968.

Newcomb, R. W., and Nelson, H.   Dermographia mediated by immunoglobulin E. *Am. J. Med.* 54:174–180, 1973.

Phanuphak, P., Schocket, A., and Kohler, R.   Treatment of chronic idiopathic urticaria with combined H-1 and H-2 blockers. *Clin. Allergy* 8:429–433, 1978.

Shumaker, J. B., Goldfinger, S. E., Alpert, E., and Isselbacher, K. J.   Arthritis and rash: Clues to anicteric hepatitis. *Arch. Intern. Med.* 133:483–485, 1974.

Soter, N. A., and Austen, K. F.   Urticaria/Angioedema: The Mast Cell, Its Diverse Mediators, and Its Role in Cutaneous Inflammation. In B. Safai and R. A. Good (eds.), *Immunodermatology*. New York: Plenum, 1981. Pp. 273–292.

Soter, N. A., Austen, K. F., and Gigli, I.   Urticaria and arthralgias as manifestations of necrotizing angitis (vasculitis). *J. Invest. Dermatol.* 63:485–490, 1974.

Warin, R. P., and Champion, R. H.   *Urticaria.* London: Saunders, 1974.

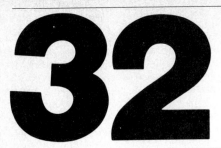

I. Definition and pathophysiology. Cutaneous abnormalities consisting of new vessel growths or vascular dilatation are extremely common; probably no individual escapes acquiring one or several throughout a lifetime. Angiomas may be most easily classified on the basis of their predominant vascular channels.

A. Capillary vessels

1. **Strawberry nevus.** This vascular malformation, present at birth or in neonates, grows for 3–12 months and begins to subside after 1 yr; 75–95% have regressed by age 5–7. Lesions that grow most rapidly usually regress most completely.

2. **Cherry angioma.** Cherry angiomas (senile angiomas) appear in early adult life and increase in number with advancing age. These asymptomatic lesions remain indefinitely.

3. **Pyogenic granuloma.** This misnamed, rapidly growing, and friable angioma often is located at a site of previous injury. Infection usually plays no part in the initiation or course of the lesion.

B. Cavernous vessels

1. **Cavernous angioma.** These vascular tumors appear first during childhood, are frequently larger and deeper than capillary angiomas, and do not subside spontaneously. They may appear as isolated lesions or may be a part of such syndromes as the Klippel-Trenaunay-Weber syndrome, blue rubber bleb nevus syndrome, or Maffucci's syndrome.

C. Disorders with vascular ectasia

1. **Port-wine stain (nevus flammeus).** These lesions, which are entirely flat and seen only as a change in skin color, are commonly found on the nuchal and eyelid areas of infants. They represent an aneurysmal dilation and ectasia of the cutaneous vascular plexus. When located in other areas, they usually occur in a unilateral or in a dermatomal distribution and may be associated with the Sturge-Weber or Klippel-Trenaunay-Weber syndrome. Most eyelid lesions disappear within the first year of life, whereas only half of those on the nuchal area (salmon patch) will have disappeared by that time. Lesions in other areas are stable and do not fade.

2. **Venous lake (venous varix).** This is a soft ectasia frequently seen on the face, lips, or ears of the elderly. The lesions persist indefinitely and occasionally thrombose and involute.

3. **Telangiectasia and spider ectasia (nevus araneus).** These lesions resemble a spider in appearance and are most commonly seen in women and children on the face and upper trunk. Acquired lesions may appear in relation to liver disease such as hepatitis or cirrhosis; changes in estrogen metabolism, as in pregnancy or in women on birth control pills; or as a part of hereditary hemorrhagic telangiectasia. Other causes of facial telangiectasia include actinic damage, the prolonged use of topical fluorinated corticosteroids, rosacea, and post-rhinoplasty "red nose" syndrome. Ectatic vessels and vasodilatation are also seen commonly on the lower extremities of women.

II. Subjective data

A. Capillary vessels

1. **Strawberry nevus.** The lesions are not painful, but large lesions may spontaneously erode or become infected.

2. **Cherry angioma.** There are no symptoms.

3. **Pyogenic granuloma.** The lesions may be painful, but the most frequent complaint relates to their friability; these angiomas bleed easily and may become secondarily infected.

B. Cavernous vessels. There are usually no symptoms.

C. Vascular ectasia. There are usually no symptoms.

Note: All angiomatous lesions may be readily visible and a cosmetic nuisance.

III. Objective data (See color insert.)

A. Capillary vessels

1. **Strawberry nevus**

   a. Bright red to purple blue lesions, which are raised, dome-shaped, or polypoid, with sharp borders.

   b. Compressible, but will not totally blanch.

2. **Cherry angioma**

   a. Bright red, raised, pinpoint to several millimeters in diameter; usually multiple and present in most profusion on the upper trunk.

   b. Will not blanch on pressure.

3. **Pyogenic granuloma**

   a. Bright red to brown, elevated, polypoid, or sessile.

   b. Usually single and found most commonly on the extremities.

   c. May be eroded, crusted, ulcerated, or infected.

B. Cavernous vessels

1. **Cavernous angioma**

   a. Small to very large, ill-defined lesion that is spongy and compressible but will slowly refill.

   b. The portions elevated above the skin's surface may be red blue to purple.

C. Disorders with vascular ectasia

1. Port-wine stain

a. Macular, pink to burgundy in color, variable in size, with distinct borders.

b. In older lesions, small, deep blue, nodular, or warty capillary or cavernous angiomas may develop.

2. Venous lake

a. Deep blue in color.

b. Soft and consists of compressible, slightly raised vessels.

3. Telangiectasia and spider ectasia

a. Bright red, discrete, usually with a central, elevated punctum and many radiating branches.

b. A pulsating center, if this is not readily seen, will become apparent on gentle pressure with a glass slide.

c. More intense pressure will obliterate the lesion entirely.

d. Other types of facial telangiectasia are present mostly over the malar regions and consist of single red blue, enlarged vessels accumulated into telangiectatic "mats."

IV. Assessment

A. Capillary vessels

1. Strawberry nevus. Measure and photograph the lesion in order to follow its evolution and subsidence.

2. Cherry angioma. How long have they been there? The most frequent lesions confused with cherry spots, particularly in the hospitalized patient, are petechiae. Small angiomas must at times be biopsied to prove their unimportant nature.

B. Cavernous vessels

1. Cavernous angioma. X-ray studies of underlying tissue may be indicated.

C. Disorders with vascular ectasia

1. Port-wine stain. Neurologic and x-ray examinations may be warranted for all but the eyelid and nuchal lesions.

2. Venous lake. No investigation needed.

3. Telangiectasia. Investigation into the underlying cause of acquired telangiectasia by history, physical examination, and serologic tests may reveal otherwise unsuspected systemic disease.

V. Therapy

A. Capillary vessels

1. Strawberry nevus

a. As almost all lesions will involute spontaneously, they should be allowed to do so. Aggressive forms of therapy most often will leave a significant cosmetic defect.

    b. Small lesions may be treated by cryosurgery with liquid nitrogen or dry ice, if warranted.

    c. Systemic corticosteroid administration may initiate involution in very large or awkward lesions (see Cavernous vessels below).

    d. Argon laser surgery has been helpful in controlling some very large lesions.

    e. X irradiation may hasten shrinking in lesions of large size or in those in awkward areas such as around orifices.

    f. Electrosurgery of small lesions or excision of large ones occasionally may be justified.

  2. Cherry angioma. Light electrodesiccation will easily remove these lesions. Argon laser treatment will destroy lesions easily.

  3. Pyogenic granuloma

    a. Curettage and electrodesiccation is the therapy of choice.

    b. Cryosurgery may work but is less effective than the foregoing.

    c. Chemical cauterants (silver nitrate stick, mono-, di-, or trichloroacetic acids) may also be efficacious.

B. Cavernous vessels

  1. Cavernous angioma

    a. Aggressive treatment of cavernous and capillary angiomas with systemic corticosteroids (prednisone 20 mg daily for several weeks, then tapered off) should be considered in the following situations:

      (1) Involvement of a vital structure

      (2) Rapid growth with cosmetic destruction

      (3) Mechanical orificial obstruction

      (4) Hemorrhage with or without thrombocytopenia

      (5) Threatened cardiovascular decompensation

    b. Excision is occasionally necessary.

C. Disorders with vascular ectasia

  1. Port-wine stain

    a. Argon laser therapy is the treatment of choice. It is most useful in adults whose lesions are a deep red blue color. In most instances the color is greatly diminished or replaced by "normal" skin tones. (Noe et al., 1980).

    b. Tattooing with flesh-colored pigments, and the application of liquid nitrogen have been used on port-wine stains with variable but not outstanding success.

    c. Often the best answer for this problem, as well as for those of other cosmetically disfiguring angiomas or other lesions, is the use of a skin-colored cosmetic that will effectively hide the lesion from public view. Covermark, which is available in a variety of colors (except very deep black) at the cosmetic counters of many stores, does this particularly well. Erace may also be useful.

2. **Venous lake.** Electrosurgery may be useful (see Telangiectasia).

3. **Telangiectasia.** Spider ectasias are simply effaced by electrosurgery. If anesthesia is used, mark the "body" of the spider before injection.

    a. Insert either a No. 30 needle or a fine electrosurgical (epilating) tip into the central punctum and deliver as small a current as possible in one or more short bursts.

    b. Destruction of the punctum will result in blanching of the entire lesion, but at times some of the radiating spokes must also be destroyed.

    c. Other ectasias may be treated in the same way, but the tip should be inserted into several areas along the vessel's course.

    d. Delivery of too much current can leave small, pitted scars.

    e. It is usually unnecessary to anesthetize the lesion; the procedure is relatively painless, and the anesthetic temporarily makes the vessels disappear, complicating the procedure.

    f. Telangiectatic vessels may also be destroyed in the same fashion by electrolysis.

    g. The argon laser is very effective in treatment of these lesions, particularly the significant number that remain after electrosurgery.

References

Arndt, K. A.   Argon laser therapy of small cutaneous vascular lesions. *Arch. Dermatol.* 118:220–224, 1982.

Arndt, K. A., Noe, J. M., and Rosen, S.   *Cutaneous Laser Surgery. Principles and Methods.* London: Wiley, 1983.

Au, Y. F.   Intralesional electrodesiccation with a 30-gauge needle. *J. Dermatol. Surg. Oncol.* 7:190–191, 1981.

Barsky, S. H., Rosen, S., Geer, D. E., and Noe, J. M.   The nature and evolution of port wine stains: A computer-assisted study. *J. Invest. Dermatol.* 74:154–157, 1980.

Bean, W. B.   *Vascular Spiders and Related Lesions of the Skin.* Springfield, Ill.: Thomas, 1968.

Bowers, R. E., Graham, E. A., and Tomlinson, K. A.   The natural history of the strawberry nevus. *Arch. Dermatol.* 82:667–680, 1960.

Braverman, I. M.   Telangiectasia as a sign of systemic disease. *Conn. Med.* 33: 42–46, 1969.

Fost, N. C., and Esterly, N. B.   Successful treatment of juvenile hemangiomas with prednisone. *J. Pediatr.* 72:351–357, 1968.

Lasser, A. E., and Stein, A. F.   Steroid treatment of hemangiomas in children. *Arch. Dermatol.* 108:565–567, 1973.

Margileth, A. M., and Museles, M.   Current concepts in diagnosis and management of congenital cutaneous hemangiomas. *Pediatrics* 36:410–416, 1965.

Noe, J. M., et al. Port wine stains and the response to argon laser therapy: Successful treatment and the predictive role of color, age and biopsy. *Plast. Reconstr. Surg.* 65:130–136, 1980.

Noe, J. M., Finley, J., Rosen, S., and Arndt, K. A. Postrhinoplasty "red nose": Differential diagnosis and treatment by laser. *Plast. Reconstr. Surg.* 67:661–664, 1981.

Rees, T. D., and Conners, D. Complications in the treatment of hemangiomas. *J. Dermatol. Surg.* 1:29–32, 1975.

Ronchese, F. Granuloma pyogenicum. *Am. J. Surg.* 109:430–431, 1965.

Whiting, D. A., Kallmeyer, J. C., and Simson, J. W. Widespread arterial spiders in a case of latent hepatitis, and resolution after therapy. *Br. J. Dermatol.* 82:32–36, 1970.

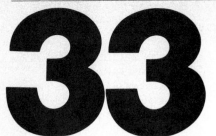

33

Warts

I. Definitions and pathophysiology. Warts are intraepidermal tumors of the skin caused by infection with the human papilloma virus (HPV). This DNA papovavirus cannot be easily cultured in laboratory animals or tissue culture systems, and thus little is known about its growth pattern or metabolism. The virus is never found below the granular level of the epidermis. It is initially within the nucleus of keratinocytes, eventually fills the entire nuclear space, and spills into the cytoplasm; in the stratum corneum, the virus lies free within the keratin mass. Virus concentration is greatest in warts of 6–12 months' duration; after that, virus particles decrease. The number of virus particles varies in warts from different locations; plantar and common warts often contain many viruses whereas condylomata acuminata and juvenile laryngeal papillomatosis contain few.

It is now clear that HPV can no longer be viewed as a single homogeneous virus producing all varieties of clinical warts. The current classification is depicted in Table 3. Infection by a single HPV type does not necessarily result in a unique lesional morphology. As noted in Table 3, common warts may contain types 2, 4, and/or 7 HPV, and types 1 and/or 4 may be isolated from plantar wart tissue. Antibody levels to HPV-1 may be found in 50% of young adults aged 5–15, are maintained until about 30, and then slowly decrease.

Both antibody and cell-mediated responses may be present in patients with active warts, and these benign tumors are more common in patients receiving immunosuppressive drugs, with immune deficiency states, or with lymphoma, chronic lymphocytic leukemia, or Hodgkin's disease. This, plus the increased frequency of cell-mediated responses and antibodies specific for viral antigens in patients with regressing or cured warts, supports a role for immunity in the resolution of warts.

Warts may be found in persons of any age but are most common between ages 12–16; in a school population in Britain the prevalence of common warts was 16.2 percent. They may be spread by contact or autoinoculation. The incubation period after inoculation into human volunteers varies from 1–12 months and averages 2–3 months. About 20–30% of all lesions will spontaneously involute within 6 months, 50% within 1 year, and 66% within 2 years. New lesions may continue to appear during this period of time and are seen 3 times more frequently in children with warts than in those without. The high rate of spontaneous involution makes it difficult to evaluate the effectiveness of suggestion or "charming," as well as the more direct methods of wart therapy.

II. Subjective data. Most warts induce symptoms only when they become awkward because of their size or appearance. Although wart tissue is not inher-

Table 3. Types of HPV and their clinical correlates

HPV Type	Associated clinical lesion(s)
1	Plantar warts
2	Common warts
3	Flat warts (including those in EV)
4	Plantar and common warts
5	Epidermodysplasia verruciformis (EV)
6	Condyloma acuminata
7	Common warts

Source: Fine and Arndt, 1982.

ently painful, condyloma acuminata (see Objective Data, **E**) may be discomforting and friable for mechanical reasons; periungual lesions may develop fissures that hurt; and plantar warts can become very painful during walking or running.

III. **Objective data (See color insert.).** There are several morphologic variants of warts:

A. **Common warts** start as small, pinhead-sized, flesh-colored, translucent papules and grow over several weeks or months to larger, raised, papillary-surfaced, flesh-colored or darker, hyperkeratotic papules. Black specks of hemosiderin pigment may be seen in thrombosed capillary loops. Paring the lesion results in punctate bleeding points. Common warts are found most often on the hands, especially in children, or on other sites often subjected to trauma but may grow anywhere on the epidermis or mucous membranes.

B. **Filiform warts** are slender, soft, thin, fingerlike growths seen primarily on the face and neck.

C. **Flat, plane, or juvenile warts** are flesh-colored or tan, soft, 1–3 mm in diameter, discrete papules appearing primarily on the face, neck, extensor aspect of the forearms, and hands.

D. **Plantar or palmar warts** are hyperkeratotic, firm, elevated or flat lesions that interrupt the natural skin lines (as opposed to calluses). Red or black capillary dots may be seen. A mosaic wart consists of the confluence of multiple lesions into one large, usually flat lesion.

E. Warts that grow in warm, moist, intertriginous areas develop into soft, friable, vegetating clusters. These **condylomata acuminata** are frequently found on the foreskin and penis, particularly in uncircumcised men, on vaginal and labial mucosa, and in the urethral meatus and perianal area. Two-thirds of women and one-third of men with genital warts may have accompanying genital infections that must be identified and treated.

IV. **Therapy**

A. Many therapeutic modalities are available for the treatment of warts. It is important to remember that warts are benign cutaneous growths and that the therapy should also be benign. Therapy should present no hazard to the patient, no scarring should result, and side effects should be minimal. It is not difficult to cause considerable pain, as well as permanent scarring, by an overly enthusiastic approach. This curative zeal must be curbed, for it is neither necessary nor warranted to remove every wart. On the other hand, the therapist should be optimistic, for most lesions can be successfully treated if warranted.

B. Data of Bunney et al. (1976) from comparative treatment trials give some indication of what may be expected from different modes of therapy. They demonstrated that 70–80% of patients with hand warts can be cured with nonblistering liquid nitrogen cryosurgery within 12 weeks, providing the interval between treatments is not more than 3 weeks; most patients require three treatments. Home treatment with salicylic acid–lactic acid paint (SAL, see p. 306) will cure as many patients within the same time period as liquid nitrogen. With simple plantar warts, SAL treatment will cure 84% of patients within 12 weeks as compared to 81% for podophyllin therapy. Mosaic warts are difficult to cure with any therapy; SAL treatment eradicated 47% within 12 weeks and was as efficient as any other method used. Throughout the study 30% of patients with hand warts, 20% of those with simple plantar warts, and 50% of those with mosaic warts were found to be resistant to treatment.

C. **Common warts** are best treated as follows:

1. Destruction by **light electrodesiccation and curettage** (see p. 205), or

2. **Cryosurgery** with liquid nitrogen. This technique, as well as electrodesiccation, carefully executed, will remove the lesion and usually will leave no scar and little or no pigmentary change (see p. 206 for details of therapy). Nonblistering therapy (5- −30-sec application) is effective. In general, cryosurgery is the best therapy.

3. **Keratolytic therapy** with paints such as 5–20% salicylic acid and 5–20% lactic acid in flexible collodion may be self-administered at home and in 60–80% of patients will lead to cures within 12 weeks on all but mosaic plantar warts. Keratolytic agents may act by mechanical removal of infected cells and wart virus and also by providing a mild inflammatory reaction that renders the virus more available to immunologic recognition and attack. Duofilm or TiFlex (17% salicylic acid, 17% lactic acid in flexible collodion) are commercially available SAL preparations; patients should be instructed to use them or other keratolytic paints as follows:

a. Wash area thoroughly with soap and water.

b. Rub surface of wart gently with mild abrasive such as emery board, pumice stone, or callus file.

c. Apply keratolytic paint to the wart with a sharpened matchstick or orange stick.

d. Allow to dry.

e. Keep bottle tightly closed.

f. Repeat each night.

g. If area becomes red or tender, discontinue therapy until this subsides and then start again. Alternatively, a keratolytic paint with a lower concentration of salicylic and lactic acids may be prescribed.

h. Do not apply paint to warts previously treated with liquid nitrogen until the inflammation has subsided.

4. Cantharidin (Cantharone), a mitochondrial poison that leads to changes in cell membranes, epidermal cell dyshesion, acantholysis, and blister formation, is also useful (see also p. 303). Thick hyper- keratotic lesions should be pared down before painting. The lesion should then be painted with cantharidin, allowed to dry, and covered with Blenderm or other nonporous occlusive tape; 40% salicylic acid plaster may be used to achieve greater activity. The tape is left on for 24 hr, or until the area begins to hurt. A blister, often hemorrhagic, will form, break, crust, and fall off in 7–14 days; at this time the lesion is pared down, and any wart remnants retreated. Since the effect of cantharidin is entirely intraepidermal, no scarring ensues. Ringlike recurrences may be seen occasionally after treatment with canthari- din or, at times, following liquid nitrogen therapy. Verrusol,* which contains 30% salicylic acid, 5% podophyllin, and 1% cantharidin, may be used in the same manner.

5. Podophyllum resin (podophyllin), a cytotoxic agent that arrests mitosis in metaphase, is used primarily for treatment of condyloma acuminata but may also be used on all other types of warts (see also p. 304). A 25% preparation in compound tincture of benzoin, or 10% podophyllum, 10% salicylic acid resin (Ver-Var) should be applied overnight when treating common nongenital warts. The effectiveness as well as the irritant potential of this medication may be increased by covering with adhesive tape or plastic tape (Blenderm).

6. Lesions may be painted weekly or more frequently with **acids** such as 50–80% trichloroacetic acid, saturated dichloroacetic acid, or 80% monochloroacetic acid. After a necrotic crust forms, it should be re- moved and the lesion retreated. This method is relatively painless and somewhat slow, but it may be carried out at home. Both the effective- ness and rapidity of therapy may be increased by covering the acid- treated lesion with a small pad of 40% salicylic plaster and adhesive tape for 12–24 hr.

D. Filiform warts are best treated by light electrosurgery or cryosurgery, or with keratolytic paints.

E. Flat warts should be treated with a short (5–15 sec) application of liquid nitrogen; by "flicking" off with a sharp curet or No. 15 blade on edge; with keratolytic paint; or with tretinoin preparations. Electrosurgery may also be used, but it may leave small, hypopigmented scars. Five percent 5- fluorouracil cream applied 1–2 times a day has been reported to clear flat facial warts within 3 weeks (Lockshin, 1979). Lesions on the male face constitute a difficult problem, as autoinoculation takes place each time the patient shaves. To avoid cosmetically damaging results it is espe- cially important to be conservative. Use of an electric shaver or of de- pilatories may decrease autoinoculation. Barely visible lesions will be- come more prominent if lightly rubbed with liquid nitrogen on a cotton tip or sprayed with a refrigerant.

---

* C & M Pharmacol, 1519 East Eight Mile Drive, Hazel Park, Michigan 48030.

F. Plantar warts are sometimes best left untreated. Unless a wart is painful, rapidly growing, or small, it is wise to recommend no therapy or nonaggressive therapy. If treatment is necessary, the following approaches can be used:

1. Enucleation by blunt dissection technique is often the therapy of choice if there is one or only a few lesions (see Heinlein, 1974; Ulbrich et al., 1974). This method of removal is also excellent for removal of verrucae vulgaris in other sites such as palms and periungual areas.

2. Intermittent flattening of the lesion with a pumice stone, callus file, or scalpel is usually enough to keep plantar lesions entirely asymptomatic.

3. Keratolytic therapy with salicylic and lactic acid paint is the most convenient and effective nontraumatic method. The patient should apply medication nightly as follows:

   a. Remove the adhesive tape from previous night's treatment.

   b. Rub the surface of the wart with an emery board, pumice stone, or callus file.

   c. Soak the foot in hot water or a bath for at least 5 min.

   d. Apply a drop of keratolytic paint to the wart. Allow to dry. If the wart is large, apply another drop.

   e. When dry, cover with a piece of adhesive tape. If the lesion is very thick or more aggressive treatment is desired, apply a piece of 40% salicylic acid plaster to the wart and then cover with adhesive tape.

   f. If soreness occurs, stop treatment and restart after it subsides. Use of "micropore" tape rather than adhesive tape may lead to less inflammation.

4. Weekly chemocautery with salicylic acid. Debride the wart to a point short of bleeding and apply a piece of adhesive tape with an orifice cut out in the shape of the wart. A duplicate-shaped felted pad is then overlaid. Pack 60% salicylic acid in petrolatum (or 40% salicylic acid plaster or 35–50% trichloroacetic acid) onto the wart and cover caustic and surrounding tapes with more waterproof tape. Remove in 1 week, cut or curet away necrotic material, and repeat.

5. Bimonthly debridement and treatment with cantharidin (see p. 303) is also effective but may be painful.

6. Liquid nitrogen freezing may produce good results, but it does cause discomfort during application; in addition, the resultant blister makes walking uncomfortable for the next several days.

7. Application of 25% podophyllin in compound tincture of benzoin under tape occlusion overnight, or nightly 15-min soaks in 3% formalin may also be of some benefit. Alternatively, the warts may be painted with 10% formalin and covered with 40% salicylic acid plaster for 3–4 days. The lesions are then debrided by patient or physician, and the formalin and dressing reapplied. This painless therapy may be continued for weeks until the lesion is gone.

8. Destructive electrosurgery, sharp scalpel excision, and radiotherapy should be avoided, because although they may remove the lesion, the resulting scar often becomes a more difficult and less easily treated problem than the wart itself.

9. It is important to correct orthopedic defects and prescribe correct footwear. Plantar warts most often occur in areas of pressure and callus, and unless the incorrect weight-bearing condition can be alleviated, it is frequently difficult either to cure the wart or to make the patient comfortable.

G. Condylomata acuminata

1. Weekly painting of the lesion with 25% podophyllum resin (see p. 304) in compound tincture of benzoin is the most effective therapy. Medication should be kept off uninvolved surrounding skin; this may be accomplished by applying a thin covering of petrolatum around the lesion before therapy. After the benzoin dries, the area should be liberally powdered to prevent undue maceration and inadvertent transfer of podophyllin from the lesions to apposing normal skin. At the start of therapy, the medication should be left on for only 1 hr and then washed off, particularly in the vulvar area and the area under the foreskin. As therapy progresses, podophyllin should be left in place 4–6 hr before it is removed. Treated lesions may become inflamed and painful during the following 2–3 days. It is wise to treat only parts of a large condyloma to prevent disabling pain, but it is important to repeat treatment every 7–10 days until all lesions are gone. If the lesions are very verrucous or bulky, remove the mass of the wart first by curettage and after healing, start podophyllum therapy. A topical anesthetic preparation is often useful during the period of pain (see p. 243).

   A standardized method based on the repeated application of 0.5% podophyllotoxin in ethanol 2id for 3 days has been described. This has the advantage of using known amounts of active ingredients and thereby limiting potential toxicity. Podophyllin can cause severe irritation and if absorbed may produce systemic toxic effects. It is inadvisable to apply it in large amounts to mucous membranes, and it is unwise to use it in pregnant women because of its possible cytotoxic action on the fetus.

2. Liquid nitrogen cryosurgery is also excellent for condylomata acuminata. The amount and intensity of therapy and the delineation of treatment margins can be better controlled than with podophyllin. Liquid nitrogen plus podophyllin (and anesthetic) may be better than either alone.

3. Occasionally it is necessary and useful to approach such lesions with electrosurgery and curettage. This is particularly true when there are large masses of warty tissue, which may then be removed in one procedure, or when painting of the lesions with podophyllin appears to lose its effectiveness. This is sometimes best carried out as an in-hospital operating room procedure.

4. Proctoscopy and treatment of rectal lesions with podophyllin or liquid nitrogen is necessary in all patients with perianal condylomata.

5. Intraurethral and meatal condylomata may be treated conservatively with podophyllin or liquid nitrogen. Alternatively, 1–5% 5-fluorouracil solution or suppositories may also be effective. Therapy must not be overaggressive if urethral stricture is to be avoided.

H. Special comments

1. If warts are recalcitrant to treatment, immunotherapy may be effective. Dinitrochlorobenzene has been most commonly employed but is difficult to use and a potential mutagenic agent. It has not been approved by the FDA for this indication. Other contact allergens such as poison oak, ivy, etc. can also be applied. Cure rates of 70–80% have been reported.

2. Intralesional bleomycin cured 99.23% of 1052 warts in a recent study (Shumack and Haddock, 1979). All varieties of skin warts were treated. Bleomycin is a cytotoxic drug used in various malignancies that acts by inhibiting DNA synthesis. The only side effect noted was moderate pain on injection of the usual dose, 0.1 ml of a 0.1% solution. Careful track of total dose over time must be kept and should probably not exceed 5 ml because of potential toxicity.

3. Therapy for children should be gentle and nonaggressive. Keratolytic solutions and applications of acids are useful and nonpainful. Cantharidin is effective and does not cause pain during application. Electrosurgery and cryosurgical procedures are often traumatic to all involved. In this age group, hypnosis appears to work well at times.

4. Treatment with keratolytic paints, liquid nitrogen, or cantharidin generally produces the best cosmetic results. Acids and electrosurgery have a greater potential for scarring.

5. Periungual lesions are best treated with either liquid nitrogen, cantharidin, or blunt dissection.

6. OTC wart remedies such as Compound W and WartAway are liquids that contain 13–14% salicylic acid (a keratolytic) and acetic acid (a caustic). The OTC corn and callus remedies are usually salicylic acid compounds.

References

Adler, A., and Safai, B.   Immunity in wart resolution. *J. Am. Acad. Dermatol.* 1:305–309, 1979.

Briggaman, R. A., and Wheeler, C. E., Jr.   Immunology of human warts. *J. Am. Acad. Dermatol.* 1:297–303, 1979.

Buckner, D., and Price, N. M.   Immunotherapy of verrucae vulgaris with dinitrochlorobenzene. *Br. J. Dermatol.* 98:451–455, 1978.

Bunney, M. H.   Viral warts: Their biology and treatment. New York: Oxford University Press, 1982.

Bunney, M. H., Nolan, M. W., and Williams, D. A.   An assessment of methods of treating viral warts by comparative treatment trials based on a standard design. *Br. J. Dermatol.* 94:667–679, 1976.

Clark, G. H. V.   The charming of warts. *J. Invest. Dermatol.* 45:15–21, 1965.

Cordero, A. A., Guglielmi, H. A., and Woscoff, A.   The common wart: Intralesional treatment with bleomycin sulfate. *Cutis* 26:319–323, 1980.

DeVillez, R. L., and Lewis, C. W. (eds.).   Verruca vulgaris seminar. *J. Assoc. Mil. Dermatol.* 1:47–54, 1975.

Epstein, W. L., and Kligman, A. M.   Treatment of warts with cantharidin. *Arch. Dermatol.* 77:508–511, 1958.

Erikson, K.   Treatment of the common wart by induced allergic inflammation. *Dermatologica* 160:161–166, 1980.

Fine, J. D., and Arndt, K. A.   Pathophysiology of Certain Viral Infections of the Skin. In H. Baden and N. Soter (eds.), *Pathophysiology of the Skin.* New York: McGraw-Hill, 1983.

Ghosh, A. K.   Cryosurgery of genital warts in cases in which podophyllin treatment failed or was contraindicated. *Br. J. Venerol. Dis.* 53:49–53, 1977.

Gibbs, R. D.   Conservative management of plantar warts by gentle chemocautery. *J. Dermatol. Surg. Oncol.* 4:915, 1978.

Habif, T. P., and Graf, F. A.   Extirpation of subungual and periungual warts by blunt dissection. *J. Dermatol. Surg. Oncol.* 7:553–555, 1981.

Kinghorn, G. R.   Genital warts: Incidence of associated genital infections. *Br. J. Dermatol.* 99:405–409, 1978.

Lockshin, N. A.   Flat facial warts treated with fluorouracil. *Arch. Dermatol.* 15:929–930, 1979.

Massing, A. M., and Epstein, W. L.   Natural history of warts: A two-year study. *Arch. Dermatol.* 87:306–310, 1963.

Oriel, J. D.   Natural history of genital warts. *Br. J. Venerol. Dis.* 47:1–13, 1971.

Pass, F.   Warts: Virology, Immunology and Therapy. In S. L. Moschella (ed.), *Dermatology Update: Reviews of Physicians.* New York: Eisener, 1982. P. 1.

Pringle, W. M., and Helms, D. C.   Treatment of plantar warts by blunt dissection. *Arch. Dermatol.* 108:79–82, 1973.

Rees, R. B.   Warts: A clinician's view. *Cutis* 28:175–180, 1981.

Rosenberg, E. W., Amonette, R. A., and Gardner, J. H.   Cantharidin in treatment of warts at home. *Arch. Dermatol.* 113:1134, 1977.

Sanders, B. B., and Smith, K. W.   Dinitrochlorobenzene immunotherapy of human warts. *Cutis* 27:389–392, 1981.

Shumack, P. H., and Haddock, M. J.   Bleomycin: An effective treatment of warts. *Australas. J. Dermatol.* 20:41–42, 1979.

Ulbrich, A. P., Koprince, D., and Arends, N. W.   Warts: Treatment by total enucleation. *Cutis* 14:582–586, 1974.

von Krough, G.   Topical treatment of penile condyloma acuminata with podophyllin, podophyllotoxin and colchicine: A comparative study. *Acta Dermatol. Venerol.* 58:163–168, 1978.

von Krough, G.   The beneficial effect of 1% 5-fluorouracil in 70% ethanol on therapeutically refractory condyloma in the preputial cavity. *Sex. Trans. Dis.* 5:137–140, 1978.

Weimar, G. W., Milleman, L. A., Reiland, T. L., and Culp, D. A.   5-fluorouracil urethral suppositories for the eradication of condyloma acuminata. *J. Urol.* 120:174–175, 1978.

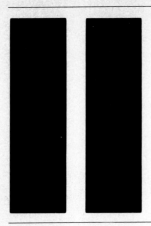

Procedures and techniques

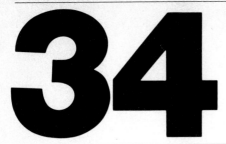

Operative procedures

Skin is uniquely available for diagnostic procedures as well as for the direct application of therapeutic agents. Single or multiple procedures can be performed within short periods of time with little discomfort to the patient. Most techniques are easily learned, easy to perform, and require only simple equipment.

Biopsy

I. Procedure

A. The punch biopsy is an extremely simple procedure that, in all but a very few cases, removes sufficient tissue for histopathologic study.

1. It is generally best to select a mature and well-developed lesion for biopsy. However, if blisters are present, choose the earliest lesion available and take care to keep the roof intact; include adjacent normal skin. Several biopsies should be obtained from evolving eruptions or those with various types of lesions (in this instance, too, biopsy of early lesions may be especially rewarding). Lesions altered by trauma or treatment or old "burned-out" areas will not yield useful information. Biopsies on the legs and feet heal more slowly, especially if the circulation is poor; if possible, choose a lesion above the knees. Choose a site entirely within the lesion; avoid including normal skin in the biopsy unless specifically desired, in which case the pathologist should be informed of its inclusion and how the specimen is to be oriented.

2. Clean the area gently with alcohol, taking care to leave scales, crusts, and vesicles intact. It is often useful to outline the small lesions before the swelling caused by injection of local anesthesia or the effect of epinephrine distorts and blanches the site.

3. Anesthetize the area by injecting into the deep dermis 0.2–0.5 ml of 0.5–2.0% lidocaine or 1–2% lidocaine with 1:100,000 epinephrine. Patients allergic to local anesthetic ether compounds (procaine, tetracaine) will tolerate use of amide compounds (lidocaine, bupivacaine) without difficulty (i.e., procaine [Novocaine] and lidocaine [Xylocaine] do not cross react; see also p. 243). The epinephrine will inhibit bleeding, increase the duration of anesthesia, and make the procedure much easier to perform. Local vasoconstriction will not become maximal before 15–20 min. Epinephrine-containing solutions should not be used when anesthetizing the distal fingers or toes, or when vasoconstriction will interfere with the histopathologic findings such as with primarily vascular (angiomatous) lesions. It is probably preferable to ring an area with anesthesia, but intradermal injection di-

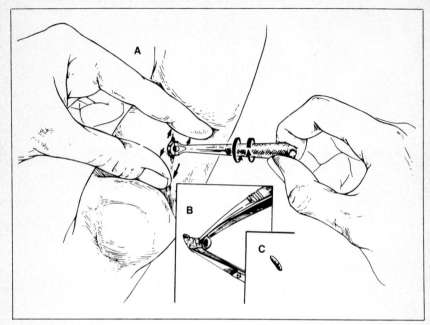

Figure 1. Punch biopsy technique. Note the oval (not round) defect left.

rectly into or below a lesion appears to cause little or no perceptible microscopic alteration.

   a. To inject with the least trauma for both the physician and the patient, a 1-ml syringe with a No. 27 or No. 30 needle should be used. The first item is available as a prepackaged, sterile, disposable syringe. No. 30 needles must be purchased separately.

   b. Ethyl chloride or other refrigerant spray is sometimes useful for dulling the pain of injection or the discomfort associated with curettage, or incision and drainage of cysts or abscesses. **Ethyl chloride spray is flammable and must not be used during electrosurgical procedures.**

  4. Biopsy punches, circular instruments with a sharp cutting edge and a handle, are available in sizes ranging from 2–8 mm in diameter; the 4-mm punch is generally the most useful. Removal of a specimen less than 4 mm in diameter may allow the histologic confirmation of a tumor, but it is inadequate for diagnosis of inflammatory processes. Sterile disposable 2-, 3-, 4-, and 6-mm punch biopsies are available.*

The skin surrounding the lesion should be stretched taut **perpendicular** to the wrinkle (relaxed skin tension) lines before the circular punch is inserted as demonstrated in Fig. 1. See endpaper figures for a

---

* Chester A. Baker Laboratories, Inc. (Division of Key Pharmaceuticals, Inc.), 50 N.W. 176th Street, Miami, Florida 33169.

guide to the most common configuration of the relaxed skin tension lines. When the punch is removed, an ellipsoidal defect will be left (Fig. 1, insets). The biopsy punch is firmly pressed downward into the lesion with a rotary back-and-forth cutting motion until it is well into the subcutaneous tissue (Fig. 1).

5. The biopsied skin plug will either pop out or lie free within its circular margin. The specimen must be gently grasped and lifted out with either forceps or a needle without applying undue pressure, the base severed with scissors or scalpel blade as deep into the fat as possible, and the tissue placed in 10% neutral buffered formalin. The amount of formalin should be at least 20 times that of the specimen by volume. If the incision is made only to the middermis, tissue will be more difficult to remove, and the wound will heal less readily and with a poor cosmetic result.

6. Simple pressure is adequate for hemostasis, and use of caustics or Gelfoam is rarely needed or warranted. Lesions will heal more rapidly and with a linear scar rather than a round defect if either a 4-0 or 5-0 nylon or silk suture is put in place (left for 3–5 days on the face, 7–14 days on the trunk) or adhesive strips are applied across the defect (left for 14–21 days).

7. The histologic interpretation of cutaneous reaction patterns requires a great deal of judgment and experience. It is wise to seek the help of a pathologist with a special interest in skin disorders.

B. A **shave biopsy** removes that portion of skin elevated above the plane of surrounding tissue and is useful for biopsying or removing many exophytic benign epidermal growths, including keratoses and viral tumors. It is also a convenient procedure for obtaining tissue diagnoses of malignant lesions such as basal cell carcinomas prior to initiating therapy. This procedure is quickly and easily performed, heals rapidly, yields a good cosmetic result, and leaves the lower levels of the dermis intact if further procedures such as curettage, electrosurgery, or cryosurgery are necessary. The decision to perform a shave biopsy requires judgment and a reasonably good impression of the preoperative diagnosis. A shave biopsy may fail to distinguish, for example, between an actinic keratosis and a squamous cell carcinoma with invasion.

1. Clean and anesthetize the area.

2. If a substantial margin of tissue surrounding and below the lesion is needed, the shave should take place immediately after injection of anesthesia, when the tissue is still elevated from the injection fluid (Fig. 2, inset, right). Tissue is removed with a lateral (horizontal) "sawing" motion of a No. 15 scalpel blade or halved Gillette Super Blue Blade on the level of the surrounding skin (Fig. 2). The latter has the potential advantages of being thinner (cutting edge a millionth-inch thick), sharper, and more flexible. When hand-held, it can be used flat or bent to the precise arc desired to conform to the shape of the lesion and the depth of biopsy. Presuming the elevated lesion alone is being removed, it is necessary before proceeding to wait a few minutes until any sublesional swelling subsides (Fig. 2, inset, left). Tissue may then be put into formalin and submitted for pathologic examination.

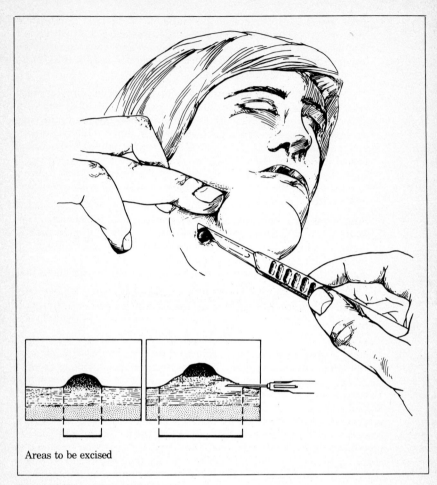

Areas to be excised

Figure 2. Shave biopsy technique.

  a. Biopsy of a flat or depressed lesion may be carried out by a saucerization technique.

  b. Pedunculated lesions may be removed by use of scissors alone.

 3. Pressure, ferric subsulfate (Monsel's solution), or electrodesiccation may be used for hemostasis.

C. Surgical excision biopsy should be considered when: (1) there are lesions with active expanding borders; (2) the junction of lesion and normal skin is important to survey; (3) the lesions are atrophic, sclerotic, or bullous; (4) it is important to acquire adequate full-thickness skin, e.g., in panniculitis and erythema nodosum; and (5) the lesion may be a melanoma.

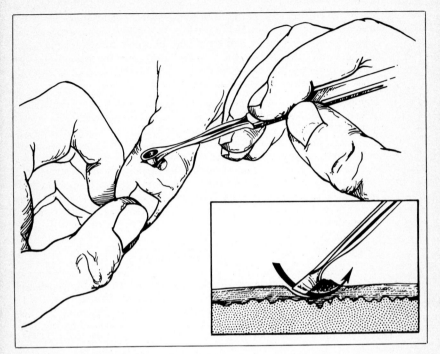

Figure 3. Curettage technique.

Curettage

I. **Discussion.** Curettage is a simple and useful technique for removing benign cutaneous lesions such as warts, molluscum, milia, and keratoses; it is also effective for treating basal and squamous cell carcinomas. The curet, a cutting instrument with a circular, loop-shaped cutting edge and a handle, is available in varying sizes. Large curets will remove masses of tissue more quickly, while smaller ones are needed to probe for small extensions of lesions into subjacent dermis; the curet 4 mm in diameter appears to be the most generally useful. A No. 15 scalpel blade used on edge with a scraping and not cutting motion can sometimes be used in place of a curet. The more friable the tissue, the easier it is to curet. Curettage is difficult to perform on normal skin or on lesions covered with a full thickness of intact skin. The curet is neither sharp enough nor does it have sufficient strength for this purpose, and the resulting tissue available for pathologic examination is usually fragmented and distorted.

II. **Procedure**

  A. Clean the area with alcohol.

  B. Anesthesia is not always necessary. The process of anesthetizing can be more painful than the surgical procedure in removal of lesions such as seborrheic keratoses, molluscum, and milia. If anesthesia is used, wait until any swelling has diminished or subsided, as it is difficult to scrape spongy tissue.

C. Apply the cutting edge of the curet to the lesions, and remove the tissue with a firm, quick, downward scoop (Fig. 3). The first tissue removed will come off relatively intact and should be submitted for pathologic examination if indicated. Scrape the base and margins of the lesion well. Normal dermis is resilient and feels rough and scratchy when scraped, while most lesions are of softer composition.

D. Hemostasis is secured by pressure, hemostatic agents (ferric subsulfate [Monsel's solution, 3.8 M ferric chloride, 35% aluminum chloride in 50% isopropyl alcohol]), caustics (trichloroacetic acid), or electrodesiccation. Use of pressure alone or with oxidized cellulose (Oxycel Cotton) yields the best cosmetic result (as with seborrheic keratoses). If electrodesiccation is used, a small spark is all that is needed for hemostasis and destruction of any remaining lesion; if there is a question of tumor, a more intense spark is used, scraping of a 3- –5-mm margin around the lesion is necessary, and curettage should be repeated at least twice to ensure complete removal of all tissue.

Electrosurgery

I. Discussion. The small electrosurgical units most often found in physicians' offices and in hospital clinics are versatile and useful tools. They deliver a high-frequency alternating current to tissue, producing an electrical field about the tip of the treatment electrode. The high resistance of tissue to this electric current causes both mechanical disruption of cells and heat. The electrode tip delivers the current but does not itself become hot.

The principal uses of electrosurgery are for: (1) the destruction of benign superficial lesions such as warts, keratoses, molluscum, and skin tags; (2) hemostasis and the ablation of vascular growths; and (3) the destruction of some malignant tumors of the skin. Patients with indwelling cardiac pacemakers (especially the demand type) should not be treated with these instruments, **because high-frequency current can deactivate a pacemaker.**

Electrodesiccation produces superficial destruction by dehydrating cells. This is a monoterminal high-voltage (2000 or more volts), low-amperage (100–1000 ma) operation in which the patient is not incorporated into the circuit. The needle is either held in contact with the tissue or kept a short distance away, and the current is transmitted through a spark. The lesion is destroyed by bursts of electric current.

Electrocoagulation produces more severe destruction, primarily by heat and secondarily by disruptive mechanical forces. This is a biterminal, relatively low-voltage (under 200 v), low-frequency, high-amperage (2500–4000 ma) operation in which the patient is grounded by being placed on a large "indifferent" electrode. The treatment needle, placed in or on the tissue, delivers an intensely hot current and literally "boils" and coagulates the lesion. Electrocoagulation produces wider and deeper damage, better hemostasis, and more scarring; it is used primarily for large lesions that require extensive destruction, some neoplasms such as basal cell carcinomas, or very vascular tumors such as pyogenic granulomas.

Electrocautery uses a red-hot wire heated by a low-voltage (5 v), high amperage (15 amp) current produced by a step-down transformer with a vari-

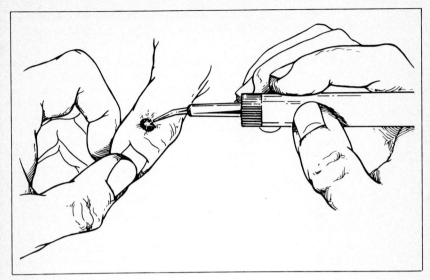

Figure 4. Electrosurgical technique.

able reactor. In this instance, the wire **is** hot, is **not** an electrode, and no current flows into the patient. Electrocautery produces excellent hemostasis in a bloody field and the extent of tissue destruction of lesions is readily apparent and sharply localized about the cautery tip.

II. Procedure

A. Clean the skin with alcohol and let dry. Alcohol, as well as ethyl chloride sprays, and some anesthetic gases are flammable. Strict asepsis is unnecessary as the procedure is itself antiseptic.

B. Infiltrate with lidocaine with epinephrine. Treatment of some lesions, such as skin tags, is so rapid that anesthesia may not be required.

C. When tissue is needed for histologic examination, first curet the lesion, removing all the accessible pathologic tissue. The difference in texture between abnormal and normal tissue becomes difficult to "feel" after a lesion has been altered by electrosurgery. Continue the curettage until the base and borders of the lesion are firm and clean and all pockets of abnormal material have been scraped away. If there is a diagnostic question, shave excision is a better method for obtaining intact tissue specimens for histologic study. It may be followed by curettage and electrosurgery, or by electrosurgery alone.

D. Apply the electrodesiccating current onto or into the tissue and deliver recurrent bursts of electricity (Fig. 4). It is never necessary to deliver a large spark, since this chars tissue, leads to greater tissue destruction, and offers no added therapeutic advantage. The area being treated should be as dry as possible.

1. Use as little current as will do the job when treating spider and other angiomas and seborrheic keratoses or when ensuring hemostasis of the base of a lesion.

2. Warts, actinic keratoses, molluscum contagiosum, and skin tags should be treated with slightly more current. The best technique for treating warts is to insert the needle electrode into the lesion and deliver current until the lesion "bubbles." The gelatinous charred tissue is removed with a curet, and a spark of less intensity is used to desiccate the base lightly. Deeper destruction will not increase the cure rate and will result in a more prolonged healing time and excessive scarring. More precise localization of destruction may be accomplished by inserting a 30-gauge needle (attached to a plastic syringe) into the lesion and then touching the active electrode to the needle shaft.

3. More intense current, repeated curettage, and a wider margin are needed when removing cutaneous neoplasms.

E. The wound produced by electrosurgery is best left open. Neither antibiotics nor dressings need to be applied. Reepithelialization takes place from the base and sides of the lesion and is complete in 1–6 weeks, depending on the size of the lesion and the amount and depth of tissue destruction.

Cryosurgery

I. **Discussion.** The application of graded degrees of cold to the skin may be used to treat many benign and neoplastic conditions. Cryogenic agents are easy to apply, usually require no anesthesia, and cause epidermal-dermal separation above the basement membrane, thus leaving no scarring after reepithelialization. The lower the boiling point of the agent, the more efficient are its freezing capabilities. The boiling point of ethyl chloride is $+13.1°C$; of Freon 114, $+3.6°C$; of Frigiderm (dichlorotetrafluoroethane), $+3.6°C$; of solid CO_2, $-78.5°C$; of liquid nitrous oxide, $-89.5°C$; and of liquid nitrogen, $-195.6°C$. Liquid nitrogen, which is readily available from medical or industrial sources, is inexpensive and noncombustible and has become a standard therapeutic agent.

Skin is relatively resistant to freezing due to its rich vascular supply and because frozen tissue itself acts as a good insulator. Although skin freezes at 0 to $-2°C$, it is necessary to cool tissue to -18 to $-30°C$ for destruction to occur. Application of liquid nitrogen to the skin with a cotton-tipped applicator stick 4 times within 60 sec will lower the temperature 2 mm below the cutaneous surface to $-18°C$. Direct spray of liquid nitrogen for an equal time period will cool the tissue to $-90°C$ and, after 120 sec, to $-125°C$ at 2 mm and $-70°C$ at 5 mm below the skin's surface. Such temperatures are needed only for cryosurgery of skin cancer. The degree of injury is roughly proportional to the intensity of freezing. Repeated freeze-thaw is more damaging than a single freeze. Rapid cooling and slow thawing produce the most damage.

The exact mechanism of injury is unclear, but the following changes, all of which take place in frozen tissue, may be operative at any time: (1) mechanical damage to cells by intracellular and extracellular ice formation; (2) osmotic changes related to dehydration of cells and increased concentration of electrolytes as a result of water withdrawal during ice crystal formation; (3) thermal shock, a term used to denote a precipitous fall in the temperature of living cells to subnormal temperatures above 0°C; (4) denaturation of lipid-protein complexes within the cell membrane; and (5) vascular stasis with resulting necrosis of tissue.

Freezing with liquid nitrogen is accompanied by a stinging, burning pain, which peaks during thawing about 2 min after treatment is over. It is usually unnecessary to use local anesthesia. Pressure, which increases both the rate and depth of freezing, should be applied only to lesions over thick, hyperkeratotic sites such as the feet. Freezing of lesions on the hands, feet, lips, ears, and eyelids is more painful than elsewhere. Within minutes of thawing, a triple response with redness, wheals, and surrounding flare will develop. A blister at the dermoepidermal junction forms 3–6 hr later, flattens in 2–3 days, and sloughs off in 2–4 weeks. Reepithelialization is under way within 72 hr of superficial freezing, and superinfection is rare. Melanocytes are more susceptible to cold injury than keratinocytes; mild hypopigmentation is sometimes seen in areas previously frozen with liquid nitrogen.

II. Procedure

A. Nitrogen is best kept in specially made vacuum flasks and may be poured into a plastic insulated cup for immediate use. Liquid nitrogen will rarely cause normal Thermos bottles to explode. An air vent must always be present in all storage apparatus.

B. Dip a loosely wrapped cotton-tipped applicator into the nitrogen and promptly place it onto the cutaneous lesion (Fig. 5). Larger fluffy swabs such as those used for sigmoidoscopy or gynecologic examination will hold greater amounts of nitrogen. When these are used, the cotton tip should be shaped into a point slightly smaller than the lesion under treatment.

Do not routinely apply pressure. Thick lesions should first be surgically pared and may be treated with moderate pressure. Small lesions are most successfully treated by interrupting contact between the applicator and skin frequently, preventing the zone of freezing from extending to a greater depth and width than necessary. Large lesions can be treated by rolling the applicator over the surface.

C. A 5-–15-sec application is adequate for small, superficial lesions, such as lentigines, especially when located on thin skin. Most other benign growths, such as warts, keratoses, and molluscum contagiosum, require a 10–20-sec application. Within seconds, the lesion begins to turn white. Nitrogen is repeatedly applied until the white freezing front extends 1–3 mm onto the margins of normal skin (see Fig. 5). The zone of frozen tissue reaches a depth of 1.5–2.0 mm within 1 min of the initiation of nitrogen application and does not advance significantly farther.

D. The posttreatment lesion requires no dressings. Avoid occlusive ointments or bandages. The blister that forms may be hemorrhagic or large. If it is uncomfortable or awkward, it may be decompressed with a sterile

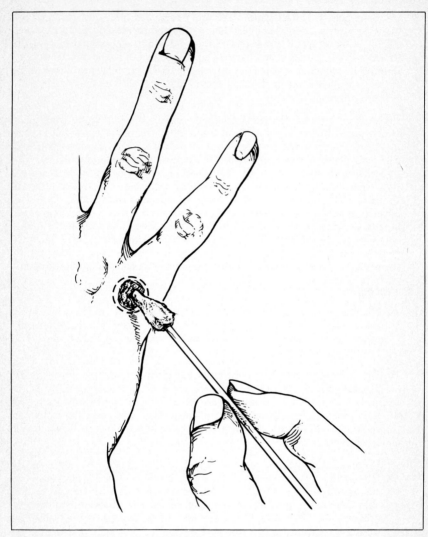

Figure 5. Cryosurgical technique. Liquid nitrogen is delivered to the lesion on a loosely wrapped cotton-tipped applicator stick (or larger cotton swab). The nitrogen should be repeatedly applied until the freezing front extends 1–3 mm around the lesion (*dotted line*).

blade or pin, leaving the roof intact. Patients with warts should be seen in 2 weeks, at which time the lesions are debrided and any remaining wart tissue is either refrozen or treated with caustics or electrodesiccation.

References

BIOPSY AND CURETTAGE

Abadir, A.   Use of local anesthetics in dermatology. *J. Dermatol. Surg.* 1:65–70, 1:68–72, 1975; 2:63–68, 1976.

Ackerman, A. B.   Biopsy: Why, where, when, how. *J. Dermatol. Surg.* 1:21–23, 1975.

Arndt, K. A., Burton, C., and Noe, J. M.   Minimizing the pain of local anesthesia. In press.

Baer, R. L., and Kopf, A. W.   Dermatologic Office Surgery. In *Year Book of Dermatology, 1963–1964*. Chicago: Year Book, 1964. Pp. 7–47.

Bart, R. S., and Kopf, A. W.   Techniques of biopsy of cutaneous neoplasms. *J. Dermatol. Surg. Oncol.* 5:979–987, 1979.

Caro, M. R.   Skin biopsy technic. *Arch. Dermatol.* 76:9–12, 1957.

Editorial.   Biopsy of skin: An underutilized laboratory "test." *N. Engl. J. Med.* 277:49–50, 1967.

Kopf, A. W., and Popkin, A. W.   Shave biopsy for cutaneous lesions. *Arch. Dermatol.* 110:637, 1974.

Mohs, F. E.   The versatile curet. *J. Dermatol. Surg. Oncol.* 4:406, 1978.

Pinkus, H.   Skin biopsy: A field of interaction between clinician and pathologist. *Cutis* 20:609–614, 1977.

Shapiro, L.   Perspectives in dermatology. *Med. Clin. North. Am.* 49:531–547, 1965.

Shelley, W. B.   The razor blade in dermatologic practice. *Cutis* 16:843–845, 1975.

Shelley, W. B.   Epidermal surgery. *J. Dermatol. Surg.* 2:125–128, 1976.

Whyte, H. J., and Perry, H. D.   A simple method to minimize scarring following large punch biopsies. *Arch. Dermatol.* 81:520–522, 1960.

ELECTROSURGERY

Au, Y. F.   Intralesional electrodesiccation with a 30-gauge needle. *J. Dermatol. Surg. Oncol.* 7:190–191, 1981.

Bodian, E. L.   Electrosurgery by bipolar modalities. *J. Dermatol. Surg. Oncol.* 4:235–241, 1978.

Burdick, K. I.   *Electrosurgical Apparatus and Their Application in Dermatology.* Springfield, Ill.: Thomas, 1966.

Jackson, R.   Basic principles of electrosurgery: A review. *Can. J. Surg.* 13:354–361, 1970.

Krull, E. A., Pickard, S. D., and Hall, J. C.   Effects of electrosurgery on cardiac pacemakers. *J. Dermatol. Surg.* 1:43–45, 1975.

CRYOSURGERY

Duperrat, B., and Bouquet, J. F.   The use of liquid nitrogen in dermatological cryotherapy. *J. Dermatol.* 12:5–9, 1971.

Finelli, P. F.   Ulnar neuropathy after liquid nitrogen cryotherapy. *Arch. Dermatol.* 111:1340–1342, 1975.

Gage, A. A.   What temperature is lethal for cells? *J. Dermatol. Surg. Oncol.* 5:459–460, 1979.

Pearson, R. W.   Response of human epidermis to graded thermal stress: A morphologic comparison of burns, cold-induced blisters and pemphigus vulgaris. *Arch. Environ. Health* 11:498–507, 1965.

Robertson, W. D.   Cryotherapy in dermatology. *Ohio State Med. J.* 64:1260–1263, 1968.

Torre, D. (ed.).   Cryosurgery (special issue). *Cutis* 16:421–518, 1975.

Zakarian, S. A. *Cryosurgery of Skin Tumors of the Skin and Oral Cavity.* Springfield, Ill.: Thomas, 1973.

Zakarian, S. A. *Cryosurgical Advances in Dermatology and Tumors of the Head and Neck.* Springfield, Ill.: Thomas, 1979.

35

Cytologic smears

I. Discussion. Cytologic techniques in dermatology are useful in the diagnosis of bullous diseases, vesicular viral eruptions, and molluscum contagiosum. Examination of the smear is not a substitute for a biopsy, but it does enable multiple lesions to be tested on repeated occasions and allows immediate confirmation of some disease processes.

II. Technique

A. Select an early lesion that shows no signs of trauma or infection.

B. Separate or remove the blister top with a scalpel or sharp scissors. Absorb excess fluid with a gauze pad.

C. Gently remove blister contents and scrape the floor of the vesicle with a No. 10 or No. 15 scalpel blade or curet. Do not provoke bleeding.

D. Make a thin smear on a clean glass slide. (With solid lesions such as molluscum, squeeze the material between 2 slides.)

E. Air dry. If the following are available, fix tissue by dipping 4–5 times in 95% ethanol or methanol or immerse the slide in these solutions for 1–2 min.

F. Stain with Wright's, Giemsa's (1 drop/1 ml water for 30 min, or undiluted Giemsa's stock for 5 min), or hematoxylin and eosin.

G. Microscopic appearance. Examine first with a low-power objective to gain an impression of cell size and depth of stain relationships; then examine with $45\times$ or oil for the morphologic details.

1. Herpes simplex, zoster, and varicella lesions contain large, bizarre, viral mononucleate and multinucleate giant cells and the degenerative nuclear changes of "ballooning degeneration." The giant cells contain 8–10 nuclei, varying in size and shape. Occasionally an intranuclear inclusion body may be identified.

2. Molluscum contagiosum bodies appear as multiple, large, oval to round, smooth-bordered masses up to 25 μ in diameter.

3. In most bullous eruptions the smear will show only inflammatory cells. In pemphigus and benign familial pemphigus, numerous rounded acantholytic epidermal cells with large nuclei and condensed cytoplasm are found.

Fungal scraping and culture

I. Discussion. Immediate confirmation of the presence of a fungal infection may be easily accomplished by microscopic identification of organisms and is more reliable than culture. All scaling lesions from the scalp, angles of the mouth, axillae, groin, inframammary area, and feet, as well as blisters on the hands and feet, should be considered for such studies.

II. Technique

A. Scraping examination

1. Skin

a. If lesions are soiled or macerated clean the skin well with alcohol or acetone and let dry.

b. Scrape with a scalpel or edge of a microscope slide at the active edge of a lesion and collect scales on a glass slide. With blistering eruptions the fungus is in the roof of the vesicle, which can be (1) gently dissected off with sharp scissors or scalpel, or (2) reflected back and the underside scraped with a No. 15 scalpel blade.

c. Small, thin fragments of tissue may be examined directly. Large pieces should be minced with a scalpel blade. Thick pieces should be discarded.

d. Gather scrapings together in the center of the slide.

e. Cover with Swartz-Medrik stain (SMS) or 10–20% potassium hydroxide (KOH) and a coverslip and heat gently, but not to boiling, for 15–30 sec.

f. SMS preparations can be examined immediately. Let KOH slides cool for 10 min (during which time the tissue is hydrolyzed and rendered clear), then press the coverslip gently to flatten the tissue and push out air bubbles.

g. Examine under a scanning lens or high-dry magnification. (It is very important to avoid getting KOH on the microscope objective, as it will etch the lens.) The diaphragm should be closed down and the condenser lowered as far as it will go. The ease of identification of hyphae varies inversely with the intensity of light passing through the slide.

h. With SMS, hyphae and spores appear blue against the red background of cells. Because the hyphae stain selectively and are more easily seen with SMS, slides may be more quickly scanned at a lower power. This stain, not commercially available, consists of two separate solutions:

(1) The fungal stain consists of a dye, a surfactant to clear the tissues quickly, and an amount of KOH (2%) less than that which will etch glass and destroy microscopic lenses.

(2) The red counterstain (rose bengal) makes it easier to identify cells.

In KOH preparations, hyphae and spores will stand out as refractile tubes and oval bodies against the background of cells and debris. It is not possible to make a species identification from tissue scrapings.

2. Hair and nails

  a. Examine the scalp with a Wood's lamp. If individual lesions fluoresce, pull out 10–15 hairs for examination. Otherwise, examine scales and 10–15 random hairs from the involved site. Altered, dystrophic, hypertrophic, or pigmented nails should be snipped off and minced on a slide. Subungual debris is less suitable for examination.

  b. Heat on a slide or in a test tube with 10–40% KOH and let cool for 15–30 min. Tissue may then be stained with SMS or examined directly.

B. Culture. In addition to direct examination of scales, scrapings from a suspicious lesion should be cultured at room temperature on Sabouraud's glucose agar, Sabouraud's agar with chloramphenicol and actidione (Mycobiotic, Mycosel), or Dermatophyte Test Medium (DTM). DTM inhibits bacteria and saprophytic molds and contains phenol red, which turns the agar from yellow to bright red when its pH becomes alkaline from dermatophyte growth. Contaminant growth does not alter the pH of the medium. Using DTM medium, if no color change takes place within 2 weeks, the culture may be discarded. If the color does change, it may be presumed that a pathogenic dermatophyte or yeast is present. Microscopic examination of the culture (culture mount) should then identify the exact species.

Wood's light examination

I. Discussion. Wood's glass, primarily barium silicate containing 9% nickel oxide, is opaque to all light except for a band extending from 340–450 nm. When light from a high-pressure mercury arc is passed through this filter, it is principally the 365-nm radiation that is transmitted as, for example, a Wood's light such as the Blak-Ray. Fluorescent bulbs (black lights) that emit a similar though slightly broader spectrum are also available. The Wood's light was first found to have medical importance in detecting fungal infections, but it is useful for many other diagnostic tasks as well. As ointments, exudates, tetracycline in sweat, makeup, deodorants, and soap may fluoresce a blue or purple color, the skin should be well cleansed before examination. The Wood's lamp may be used in the following situations:

A. Detection and control of scalp ringworm. Hairs infected with *Microsporum audouini* or *M. canis* fluoresce a bright blue green. Fluorescent hairs may be selected for microscopic examination and culture. Pteridine compounds have been postulated as the cause of this fluorescence. As normal hair regrows, a band of nonfluorescent hair will emerge. Large school populations may be screened with the Wood's lamp for tinea capitis caused by organisms acquired from humans or animals. Infections acquired from soil fungi will not fluoresce, however.

B. Detection of other fungal infections. Tinea versicolor may fluoresce a golden yellow color. Although this is often imperceptible, Wood's light examination nevertheless allows the accompanying pigmentary changes to be seen more vividly.

C. **Detection of bacterial infections**

1. Erythrasma, an intertriginous infection caused by *Corynebacterium minutissimum,* fluoresces a brilliant coral red or pink orange. The fluorescent substance is a water-soluble porphyrin and therefore may not be present if the area has been washed recently.

2. *Pseudomonas aeruginosa* infections give off a yellowish green fluorescence due to pyocyanin. Fluorescence due to fluorescin is detectable before obvious purulence appears and is useful in screening burn patients for infections.

D. **Delineation of pigmentary disorders.** Long-wave UVL is transmitted into the dermis where it gives a white to blue white fluorescent color. Melanin present in the epidermis (but not dermis) acts to absorb long-wave UVL and thus prevents this "white" color. Under Wood's light variations in epidermal pigmentation (freckles, melasma, vitiligo) are more apparent, and variations in dermal pigmentation (Mongolian spot, some instances of postinflammatory hyperpigmentation) are less apparent or unchanged compared to their appearance in ambient visible light. The Wood's light accentuates contrast between pigmented and nonpigmented skin, but, of more importance, it separates hypopigmented from totally amelanotic areas (the latter have true white to blue white fluorescence). It is used for examining patients with vitiligo, albinism, leprosy, and other disorders of hypopigmentation and is also useful as a screening procedure in nurseries to look for the small, ash leaf-shaped, white macules indicative of tuberous sclerosis.

E. **Detection of porphyrins.** Acidified urine, feces, and, rarely, blister fluid from patients with porphyria cutanea tarda will fluoresce a brilliant pink orange.

F. **Drug detection.** The teeth of people who took tetracycline in childhood while deciduous teeth were forming will fluoresce yellow, as will the nails and bones of adults taking that antibiotic. Patients applying topical tetracycline lotions will have skin fluorescence in those sites when viewed under long-wave UVL lamps.

G. **Miscellaneous.** Fluorescent ingredients or markers in cosmetics, medications, or industrial compounds may be detected with the Wood's lamp.

Patch testing

I. **Discussion.** Patch testing is used to document and validate a diagnosis of allergic contact sensitization and identify the causative agent. It may also be of value as a screening procedure in some patients with chronic or unexplained eczematous eruptions (e.g., hand and foot dermatoses). It is a unique means of in vivo reproduction of disease in diminutive proportions, since sensitization affects the whole body and may therefore be elicited at any cutaneous site. The patch test is easier and safer than a "use test" because test items can be applied in low concentrations on small areas of skin for short periods of time.

II. **Technique**

A. Delay patch testing until any acute inflammation has subsided. Reexposure to the antigen may cause the eruption to flare up. Neither low-dose systemic steroids nor antihistamines will influence the results.

B. Test only with potential allergens. There are no methods available for easily assaying primary irritants.

C. Be certain that the substances being tested will not irritate the skin. Cosmetics may be applied full strength, but items of unknown irritant potential should be diluted to 1–2% in petrolatum, mineral oil, or, less preferably, water. Standard patch test trays are available from Hollister-Stier Laboratories and through the American Academy of Dermatology. Suitable dilution and vehicle data are available in the references cited at the end of this chapter and in the textbooks mentioned previously (see Preface and p. 55).

D. Apply test substances to a disk of filter paper bound to plastic-coated aluminum (Al-Test) and attach to the skin with occlusive tape. The Al-Test is the standard utilized by the North American and International Contact Dermatitis groups. Alternatively, one can use a 1 cm square piece of soft cotton (Webril) and cover with occlusive tape (Blenderm) or cellophane and tape. A smaller patch, which may be slightly less effective, may be applied with a ¼-in. piece of gauze, linen, cotton, or filter paper and covered with Elastopatch and tape (or Dermicel for those who cannot tolerate tape). Liquids and ointments may be applied directly to the cotton or gauze. Volatile liquids should be applied directly to the skin and allowed to dry before being covered. Solids must be powdered prior to application. Moisten powders and fabrics with water before application. The site of application should be normal hairless skin on the back or inner arms.

E. Leave the patches in place for 48 hr. If pain, pruritus, or irritation under a patch is noted, the patient should remove it at once. Readings should not be made until the patches have been off at least 20–30 min, as positive reactions may not show immediately. Delayed reactions are not uncommon and a final reading should be made at 4 days (96 hr).

F. The results are interpreted and noted as follows:

?+ = Doubtful reaction.
+ = Weak (nonvesicular) reaction—erythema and/or papules.
++ = Strong (edematous or vesicular) reaction—erythema papules and/or small vesicles.
+++ = Extreme reaction—all of the foregoing plus large vesicles, bullae, and, at times, ulceration.
IR = Irritant reaction.

A positive patch test proves only that the patient has a contact sensitivity, but not necessarily that the eliciting substance is the cause of the clinical eruption.

G. False-negative tests may be caused by:

1. Low concentration or insufficient amount of antigen.

2. Improper testing, including inadequate occlusion, inappropriate vehicle, wrong site, incorrect reading times, or deteriorating substances.

3. Depressed reactivity due to administration of high amounts of systemic steroids or recent and aggressive topical steroid application.

4. Failure to reproduce the true conditions of exposure to antigen and lack of heat, friction, trauma.

H. False-positive tests may be related to:

1. Primary irritant reactions.

2. Tape reactions and pressure effects.

3. Reactions to occlusion: maceration, miliaria, folliculitis.

4. Contamination from another site.

5. Presence of impurities in the test material.

I. Positive reactions may sometimes take several weeks to subside. A topical corticosteroid will decrease local symptoms at test sites with active or prolonged inflammation and also shorten the healing time.

Ultraviolet light therapy

I. Discussion. (Units of wavelengths: 1 cm = 10^8 angstrom [Å] = 10^7 nanometer [nm].) Ultraviolet radiation (UVL), that part of the electromagnetic spectrum that begins next to the violet end of the color spectrum (400 nm) and extends to the beginning of the x-ray region (200 nm), is often used in the therapy of psoriasis, acne, pityriasis rosea, and chronic eczematous eruptions; it may also be used in conjunction with psoralen administration for photochemotherapy of psoriasis and vitiligo. UVL causes temporary suppression of epidermal basal cell division, followed by a later increase in cell turnover. The UVL spectrum is subdivided into three bands: UVC (200–290 nm), UVB (290–320 nm), and UVA (320–400 nm). Each region has different photobiologic characteristics and will be discussed here separately.

II. Sources and techniques

A. Sunlight is often the optimal source of UVL. It is the least expensive and most effective under most circumstances. Sun emits radiation with a continuous emission spectrum. The ozone layer in the upper atmosphere acts as a filter and absorbs virtually all UVL shorter than 290 nm. The erythema dose for a fair-skinned person is 20 min at latitude 41° (Boston) at midday in June. The disadvantages of sunlight radiation are its variable absorption by clouds and the difficulty in controlling or monitoring its intensity.

B. UVC radiation from artificial sources is present in operating room germicidal lamps and in cold quartz lamps. These lamps, low-pressure, low-temperature mercury arcs, emit a band of radiation predominantly at 253.7 nm through a quartz envelope filter. The erythema dose is 30 sec at 25 cm. Advantages are that (1) little or no pigmentation follows the erythema, and (2) severe burns cannot occur, since large increases in exposure time lead to only minimal increases in redness. Cold quartz radiation is sometimes used to produce erythema and desquamation in acne patients, particularly in pigmented individuals who wish to avoid more intense melanin pigmentation. UVC radiation can cause a painful conjunctivitis after only seconds of exposure. No one should ever look directly into these lamps or spend much time around the lamp without adequate protection (protective clothing, glasses, or sunscreens [see pp. 176, 311]).

C. UVB radiation is probably most responsible for most of the beneficial effects of sunlight and conventional artificial UVL therapy. Detailed protocols for aggressive UVB phototherapy of psoriasis have been developed and are very effective (see p. 145). They are best administered in hospital or office settings using UVB fluorescent-bulb-lined phototherapy booths. Occasionally, patients may want to treat acne or small areas of psoriasis at home. There are several sources of UVB for clinical use:

1. **UVB sources**

   a. **Fluorescent sunlamp bulbs** (FS40), low-pressure, low-temperature mercury arc sources, emit a continuous spectrum with a peak at 313 nm. The radiation is filtered through calcium, zinc, and thallium phosphate phosphor in the glass envelope. The erythema dose is 90–120 sec at 25 cm. These lamps are easily obtainable, relatively inexpensive, and good sources of sunburn radiation (290–320 nm). They are usually used as a bank of four bulbs for home use, or constructed into a light box lined by reflecting metal and many 2-, 4-, and/or 6-ft lamps for office or clinic.

   b. **Sunlamp bulbs** or units are low-pressure mercury lamps that emit UVL in the sunburn spectrum. They are inexpensive and readily available (GE, Sylvania, or Westinghouse R-S [rapid start] bulbs; Hanovia or Sperti lamps).

   c. **Hot quartz lamps,** high-pressure, high-temperature mercury arc sources, emit a discontinuous UVL spectrum with bands at 254, 265, 297, 303, 313, and 365 nm but with particular effectiveness in the erythema-producing midrange. The erythema dose is 30–60 sec at 46 cm. Overexposure can lead to severe burns. These large lamps (Hanovia) are expensive and have been used primarily for in-hospital and office or clinic patient care. Booths containing fluorescent bulbs emitting UVB or UVA have generally supplanted use of hot quartz lamps.

2. **General instructions for the patient using small UVB lamps for home treatment of acne or psoriasis.**

   a. Protect the eyes with special sun goggles or moist cotton to prevent sunburn to the eyes.

   b. Use a dependable timer or have someone in the room during therapy. If UVL is to be self-administered, do not use it when tired. The primary danger of sunlamp therapy is overexposure. In most instances this occurs when patients turn on the unit before going to bed and then fall asleep under the pleasant warmth of the lamp.

   c. Allow the lamp to warm up for 5 min.

   d. Administer UVL every day or every other day.

   e. If excessive and painful erythema develops, discontinue UVL treatment until the redness completely subsides and then resume therapy at one-half the last exposure time. The object of therapy is to produce a minimal but noticeable erythema that subsides within 24 hr. Mild dryness and desquamation will follow within 1–2 days.

3. Specific instructions for the patient

a. Sunlamp (R-S) therapy to the face

(1) Place lamp 12 in. from the face.

(2) Treatment consists of three separate exposures of the face: left side, front, right side.

(3) Start therapy at 30-sec exposure to each aspect of the face. Increase each treatment by 30 sec a day until an erythema dose is reached, after which it is often possible to administer the same minimal erythema dose for some time. However, tanning and accommodation to UVL usually make it necessary to raise the amount of UVL exposure eventually by 30-sec increments in order to continue achieving an erythema response. Patients with darker skin may begin with a 1-min exposure and increase by 1-min increments a day until the erythema dose is reached, then revert to the other schedule. After reaching a 10-min exposure, continue without further increase in exposure time.

b. Sunlamp (R-S) therapy to the body

(1) Position the bulb 30 in. from the supine, unclothed body.

(2) Deliver UVL to four areas: upper trunk and face, lower trunk and legs, upper back, buttocks and lower legs. It is often useful to drape that half of the body not receiving light with a sheet to control dosage more accurately.

(3) Begin with an exposure time of 1 min to each area and increase by 30 sec daily until a minimal erythema dose is reached. Depending on the erythema response, the UVL exposure is either kept stable or increased by 30-sec increments until a 5-min exposure to each area is reached, then increased by 1 min each time until a 15–20 min exposure is reached.

c. Hot quartz lamp therapy is never self-administered. The attendant and patient must use goggles at all times.

(1) The lamp should be 30 in. away from the area being irradiated.

(2) Start with 30 sec for each exposure and increase by 30 sec daily. Hold treatment at the dose that produces a moderate erythema 24 hr later.

(3) Isolated areas may be irradiated by shielding all the surrounding area with sheeting or towels and exposing as described, but at one-half the distance. This will greatly increase the intensity of light, as the intensity is inversely proportional to the square of the distance; i.e., at one-half the distance there will be 4 times as much light energy delivered (from a point source).

D. UVA radiation from sunlight or fluorescent tubes will not, by itself, cause erythema or pigmentation except with extremely large doses. However, in the presence of a circulating photosensitizer such as psoralen compounds, the long-wave UVL spectrum becomes an excellent therapeutic tool. This combination of light and drug has been termed photochemotherapy, or PUVA (*p*soralen plus *u*ltraviolet A) therapy (see also p. 146). In the doses used, neither the drug alone nor the light alone has any biologic activity. Absorption of electromagnetic energy in the UVA waveband in the presence of psoralens results in transient inhibition of DNA synthesis. This is presumably the mode of action of PUVA therapy for psoriasis. At this time, PUVA treatment is primarily useful in severe psoriasis and is also effective for some patients with vitiligo and mycosis fungoides. It is sometimes helpful in treating atopic dermatitis and other inflammatory dermatoses.

1. UVA sources

a. **Fluorescent blacklight lamp** (FS40BL), low-pressure, low-temperature mercury arcs, emit a spectrum of 320–450 nm (peak 360 nm) filtered through the barium disilicate phosphor in its glass envelope. The peak is at 360 nm. Use of these bulbs is limited because of the low intensity of UVA emission.

b. **High-intensity UVA fluorescent bulbs** were developed by GTE Sylvania and it is these and similar bulbs that are best used in PUVA light boxes.

c. **PUVA treatment boxes** are used in hospital clinics and in some dermatologists' offices. Two hours after ingestion of 0.5–0.8 mg/kg of 8-methoxypsoralen, patients are exposed to incremental doses of UVA, starting at 1–5 joule/sq cm (approx. 2–10 min) depending on degree of melanization and skin type (see p. 175) determination of a minimal phototoxic dose (MPD). The treatment protocols are complicated, should be administered only under the direction of dermatologists experienced in their use, and will not be discussed here.

d. Sunlight-produced UVA can be used with psoralens for the treatment of vitiligo and psoriasis (see pp. 110, 146 for method). This technique is potentially dangerous because it is nearly impossible to gauge UVL exposure accurately and thus severe burns can result.

2. Biologic reaction to PUVA

a. PUVA redness may be absent or minimal at 12–24 hr after exposure (when UVB erythema is most intense) and may peak at 48–72 hr or later. Severe PUVA burns can continue to intensify for up to 1 week after exposure and can be treated with prednisone (see p. 176).

b. PUVA pigmentation, which appears clinically and histologically similar to normal UVB-induced melanogenesis (tanning) maximizes about 5–7 days after exposure, may become very intense after repeated PUVA treatments, and lasts longer than a normal suntan—weeks to many months.

c. Repeated high-dose UVA or PUVA exposure of laboratory animals causes cataracts and skin cancer just as UVB or sun exposure does. An increased number of basal cell carcinomas and squamous cell carcinomas have been found in long-term PUVA psoriasis patients who have previously had skin cancer or were exposed to carcinogens. Patients must be carefully observed for evidence of accelerated actinic damage, and UVA-blocking sunglasses should be worn on PUVA treatment days to decrease UVA exposure to the lens of the eye (see p. 110).

References

CYTOLOGIC SMEARS

Blank, H., and Burgoon, C. F.   Abnormal cytology of epithelial cells in pemphigus vulgaris: A diagnostic aid. *J. Invest. Dermatol.* 18:213–223, 1952.

Blank, H., Burgoon, C. F., Baldridge, G. D., McCarthy, P. L., and Urbach, F.   Cytologic smears in diagnosis of herpes simplex, herpes zoster and varicella. *J.A.M.A.* 146:1410–1412, 1951.

FUNGAL SCRAPING AND CULTURE

Rebell, G., and Taplin, D.   *Dermatophytes: Their Identification and Recognition* (rev. ed.). Coral Gables, Fla.: University of Miami Press, 1970.

Swartz, J. H., and Lamkins, B. E.   A rapid simple stain for fungi in skin scales, nail scrapings and hairs. *Arch. Dermatol.* 89:89–94, 1964.

Swartz, J. H., and Medrik, T. F.   Rapid contrast stain as a diagnostic aid for fungus infections. *Arch. Dermatol.* 99:494–497, 1969.

Taplin, D., Zaias, N., Rebell, D., and Blank, H.   Isolation and recognition of dermatophytes on a new medium (DTM). *Arch. Dermatol.* 99:203–209, 1969.

WOOD'S LIGHT EXAMINATION

Caplan, R. M.   Medical uses of the Wood's lamp. *J.A.M.A.* 202:1035–1038, 1967.

Gilchrest, B. A., Fitzpatrick, T. B., Anderson, E., and Parrish, J. A.   Localization of melanin pigmentation in the skin with Wood's lamp. *Br. J. Dermatol.* 96:245–248, 1977.

Task Force Report.   Report on ultraviolet light sources. *Arch. Dermatol.* 109:833–839, 1974.

Ward, C. G., Clarkson, J. G., Taplin, D., and Polk, H. C., Jr.   Wood's light fluorescence and *Pseudomonas* burn wound infection. *J.A.M.A.* 202:1039–1040, 1967.

PATCH TESTING

Adams, R. M.   *Occupational Contact Dermatitis.* Philadelphia: Lippincott, 1969.

Agrup, G., Dahlquist, I., Fregert, S., and Rorsman, H.   Value of history and testing in suspected allergic contact dermatitis. *Arch. Dermatol.* 101:212–215, 1970.

Baer, R. L., Ramsey, D. L., and Biondi, E.   The most common contact allergens 1968–1970. *Arch. Dermatol.* 108:74–78, 1973.

Cronin, E.   *Contact Dermatitis.* Edinburgh: Churchill-Livingstone, 1980.

Epstein, E.   Simplified patch test screening with mixtures. *Arch. Dermatol.* 95:269–274, 1967.

Fisher, A. A.   Contact Dermatitis (2nd ed.). Philadelphia: Lea & Febiger, 1973.

Hjorth, N.   Contact dermatitis: 1980. *Br. J. Dermatol.* (Suppl. 18) 103:19–20, 1980.

Kligman, A. M.   The identification of contact allergens by human assays: I. A critique of standard methods: II. Factors influencing the indication and measurement of allergic contact dermatitis: III. The maximization test: A procedure for screening and rating contact sensitization. *J. Invest. Dermatol.* 47:369–374, 375–392, 393–409, 1966.

Mailbach, H. I.   Patch testing: An objective tool. *Cutis* 13:613–619, 1974.

Rudner, E. J., et al.   Epidemiology of contact dermatitis in North America: 1972. *Arch. Dermatol.* 108:537–540, 1973.

Shelley, W. B.   The patch test. *J.A.M.A.* 200:874–878, 1967.

ULTRAVIOLET LIGHT THERAPY

Adrian, R. M., Parrish, J. A., Momtaz, T. K., and Karlin, M. J.   Outpatient phototherapy of psoriasis: A new protocol for thrice weekly treatments. *Arch. Dermatol.* 117:623–626, 1981.

Current status of oral PUVA therapy for psoriasis. *J. Am. Acad. Dermatol.* 1:106–117, 1979.

Monash, S.   Composition of sunlight and a number of ultraviolet lamps. *Arch. Dermatol.* 91:495–496, 1965.

Parrish, J. A., Fitzpatrick, T. B., Tannenbaum, L., and Pathak, M. A.   Photochemotherapy of psoriasis with oral methoxsalen and long wave ultraviolet light. *N. Engl. J. Med.* 291:1207–1212, 1974.

Stern, R. S., Thibodeux, L. A., Kleineman, R. A., Parrish, J. A., and Fitzpatrick, T. B.   Risk of cutaneous carcinoma in patients treated with oral methoxsalen photochemotherapy for psoriasis. *N. Engl. J. Med.* 300:809–813, 1979.

Task Force Report.   Report on ultraviolet light sources. *Arch. Dermatol.* 109:833–839, 1974.

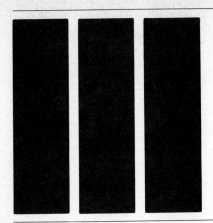

Treatment principles and formulary

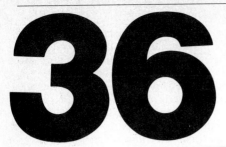

36

Treatment principles

Dermatologic prescriptions and drug costs

The writing of dermatologic prescriptions has changed radically over the past decades. In the past, most topical preparations were compounded according to the specific instructions of the physician. Currently, there are numerous, single-component medications and fixed-composition compounds available both as prescription and over-the-counter (OTC) nonprescription drugs. As opposed to most fixed-dose medications for systemic use, where the drug ratios are often not optimum, or unnecessary medications are included, the topical agents containing several ingredients are frequently efficacious. However, there may be an enormous variance in price between many items of approximately equal benefit to the patient—and it is essential to know not only the ingredients of the topicals prescribed but also the cost to the patient; at times, the cost does and should make the difference between whether a questionably effective topical or systemic medication is prescribed or discarded. Small package sizes (5–15 gm) are relatively much more costly than larger amounts (60 gm, 120 gm, 480 gm).

All drugs carry two names: the official **(generic)** and the brand **(trade,** or **proprietary)** name. The brand name is made almost universally more attractive, as it is both pronounceable and frequently carries a suggestion of the drug's alleged effects. For the first 17 years of patent monopoly on a new drug, only one company's product is available by either name unless other pharmaceutical firms have also been licensed to market the drug. Thereafter, the drug may be manufactured by several pharmaceutical houses, but the original trade name is protected forever by trademark laws and cannot be borrowed. Furthermore, pharmacies in some states are prohibited by law from substituting the generic drug when trade names are prescribed, even though the medications are identical but the costs radically different. By referring to drugs by their generic names, physicians are sometimes able to make the treatment of dermatologic disorders far less expensive. Writing "interchange permitted" on a prescription will instruct the pharmacist to dispense the generic equivalent for a brand name drug and will save the patient money. For example, the average wholesale cost to the druggist for 1000 4-mg Chlor-Trimeton is $40.00, 1000 Chlor-Trimeton 12-mg Repetabs $126.00, and 1000 50-mg Benadryl $75.00; the cost of their generic equivalents is $2.00, $6.00, and $7.50 respectively.

The cost of drugs to the pharmacist is easily available and is published yearly in the *Drug Topics Red Book* and *American Druggist Blue Book*. The actual cost to the patient varies, depending on the pricing policy of the pharmacy involved. Many pharmacies simply add a fee of $2.00–2.50 to the cost of the medication, while others mark up each item by 33% or 50% based on cost (66–100% based on selling price) in order to cover overhead costs and earn a profit. If the pharmacy cost of a drug is $6.00, the patient cost would be around $8.50 if a fee is charged, or $10.00 if computed by cost plus one-third cost. There is usually a minimum fee of $1.50–2.00 for any prescription filled. This obviously makes it important not to write prescriptions for OTC products, which may then become more costly to the patient, and never to write repeated prescriptions for small amounts of medication. It is quite costly to compound topical medications simply because it takes the pharmacist considerable time, which is usually charged at $15.00/hr. Thus, if a few inexpensive antipruritic agents, such as menthol and/or phenol (cost: 20–40¢) are added to 6.5 oz (195 gm) of Keri lotion (cost to pharmacy: $2.75–3.00) or to 1 lb (454 gm) of Eucerin cream (cost to pharmacy: $3.25), the total cost to the patient will be $10–15. Last, all drugs should always be clearly labeled as to ingredients and instructions for use. If necessary, the prescription should contain explicit instructions to the pharmacist to label all medications.

Types of topical medications
(see also *Dermatologic Topical Preparations and Vehicles,* Ch. 37, p. 297)

It is important to note that there are two variables in topical therapy. Both the medication and the vehicle chosen must be appropriate for the condition being treated. In general, acute inflammation is treated with aqueous drying preparations, and chronic inflammation is treated with greasier, more lubricating compounds, as noted in the following.

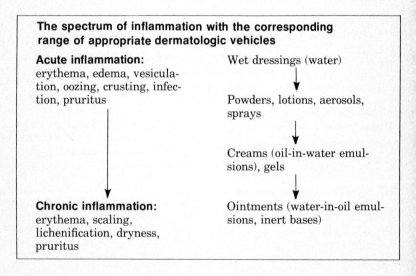

The spectrum of inflammation with the corresponding range of appropriate dermatologic vehicles

Acute inflammation:
erythema, edema, vesiculation, oozing, crusting, infection, pruritus

Wet dressings (water)
↓
Powders, lotions, aerosols, sprays
↓
Creams (oil-in-water emulsions), gels
↓

Chronic inflammation:
erythema, scaling, lichenification, dryness, pruritus

Ointments (water-in-oil emulsions, inert bases)

I. **Open wet dressings.** These types of dressings cool and dry through evaporation. They thus cause vasoconstriction, decreasing the vasodilatation and augmented local blood flow present in inflammation. In addition, wet dressings cleanse the skin of exudates, crusts, and debris and help maintain drainage of infected areas. They are indicated in the therapy of acute inflammatory conditions, erosions, and ulcers. Although various medicaments and antibacterial substances may be added for specific causes, water is by far the most important ingredient of wet dressings. Wet dressings covered by an impermeable cover **(closed wet dressings)** retain heat, prevent evaporation, and cause maceration, which may not be desirable (see Formulary, p. 313, for the technique of application).

II. **Powders.** Powders promote drying by increasing the effective skin surface area. They are used primarily in intertriginous areas to reduce moisture, maceration, and friction. Powders may be inert or may contain active medications (see p. 301).

III. **Liquids. Lotions** consist of suspensions of a powder in water (see p. 298). **Tinctures** are alcoholic or hydroalcoholic solutions. As lotions and tinctures evaporate, they cool and dry; lotions leave a uniform film of powder on the skin. **Sprays** and **aerosols** act in a similar manner. Active agents are often incorporated into the aqueous phase.

IV. **Creams. Creams** are semisolid emulsions of oil in water (O/W). As the proportion of grease increases and the proportion of water decreases, the preparation becomes more viscous and at some undefined ratio will no longer be considered a cream, entering the classification of ointments. A **gel** is a transparent and colorless semisolid emulsion that liquifies on contact with the skin, drying as a thin, greaseless, nonocclusive, nonstaining film. Aqueous, acetone, alcohol, or propylene glycol gels of organic polymers such as agar, gelatin, methylcellulose, pectin, and polyethylene glycol are primarily used.

V. **Ointments.** These consist of water droplets suspended in the continuous phase of oil (W/O) or of inert bases such as petrolatum. Ointments are of three types: those soluble in water, those that will emulsify with water, and those completely insoluble in water (see p. 299).

VI. **Pastes.** Pastes, which are little used today, are mixtures of a powder and an ointment.

VII. **Lubricants, bases, and protective coverings**
The following preparations are most often used as lubricants, bases in which to incorporate drugs, and protective coverings for the skin:

A. The **oil-in-water creams,** which are water-washable ("vanishing cream") and cosmetically pleasing, account for the majority of topical items prescribed.

B. **Water-in-oil emulsions,** which are better lubricants than oil-in-water creams, retain heat, impede water loss, increase hydration, and may thereby encourage percutaneous absorption. Because W/O preparations are occlusive, they are best not used in oozing or infected areas. To provide smooth mixtures, dispersing and emulsifying agents, surfactants, and detergents are usually added to these emulsions.

C. **Lotions, sprays, and O/W emulsions** are most easily applied to hirsute areas and scalp.

Amount to dispense
(see Table 5)

It will become apparent on long-term patient follow-up that, when inadequate amounts of medication are dispensed, the patient will tend to apply too little, will use the drugs less frequently than prescribed (often not frequently enough to provide adequate therapy), will soon run out of medication, and then may not refill the prescription. If a medication is known to be effective and is to be used on a long-term basis, dispensing large quantities will be more economical and will ensure continuous supply, resulting in better treatment.

One gm of cream will cover an area of skin approximately 10 cm × 10 cm, or about 100 sq cm. This assumes a layer 100 μ in thickness. The same amount of ointment will cover an area 5–10 percent larger. Table 5 in the Appendix gives conservative figures for the amounts needed for a single application of an ointment or cream and for application 3id for a 2-week period. If a lotion is to be used, the amounts should be doubled.

General principles of normal skin care

Recommendations for the care of normal skin are based on principles of moderation and common sense as well as on knowledge derived from study of skin structure and function. Routine daily care is far more simple than one may be led to believe by the profusion of astounding advertising claims. While much is known about adverse reactions to cosmetics and other products for topical use, well-controlled scientific studies related to the care and maintenance of healthy skin are either so limited or so rudimentary as to preclude precise recommendations in most instances. "Normal" skin refers to skin that is not affected by any disease process. Within "normal" there is obviously a wide variation of skin textures, complexions, and appearances. The principles below are applicable to almost everyone within this category, whether the skin is on the "dry" or "oily" end of the spectrum. The various systems and categorizations of skin types so readily available at cosmetic counters of department stores yield little useful information, are not based on any basic pathophysiologic principles, and are useful primarily for the cosmetic company whose products are subsequently recommended.

It is not at all clear that normal skin benefits from much, if anything at all, in the way of specific care, except for protection from harsh chemical and physical agents (especially sunlight). On the other hand, many products used for skin care or cosmetic purposes can occasionally produce adverse reactions, such as allergic and irritant contact dermatitis, phototoxic and photoallergic reactions, and induction of acne (acne cosmetica). Neither price range nor brand name provides absolute assurance that a given product will be of high quality or will not cause adverse reactions. The area of skin care is beset with an amazing number of unsubstantiated claims, "secret" ingredients, and fads. It is beyond the scope of this book to address all of them, and for more complete and detailed information, the reader is referred to the references at the end of the section.

I. Protection

A. Changes induced by sunlight are the major factor in causing alterations in the skin that contribute to the appearance of aging. Sunscreens and sunblocking agents can prevent or retard these changes. The more fair the skin, the stronger the indication for a stronger sun-protective agent (see p. 176).

    1. *No other form* of intervention either taken internally or applied externally will alter the cutaneous aging process. A variety of topical agents can camouflage the appearance of aging or induce transient changes that make the skin look or feel "younger." For example, mild irritation caused by certain chemicals in "rubefacient" masks accomplishes this by inducing mild erythema and edema. Aside from cosmetic surgical techniques, the same applies to remedies for wrinkles and for sagging.

B. Efforts to protect the skin from harsh chemicals (e.g., strong acids and alkalis) and physical agents (e.g., cold, wind, and extreme dryness) that may damage the skin are also sensible and desirable (see p. 51).

II. Nutrition

A. The normal epidermis, hair follicles, and nail matrices receive their nutrition from the cutaneous (dermal) vasculature, and there is no evidence that any topically applied "nutrient" can enhance their performance. Except in bona fide nutritional disorders such as avitaminoses (e.g., pellagra) there is no convincing proof that any dietary supplement can enhance skin, hair, or nail growth.

B. Since the stratum corneum, hair, and nails consist of dead cells, there is no evidence or reason to believe that external application of "protein," "amino acids," "collagen," "elastin," "RNA," "nucleic acids," or the like will have anything more than a transient effect on the appearance or texture of the skin or its appendages.

    1. The percutaneous penetration of these molecules is nil, as is the likelihood of linking with epidermal proteins.

III. Cleaning the skin; "facials"

A. Soap is not inherently harmful to the skin. Washing several times daily will not lead to dryness. Use of cleansing creams instead of soap has no benefits and may induce acneform lesions.

B. *Excessive* washing with water and with soap or detergents can lead to dryness of the skin. Also, exposure to air with low relative humidity in either a warm or cold environment permits a significant degree of moisture loss from the skin (see p. 67).

C. The use of a "mild" soap or detergent bar, and a reduction in the number of washings per day (to once, twice, or at most three times) will minimize the drying effects of washing. A recent study showed that the soaplike cleanser Dove was the least irritating among 18 soaps and detergent bars tested (see p. 294).

1. People who are obliged to wash their hands frequently are well advised to use as little soap as possible and to apply an emollient such as petrolatum or an O/W lubricant after washing (see p. 298).

D. The pH of normal skin at its surface is about 6.8. Most soaps and shampoos are alkaline. While extremes of acid or alkaline pH may be harmful to hair or skin, no skincare or cosmetic product—even inexpensive ones—achieves such extremes. For the most part, products that claim to be "pH balanced" offer no particular advantage over other products on that score alone.

E. Facial massage, saunas, mudpacks, pore-cleaning, "facials," etc. may feel pleasant and may temporarily improve the appearance of the skin, but have not been shown to have any short- or long-term beneficial effects other than those that can be attributed to looking and feeling good (which may be substantial).

IV. Astringents; facial masks; clarifiers; large pores

A. "Large pores" can be camouflaged or temporarily altered but cannot be permanently changed or prevented. To say that large pores look much worse to the observer with a magnifying mirror than they do to anyone else is a truism worth mentioning.

B. Astringents, also called skin bracers or after-shave lotions in products for men, contain water (as much as 50%), and alcohol or witch hazel. As the alcohol evaporates, it cools the skin, which is interpreted as feeling refreshed.

1. Astringents with aluminum salts (alum) added are called refiners. Alum irritates the skin and causes mild erythema and edema which makes the face rosy and the pores look transiently smaller.

C. Clarifiers are meant to act as keratolytics. The lotions may contain resorcinol or salicylates, and the cleansers contain grains that are scrubbing agents (see pp. 8, 240). They are meant to thin the stratum corneum in order to leave the skin rosy and refreshed.

D. Masks, which may contain an absorbent clay or synthetic resin, form a film that tightens on the skin as it dries. This produces mild irritation and some effects as noted for astringents.

V. Lubricating the skin

A. Water is the most important plasticizer of the epidermis. Used appropriately, emollients or "moisturizers" can restore water to the skin for a short period of time or can help the skin to retain moisture when applied after bathing.

1. Emollients may make the skin look better or feel more supple transiently, but there is *no* evidence that aging or wrinkling can be slowed down or prevented by such measures. Furthermore, some emollients can cause or exacerbate acne (see p. 234).

2. The most effective lubricants are usually the least cosmetically acceptable—petrolatum, mineral and "baby" oil, Albolene or Eucerin. Next most helpful are O/W emulsions such as cold creams and Nivea Skin Oil, which contain oils, fatty alcohols, and waxes with emulsifiers and humectants. Least effective but most comfortable to

use are W/O creams and "moisturizers" which are principally water along with emulsifiers, colors, fragrances, preservatives, and humectants (see p. 298).

B. Certain lipids and oils are thought to lubricate the skin by reducing surface friction between lamellae of the stratum corneum. "Humectants" such as lactic acid and urea may enhance the water-bearing capacity of the stratum corneum and hold water in the skin for prolonged times (see pp. 69, 308).

C. A variety of compounds such as aloe, jojoba oil, and vitamin E are receiving increasing attention as lubricants, for cosmetic use, and as home healing aids. Some have been in use as folk remedies for many years. How they will stand rigorous testing remains to be seen; an open mind is in order. On the other hand, cases of allergic sensitization to such substances have been reported.

VI. Hair care

A. Daily shampooing of normal scalp and hair will not ordinarily cause dryness or other damage and will remove exfoliated skin and debris.

   1. If hair becomes *too* alkaline, the cuticular cells may become rough and the hair catches and looks dull.

   2. Detergents may be more alkaline than soaps. Sodium lauryl sulfate and ammonium lauryl sulfate are the strongest; laureth sulfate detergents are less alkaline; the amphoterics, which are in some baby shampoos, are mildest.

B. Use of electric rollers, curling irons, hot combs, and exposure to permanent waving solutions can alter and "dry out" hair and make it more brittle. This damage affects only hair that has already grown out of the follicle, i.e., hair growth is not altered.

C. Physical abuses to hair, such as some straightening techniques, and hair styles that promote prolonged traction on hair can cause follicular scarring and permanent alopecia.

D. Acid hair rinses counteract the temporary effects of the alkaline shampoos, smooth down cuticular cells, and reduce swelling of the hair shaft so that the hair looks smooth and shiny.

   1. They also change the electrical charge on the hair and remove mineral deposits left by soaps.

E. Conditioning rinses put an oily coating back on the hair to replace that removed by the shampoo. In addition to ingredients to change the electrical charge, they also contain emollients, thickeners, preservatives, humectants, fragrances, colors, and sometimes an alkali to make the hair swell so the conditioner can penetrate.

   1. These rinses are useful for hair damaged by chemical treatments, physical abuse, or excessive exposure to ultraviolet light or harsh weather.

VII. "Hypoallergenic" and "noncomedogenic"

A. "Hypoallergenic" cosmetics are theoretically designed to eliminate the most common and notorious allergy-producing compounds, but still contain components allergenic to some individuals. The term "hypoallergenic" means only that all product ingredients are pure, but does not necessarily imply that there are fewer antigens present. Any product may legally call itself hypoallergenic.

1. Even inexpensive cosmetics are usually screened and tested quite thoroughly in order to eliminate potential allergens. The rate of adverse reactions to cosmetics of all types is quite low.

B. A long history of problem-free use is no guarantee that a particular product is not the cause of an allergic reaction. It is possible for an individual to become allergic to a compound even if it has been applied to the skin for years without difficulty. Furthermore, manufacturers may change the ingredients in a preparation without concomitant labeling changes.

1. The investigation and prevention of allergic contact dermatitis from cosmetic products may be complex, and require dedication on the part of patient and physician. A single fragrance or scent may contain more than 200 chemicals. It is often necessary to discontinue use of *all* cosmetics.

C. Persons with suspected allergies to cosmetic ingredients will often benefit from patch testing so that the knowledge of sensitivity to particular compounds can help in the choice of alternative products. In some instances it is wise for individuals with multiple sensitivities or with sensitivity to an undetermined compound to perform pre-use open patch tests (see p. 216).

D. Acne cosmetica is not an allergic reaction, but is caused by the inclusion of comedogenic substances that can be found in many cosmetic products, especially emollients and oil-based makeups (see p. 5). "Hypoallergenic" does *not* mean "noncomedogenic." Some notable comedogenic compounds are sodium lauryl sulfate, isopropyl isostearate, isopropyl myristate, butyl stearate, hexadecyl alcohol, lauryl alcohol, oleic acid, lanolin, cocoa butter, and petrolatum.

E. Water-based, rather than oil-based, cosmetics should be used to decrease the risk of acne cosmetica in susceptible individuals. "Oil-free" cosmetics are not necessarily noncomedogenic, and may contain certain comedogenic organic oils. Some soaps also contain comedogenic materials; certain "creamy" or "moisturizing" soaps should be avoided by individuals with acne.

VIII. It is difficult to recommend specific products. Except for advice to be on the lookout for adverse reactions, trial and error in combination with individual preference is about the only rational way for people with normal skin to choose among most cosmetic products.

References

DERMATOLOGIC PRESCRIPTIONS AND DRUG COSTS

Cost of prescription drugs. *Med. Lett. Drugs Ther.* 17:5–6, 1975.

TYPES OF TOPICAL MEDICATIONS

Hadgraft, J. W.   Recent progress in the formulation of vehicles for topical applications. *Br. J. Dermatol.* 87:386–389, 1972.

Hellier, F. F.   Creams, ointments and lotions. *Practitioner* 202:23–26, 1969.

AMOUNT TO DISPENSE

British Medical Association. *British National Formulary*. London: Pharmaceutical Society of Great Britain, 1968. P. 13.

Schlager, C., and Sanborn, E. D.   The weights of topical preparations required for total and partial body inunction. *J. Invest. Dermatol.* 42:253–256, 1964.

GENERAL PRINCIPLES OF NORMAL SKIN CARE

Conry, T.   *Consumer's Guide to Cosmetics*. Garden City, N.Y.: Anchor Books, 1980.

Cronin, E.   *Contact Dermatitis*. Edinburgh: Churchill-Livingstone, 1980.

Estrin, N. F., Crosley, P. A., and Haynes, C. R.   *CFTA Cosmetic Ingredient Dictionary*. Washington, D.C.: Cosmetic, Toiletry and Fragrance Association, Inc., 1982.

Fisher, A. A.   Cutaneous Reactions to Cosmetics. In A. A. Fisher (ed.), *Contact Dermatitis*. Philadelphia: Lea & Febiger, 1973. Pp. 217–241.

Fisher, A. A.   New advances in contact dermatitis. *Int. J. Dermatol.* 16:552–566, 1977.

Fisher, A. A.   Cosmetic actions and reactions: Therapeutic, irritant and allergic. *Cutis* 26:22, 1980.

Frosch, P. J., and Kligman, A. M.   The soap chamber test: A new method for assessing the irritancy of soaps. *J. Am. Acad. Dermatol.* 1:35–41, 1979.

Kligman, A. M., and Kwong, T.   An improved rabbit ear model for assessing comedogenic substances. *Br. J. Dermatol.* 100:699–702, 1979.

Kligman, A. M., and Mills, O. H.   Acne cosmetica. *Arch. Dermatol.* 106:843–850, 1972.

Morrow, D. M., Rapaport, M. J., and Strick, R. A.   Hypersensitivity to aloe. *Arch. Dermatol.* 116:1064–1065, 1980.

Parrish, J. A., Gilchrest, B. A., and Fitzpatrick, T. B.   *Between You and Me: A Sensible and Authoritative Guide to the Care and Treatment of Your Skin*. Boston: Little, Brown, 1978.

Rinzler, C. A.   The new and improved chemistry of cosmetics: They used to sell dreams, now they're selling science. *Science* 82:54–61, 1982.

Rook, A., and Dawber, R.   Hair Cosmetics. In *Diseases of the Hair and Scalp*. Oxford: Blackwell, 1982.

Scher, R. K.   Cosmetics and ancillary preparations for the care of nails: Composition, chemistry, and adverse reactions. *J. Am. Acad. Dermatol.* 6:523–528, 1982.

Schoen, L. A. (ed.).   *Skin and Hair Care*. Hammersmith: Penguin, 1978.

Scott, M. J., and Scott, M. J.   Jojoba oil. *J. Am. Acad. Dermatol.* 4:545, 1982.

Spoor, H. J.   Supplemental hair care. *Cutis* 22:17, 1978.

Zizmor, J., and Foreman, J.   *Dr. Zizmor's Brand Name Guide to Beauty Aids and Everything You Want to Know about Them and Whether There's Anything There That'll Hurt You and Most of All Whether They Really Do All (or Even Some) of the Things for You that the Labels Say They Do*. New York: Harper & Row, 1978.

37

Formulary

This section includes the topical and systemic medications most useful for treating cutaneous disease. Drugs are listed alphabetically in each instance. This is not a complete listing of all the pharmaceutical preparations available for dermatologic use, and many useful products may have been omitted. No sustained-release capsules and few aerosols or antibiotic-steroid combinations are cited here. For uniformity and ease of conversion, all package sizes are listed in metric terms (see Table 6). Costs shown are average retail cost per item to the patient, based on the usual pharmacy markup of cost + two-thirds of cost (computed as cost/0.66), or manufacturer's recommended cost. Prices to the pharmacist are those listed as Average Wholesale Price (AWP) in the *Drug Topics Red Book* or *American Druggist Blue Book*. Although pharmacists can buy some drugs directly from the manufacturer at a slightly lower price ("direct price"), some manufacturers do not distribute any drugs directly and others have minimum requirements for direct orders that may exclude small orders or those from small-volume pharmacies. Thus, of the total pharmacy charge, in most instances 60% is drug cost and 40% pharmacy cost. The prices given here should be viewed only as a general guide to comparative costs and are, of course, constantly subject to change. Prices currently increase by approximately 10% per year. The medication costs noted in this formulary average 50–100% more than in the previous 1978 edition. Medications that require a prescription are so noted (R_x).

Acne preparations

I. **Discussion.** See Acne, p. 3.

II. **Prescription drugs (R_x)**

    A. Isotretinoin (13-*cis*-retinoic acid; Accutane)

        1. Structure: *cis*-isomer of tretinoin (see below **B.1**).

        2. Indications and pharmacology. Isotretinoin is a retinoid that inhibits sebaceous gland function and keratinization. It is approved for the treatment of severe cystic acne that is unresponsive to conventional therapy (see p. 11). It has also been found to be very useful in the therapy of disorders of keratinization such as pityriasis rubra pilaris, lamellar ichthyosis and epidermolytic hyperkeratosis, Darier's disease, and keratosis palmaris et plantaris. Some patients with X-linked ichthyosis, congenital ichthyosiform erythroderma, and ichthyosis vulgaris have improved. Good clinical results have been obtained in the treatment of severe rosacea and gram-negative folliculitis, dissecting cellulitis of the scalp, and some cases of hidradenitis suppuritiva.

This drug probably has multiple modes of action, including (1) alteration in keratinization both in epidermis and within the pilosebaceous follicle, (2) inhibition of sebaceous gland activity, (3) inhibition of the growth of *P. acnes* within follicles, although isotretinoin is not antibacterial, and (4) inhibition of inflammation.

3. **Adverse effects**

   a. Hypertriglyceridemia develops in 25% of patients with about 10% having an elevation above 500 mg%. About 15% show mild to moderate decrease in serum high density lipoprotein (HDL) levels, and 7% elevations of serum cholesterol.

      (1) Pretreatment and follow-up lipids should be obtained under fasting conditions and at least 36 hours after alcohol was last consumed. These tests should be performed biweekly until the lipid response of the drug is established.

      (2) If elevated triglycerides develop either the drug should be discontinued or levels should be decreased by restriction of dietary fats and alcohol, weight reduction, or dosage reduction.

   b. Cheilitis occurs in more than 90% of patients, dry skin, itching, and/or epistaxis in 80%, conjunctivitis in 40%, musculoskeletal symptoms in 16%, rash or hair thinning in 10%, and peeling of palms and soles, GI symptoms, headaches, and sunburn sensitivity in 5%.

      (1) Most reactions are dose related and reversible when treatment is decreased or discontinued.

   c. Isotretinoin is teratogenic in animals and is contraindicated in women who are pregnant or intend to become pregnant while undergoing therapy. Women of childbearing potential should not be given isotretinoin unless effective contraception is used, and possible risks to the fetus should they become pregnant must be fully explained.

   d. Patients sensitive to parabens will also react to Accutane, which contains these agents as preservatives. Supplementary vitamins containing vitamin A are contraindicated to avoid additive toxic effects.

   e. Side effects may appear before therapeutic effects. Concomitant use of topical drying agents should be avoided. Initial flares in acne lesions are common.

4. **Dosage.** 1–2 mg/kg, given in 2 divided daily doses for 15–20 weeks.

   a. If the acne cyst count is reduced by 70% prior to this time, the drug may be discontinued.

   b. If severe cystic acne is persistent, a second course may be initiated after 2 months off therapy.

   c. Individuals with lesions primarily on chest and back or those weighing more than 70 kg may require doses at the higher end of the range.

5. **Packaging and cost:**

   a. 40-mg soft gelatin capsules: as Accutane, 100/$175.00

B. Tretinoin (vitamin A acid; Retin-A)

1. Structure

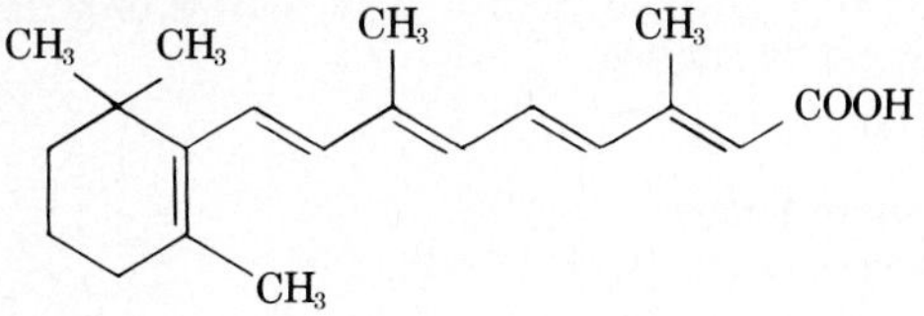

Tretinoin

2. Contains: 0.05% tretinoin (vitamin A acid) in the solution and swabs, 0.1% or 0.05% in the cream, and 0.01% and 0.025% in the gel. The 0.05% cream or the 0.01% gel is usually the least irritating. Tretinoin does not function as a vitamin in this therapy.

3. Use: See p. 8.

4. Packaging and cost:
0.05% liquid: 28-ml bottle/$8.50
0.05% cream: 20-gm tube/$8.50
0.05% cream: 45-gm tube/$14.75
0.1% cream: 20-gm tube/$9.75
0.01% gel: 15-gm tube/$7.00
0.01% gel: 45-gm tube/$15.00
0.025% gel: 15-gm tube/$8.00
0.025% gel: 45-gm tube/$16.75

C. Benzoyl peroxide preparations

1. Structure

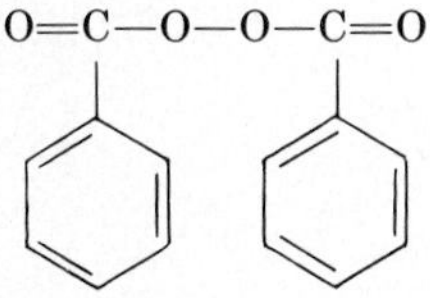

Benzoyl peroxide

2. Contain: 2.5%, 5%, or 10% benzoyl peroxide, oil base lotion (Benoxyl, Persadox; no R_x for either); alcohol gel base (Benzagel, Pan Oxyl); acetone gel base (Persa-Gel); aqueous gel base (Desquam-X).

3. Use: See p. 6.

4. Packaging and cost:
Benoxyl 10: 30 ml/$4.50
              60ml/$6.75
Desquam-X 5 & 10: 45 gm/$4.50
                   90 gm/$7.50
Desquam-X Wash (5 or 10%): 150 ml/$7.00
Pan Oxyl AQ 2.5: 60 gm/$4.25

D. Topical antibiotics

1. Clindamycin phosphate

   a. Contains: 10 mg/ml clindamycin in 50% isopropyl alcohol and propylene glycol solution.

   b. Use: See p. 7.

   c. Packaging and cost:
   1% solution (Cleocin T): 60 ml/$15.00

2. Erythromycin base solution

   a. Contains: erythromycin base in propylene glycol and alcohol solution. The alcohol content is 60% (A/T/S), 55% (Staticin), and 77% (Ery Derm).

   b. Use: See p. 7.

   c. Packaging and cost:
   1.5% solution (Staticin): 60 ml/$10.25
   2% solution (A/T/S/): 60 ml/$8.75
   2% solution (EryDerm): 60 ml/$11.75

3. Meclocycline sulfosalicylate cream

   a. Contains: 1% meclocycline sulfosalicylate.

   b. Use: See p. 7.

   c. Packaging and cost:
   Meclan: 20-gm tube/$10.00

4. Tetracycline hydrochloride solution

   a. Contains: 2.2 mg/ml tetracycline hydrochloride in 40% ethanol solution.

   b. Use: See p. 7.

   c. Packaging and cost:
   Topicycline: 70-ml applicator bottle/$12.25

III. Over-the-counter (OTC) drugs

A. Structure of common ingredients

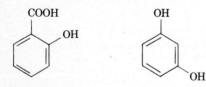

Salicylic acid   Resorcinol

B. Abrasive soaps

1. Brasivol

   a. Contains: aluminum oxide particles.

   b. Use: See p. 8.

   c. **Packaging and cost:**
   Fine grain: 153-gm tube/$5.00
   Medium grain: 180-gm tube/$5.00
   Rough grain: 195-gm tube/$5.00

2. **Pernox**

   a. **Contains:** polyethylene granules, 2% sulfur, 1.5% salicylic acid.

   b. **Use:** See p. 8.

   c. **Packaging and cost:**
   60 gm/$3.50
   120 gm/$5.50

C. **Cleansers**

1. **Fostex cake, cream, cleanser**

   a. **Contain:** 2% sulfur, 2% salicylic acid.

   b. **Use:** See p. 7.

   c. **Packaging and cost:**
   112-gm cake/$2.25
   120-gm cream/$4.25
   150-gm cleanser/$3.50

2. **Seba-Nil**

   a. **Contains:** 49.7% alcohol, acetone, polysorbate in saturated towelette.

   b. **Use:** prn for oily skin.

   c. **Packaging and cost:**
   Box of 24/$3.00
   Liquid: 240 ml/$3.75

D. **Other drying and antiseptic topicals.** Although benzoyl peroxide, ret-inoic acid preparations, or topical antibiotics are the drugs of choice, a few other acne medications are listed here for comparison of ingredients and price.

1. **Acne-Aid cream and lotion**

   a. **Contain:** 2.5% sulfur, 1.25% resorcinol (cream); 10% sulfur, 10% alcohol in clear or tinted base (lotion).

   b. **Use:** Apply 1–2 times a day.

   c. **Packaging and cost:**
   Cream: 54 gm/$3.25
   Lotion: 30 ml/$2.50
        60 ml/$4.00

2. **Acnomel cream**

   a. **Contains:** 8% sulfur, 2% resorcinol, 11% alcohol in tinted vehicle.

   b. **Use:** Apply 1–3 times a day.

   c. **Packaging and cost:**
   30 gm/$3.00

3. **Fostril lotion**

   a. **Contains:** 6% polyoxyethylene lauryl ether, 2% sulfur in tinted base.

   b. **Use:** Apply 1–3 times a day.

   c. **Packaging and cost:**
   30 ml/$3.75

4. **Komed lotion**

   a. **Contains:**

Mild	Regular	
2%	8%	Sodium thiosulfate
1%	2%	Salicylic acid
1%	2%	Resorcinol
25%	25%	Alcohol

   b. **Use:** Apply 1–3 times a day.

   c. **Packaging and cost:**
   60 ml/$4.75
   with 1% hydrocortisone (R_x): 60 gm/$9.25

5. **Liquimat lotion**

   a. **Contains:** 5% sulfur, 22% alcohol in tinted lotion in 9 shades.

   b. **Use:** Apply 1–3 times a day.

   c. **Packaging and cost:**
   45 ml/$3.00

6. **Transact gel**

   a. **Contains:** 6% polyoxyethylene lauryl ether, 2% sulfur, 40% alcohol.

   b. **Use:** Apply 1–3 times a day.

   c. **Packaging and cost:**
   30 gm/$4.00

7. **Vlemasque**

   a. **Contains:** 6% sulfurated lime solution, 7% alcohol in drying clay mask.

   b. **Use:** Apply for 20 min daily.

   c. **Packaging and cost:** 120 gm/$7.00

E. **Hot drying compresses**

   1. **Vlem-Dome liquid concentrate**

      a. **Contains:** 60.5% calcium polysulfide, 4.5% calcium thiosulfate, 4.5% sulfur (Vleminckx solution).

      b. **Use:** Dissolve package with 1 pint hot water and apply for 15 min nightly.

      c. **Packaging and cost:**
      Box of six 4-ml packets/$7.00

Anesthetics for topical administration (see also pp. 289–293)

I. Discussion. Topical anesthetics are useful therapeutic agents only in rare instances but are very commonly used as OTC antipruritic and analgesic agents. They usually are not helpful because (1) they are ineffective if applied to epidermis that has an intact barrier layer (stratum corneum); (2) even on inflamed (e.g., sunburned) skin, only agents containing benzocaine have been shown to be possibly useful, and (3) the more effective drugs (e.g., benzocaine) are potential allergic sensitizers. A large trial on volunteers with intact or sunburned skin has shown that the wide range of local anesthetics commercially available were all useless in relieving burn discomfort or preventing experimental pain except for ≥10% benzocaine. Mucosal surfaces lack a stratum corneum and thus topical anesthetics can be both effective and useful in some oral or anogenital disorders. Topical anesthetic use may be considered for (1) primary or recurrent herpes simplex infection of mouth or genital areas, (2) pain induced by podophyllin or alternative therapy for genital warts, and (3) aphthous stomatitis. They may also be useful on episiotomy wounds, after rectal surgery, for anesthesia of the urethra prior to cystoscopy, and for gingival anesthesia prior to injections.

Amides
Dibucaine (Nupercainal)
Lidocaine (Xylocaine)

Aminobenzoate esters
Benzocaine (Americaine)
Butamben picrate (Butesin)
Tetracaine hydrochloride (Pontocaine)

Nonamide, nonaminobenzoate esters
Benzyl alcohol (Topic: see p. 292)
Cyclomethycaine sulfate (Surfacaine)
Dimethisoquin hydrochloride (Quotane)
Diperodon (Diothane)
Dyclonine hydrochloride (Dyclone)
Pramoxine hydrochloride (Prax; Tronothane)

Local anesthetics by chemical structure. Selected brand names are given, but some agents are available as generic products.

II. Prescription drugs

A. Dyclonine HCl is a synthetic organic ketone agent related in structure to antihistamines. Onset of action is within 2–10 min and anesthesia lasts for 30–60 min.

1. Structure

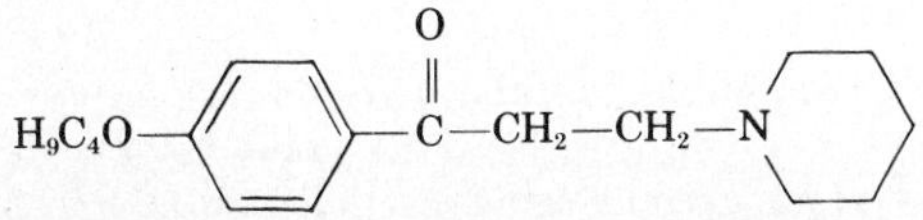

Dyclonine

   2. **Packaging and cost:**
      Dyclone, 0.5% solution: 30 ml/$6.00
      Dyclone, 1.0% solution: 30 ml/$8.00
      Resolve, 1.0% gel: 3 gm/$3.50

B. Dibucaine HCl is an amidelike quinoline derivative and is one of the most potent and longest acting of the commonly used local anesthetics.

   1. **Structure**

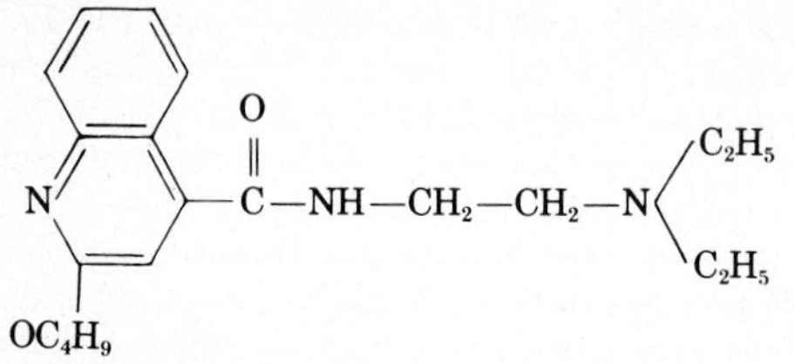

     Dibucaine

   2. **Packaging and cost:**
      1.0% ointment: 30 gm/$1.25
      As Nupercainal, 1% ointment: 30 gm/$2.75

C. Diphenhydramine HCl (Benadryl) is an effective topical agent. See pp. 20, 246 for further discussion.

D. Lidocaine is an amino acyl amidelike local anesthetic. Allergic reactions to lidocaine are rare, but do occur. Duration of anesthesia is relatively short (less than 1 hr). A lidocaine-prilocaine cream applied under occlusion for 1 hr has been found to produce effective anesthesia adequate for minor surgical procedures or dermabrasion.

   1. **Structure**

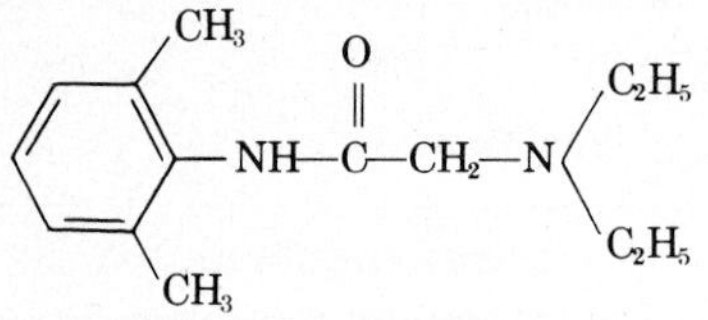

     Lidocaine

   2. **Packaging and cost:**
      Xylocaine, 2% jelly: 30 ml/$5.50
      Xylocaine, 2.5% ointment (no R_x): 35 gm/$2.75
      Xylocaine, 5.0% ointment: 35 gm/$5.00
      Generic, 5.0% ointment: 35 gm/$2.00
      Xylocaine, 2% viscous: 100 ml/$6.25

III. Nonprescription drugs

A. Benzocaine (ethyl aminobenzoate), a para-aminobenzoate (PABA) derivative, is poorly soluble in water and used only for topical anesthesia. About one-fourth of benzocaine-sensitive individuals are also sensitive to paraphenylenediamine, sulfonamides, hydrochlorothiazide, and the sunscreens based on PABA esters (see p. 311). Such patients may also show cross reactions for other local anesthetics based on PABA: dibucaine and cocaine, and the injectable agents procaine (Novocaine), butethamine (Monocaine), tetracaine (Pontocaine), and propoxycaine (Ravocaine). Injection of such local anesthetics into benzocaine-sensitive subjects may lead to local swelling, or rarely, urticaria or anaphylaxis. Non–cross-reacting local anesthetics include lidocaine, mepivacaine, and prilocaine. Benzocaine's anesthetic action is of short duration.

1. Structure

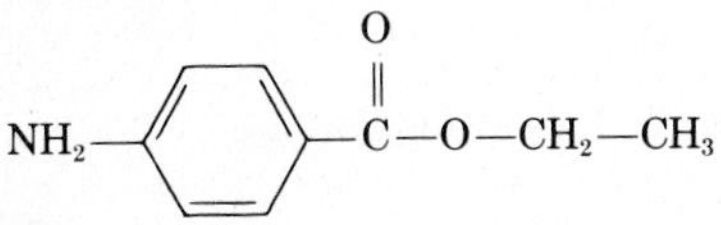

Benzocaine

2. Packaging and cost:

Benzodent, 20% benzocaine with 0.4% eugenol and 0.1% hydroxyquinoline sulfate in a denture-adhesive-like base: 30 gm/$4.00

Generic, 5% cream: 30 gm/$1.00

Americaine, 20% ointment: 22 gm/$2.25

Generic, 20% spray: 210 gm/$4.50

Americaine, 20% spray: 120 gm/$5.50

Burntame, 20% spray: 100 gm/$6.60

B. Dimethisoquin is an active etherlike surface anesthetic of value for treatment of cutaneous lesions. It is less sensitizing than drugs based on an antihistamine structure, and along with a similar compound, **pramoxine** (Prax, Tronothane), is especially useful in patients sensitive to esterlike or amidelike agents. Pramoxine is also available as a lotion or cream with 0.5% or 1.0% hydrocortisone (Pramosone) or as foam with 1% hydrocortisone (Proctofoam-HC). Onset of anesthesia is within a few minutes and its duration is 2–4 hr. Either of these two agents is the topical anesthetic of choice in most situations.

1. Structure

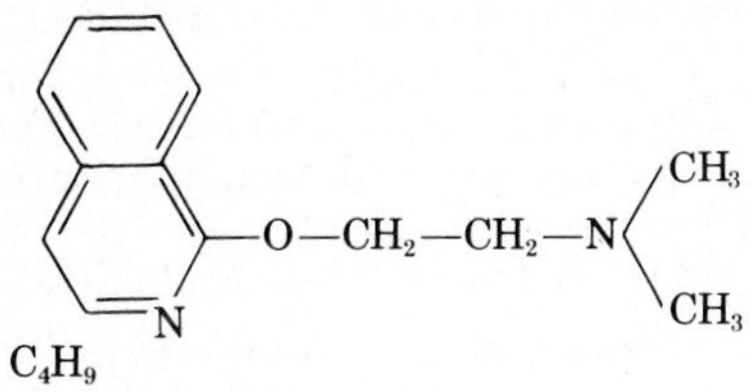

Dimethisoquin

2. Packaging and cost:

Quotane, 0.5% ointment: 30 gm/$3.00

Tronothane, 1% pramoxine cream or jelly: 30 gm (R_x)/$3.25

Prax, 1% pramoxine lotion: 15 ml/$2.00

Prax, 1% pramoxine lotion: 120 ml/$5.25

References

ANESTHETICS FOR TOPICAL ADMINISTRATION

Dalili, H., and Adriani, J.   The efficacy of local anesthetics in blocking the sensations of itch, burning, and pain in normal and "sunburned" skin. *Clin. Pharmacol. Ther.* 12:913–919, 1971.

Fisher, A. A.   Allergic reactions to topical (surface) anesthetics with reference to the safety of tronothane (Pramoxine hydrochloride). *Cutis* 25:584–591, 1980.

Juhlin, L., Evers, H., and Broberg, F.   A lidocaine-prilocaine cream for superficial skin surgery and painful lesions. *Acta Dermatol. Venerol.* 60:544–546, 1980.

Lamid, S., and Wang, R. H.   The range of local anesthetics. *Drug Ther.* 103–113, Aug. 1975.

Antihistamines

I. **Discussion.** There are two types of histamine receptors on many cells, and two types of antihistamines. These drugs antagonize the pharmacologic actions of histamine by occupying histamine receptor sites, but only if histamine has not yet reached its target receptors (competitive inhibition). Antihistamines are able to do this because they bear a close structural resemblance to histamine:

Histamine   Most antihistamines

They do not elicit any direct effect at the receptor sites, do not affect antibody production, antigen-antibody interactions, do not react chemically with histamine, and do not prevent its release. In addition, they may diminish capillary permeability to substances other than histamine and may also have a mild local anesthetic effect. Classic antihistamines (H1 blockers) do not alter gastric acid secretion; H2 antagonist drugs that are able to block specific cell wall receptors not affected by the older H1 compounds affect acid secretion and have been shown to be effective in treatment of gastric ulcers. Skin blood vessels possess both histamine H1 and H2 receptors and under experimental conditions combined H1 and H2 blockade has a greater effect on the response to histamine injected into the skin than either substance alone. Simultaneous use of H1 and H2 antihistamines has been found to be clinically effective in treatment of dermatographism, cold urticaria, and the flush associated with metastatic carcinoid (see p. 182). There are conflicting results from studies on combined H1-H2 antihistamine treatment of chronic urticaria.

The classic H1-blocking antihistamines are most effective in the management of acute urticaria and seasonal rhinitis. They are also currently the drugs of choice in the therapy of chronic urticaria, angioedema, and other allergic cutaneous reactions, including drug reactions. They are, however, of only limited value when given systemically for the relief of itching. Antihistamines have been shown to be no more effective than aspirin or a placebo for relief of nonhistamine-related itching (i.e., eczematous eruptions, as opposed to urticaria), but apparently there is an enormous placebo effect; in dealing with patients bothered by pruritus, the magnitude of this beneficial phenomenon should not be overlooked.

The several chemical classes of antihistamines show only minor variations in their properties. However, individuals frequently react differently to these preparations, and one or several antihistamines of different types may have to be tried, occasionally in combination, before the best therapeutic-sedative ratio is reached. Hydroxyzine appears to be the most effective drug in suppressing histamine-induced pruritus. In one experimental system, cyproheptadine and placebo administration necessitated a fivefold increase in the intradermal histamine dose required to produce pruritus compared to a tenfold increase following diphenhydramine and a 750-fold increase following hydroxyzine HCl.

Antihistamines are rapidly absorbed after oral or parenteral administration. Following an oral dose, symptomatic relief is noted within 15–30 min and usually lasts 3–6 hr. These drugs are metabolized mainly in the liver and excretion by the kidney is nearly complete in 24 hr. Antihistamines are also used topically in antipruritic lotions, but whatever small benefit might result is greatly overshadowed by the risk of inducing an allergic contact dermatitis, and this route should be avoided. The most common untoward systemic effect is sedation, and ambulatory patients must be warned of this, especially if driving is contemplated. Gastrointestinal side effects can also be seen. Because H1 antihistamines are structurally similar to atropine, they all produce atropinelike peripheral and central anticholinergic effects, including excitation, dry mouth, blurred vision, and urinary retention. Patients should be cautioned about taking alcoholic beverages or barbiturates during antihistamine therapy since the depressant action of these drugs is additive.

To be used most effectively, antihistamines should be gradually increased until either clinical remission occurs or side effects (most often sedation) become significant. It is usually unwise to start at too high a dose, and often the optimal course is to begin at 1 tablet q4h and to increase the number of tablets administered as long as the dosage remains ineffective. It is rarely necessary to exceed 4 tablets q4h but the interval between doses may be decreased if necessary. For general use, chlorpheniramine maleate and/or hydroxyzine hydrochloride or hydroxyzine pamoate have proved consistently effective.

II. Specific agents (all R$_x$)

A. Ethanolamine derivatives are potent antihistamines. However, there is a high incidence of sedation among patients who take them, and they have an additive effect with hypnotics and sedatives. With doses of 100 mg or more, hypertension, tachycardia, T-wave changes, or shortened diastole may further complicate the clinical picture.

1. Diphenhydramine hydrochloride (Benadryl)

a. Structure

Diphenhydramine

    b. Dosage: 50 mg (or 1 tsp) PO q4h.

    c. Packaging and cost:
        50-mg capsules: as diphenhydramine, 1000/$11.50
                      as Benadryl, 1000/$120.00
        Elixir (10 mg/4 ml): as diphenhydramine, 480 ml/$2.75
                      as Benadryl, 500 ml/$11.24

  2. Other ethanolamine antihistamines include bromodiphenhydramine hydrochloride (Ambenyl), carbinoxamine maleate (Clistin), clemastine fumarate (Tavist), dimenhydrinate (Dramamine), doxylamine succinate (Decapryn), and diphenylpyraline hydrochloride (Diafen, Hispril).

B. Ethylenediamine derivatives cause less drowsiness but more gastrointestinal side effects. These antihistamines must be avoided in individuals with contact allergy to ethylenediamine. Because of structural similarities it would also be wise to avoid piperazine and hydroxyzine antihistamines as well in these patients.

  1. Tripelennamine hydrochloride (Pyribenzamine)

    a. Structure

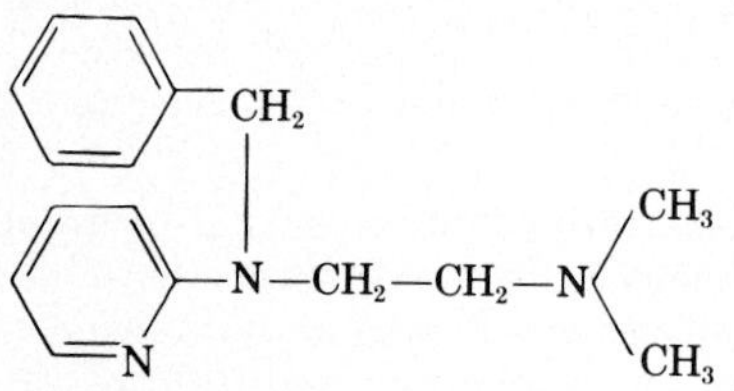

    Tripelennamine

    b. Dosage: 50 mg PO q4h.

    c. Packaging and cost:
        50-mg tablets: as tripelennamine, 1000/$9.00

  2. Other ethylenediamine antihistamines include methapyrilene hydrochloride (Histadyl), pyrilamine maleate (Fiogesic, Ryna).

C. The hydroxyzine antihistamines, hydroxyzine hydrochloride (Atarax), or hydroxyzine pamoate (Vistaril), are commonly also used for mild calming effects as tranquilizers.

  1. Structure

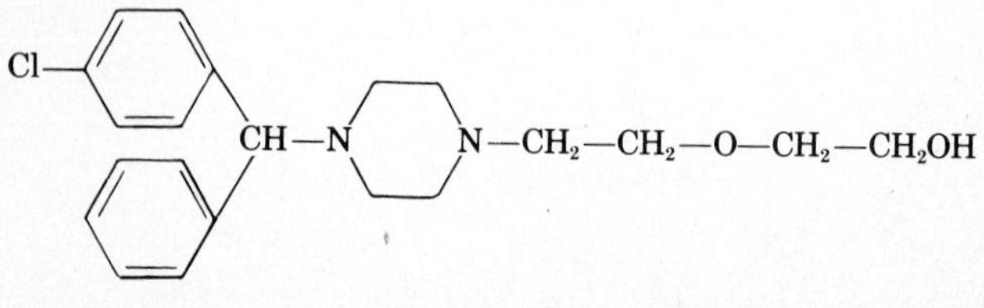

    Hydroxyzine

2. **Use:** These are the drugs of choice for therapy of dermatographism and cholinergic urticaria, and are also effective alone or in combination with other antihistamines in the therapy of acute and chronic urticaria and pruritus.

3. **Dosage:** 25 mg PO q4h.

4. **Packaging and cost:**
   10-mg tablets: as Atarax, 100/$18.00
   25-mg tablets: as Atarax, 100/$30.00
        as generic, 100/$12.00
        syrup, 500 ml/$20.00

D. Alkylamine derivatives include some of the most active antihistamines effective in low dosage. As there is no variation in the effectiveness of members of this antihistamine class, particular emphasis should be placed on the lower cost and easy availability of chlorpheniramine.

1. **Brompheniramine maleate (Dimetane).** The only difference between this and chlorpheniramine is the substitution of a bromine for a chlorine atom in the first.

   a. **Dosage:** 4 mg PO q4h; 1 tsp (2 mg) q4h.

   b. **Packaging and cost:**
   4-mg tablets: as brompheniramine, 100/$2.00
       as Dimetane, 100/$5.25
   Elixir (4 mg/5 ml): as brompheniramine, 500 ml/$3.00
         as Dimetane, 500 ml/$6.75

2. **Chlorpheniramine maleate (Chlor-Trimeton)**

   a. **Structure**

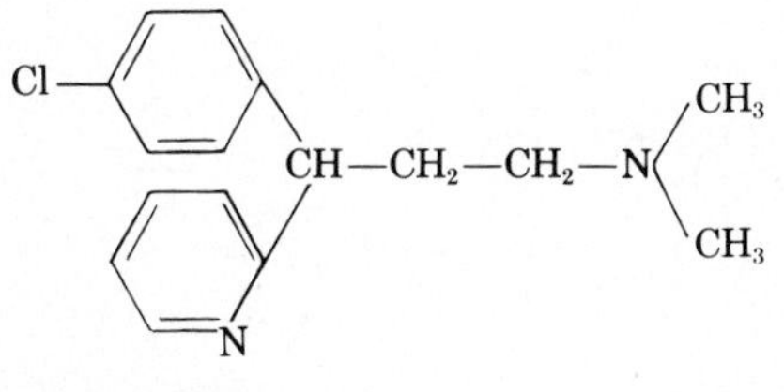

   Chlorpheniramine

   b. **Dosage:** 4 mg PO q4h.

   c. **Packaging and cost:**
   4-mg tablets: as chlorpheniramine, 1000/$3.50
       as Chlor-Trimeton, 1000/$67.00
   Chlor-Trimeton and chlorpheniramine maleate, 4 and 8 mg, are available as nonprescription OTC drugs.

3. **Dexchlorpheniramine maleate (Polaramine)** is the dextrorotatory isomer of chlorpheniramine.

   a. **Dosage:** 2 mg PO q4h.

   b. **Packaging and cost:**
   2-mg tablets: as Polaramine, 100/$9.00

4. Other alkylamine antihistamines include dimethindene maleate (Forhistal maleate, Triten), triprolidine hydrochloride (Actidil), and dexbrompheniramine maleate (Disomer).

E. Phenothiazine derivatives are used primarily as central nervous system depressants, but some are useful as antihistaminics.

   1. Promethazine hydrochloride (Phenergan)

      a. Structure

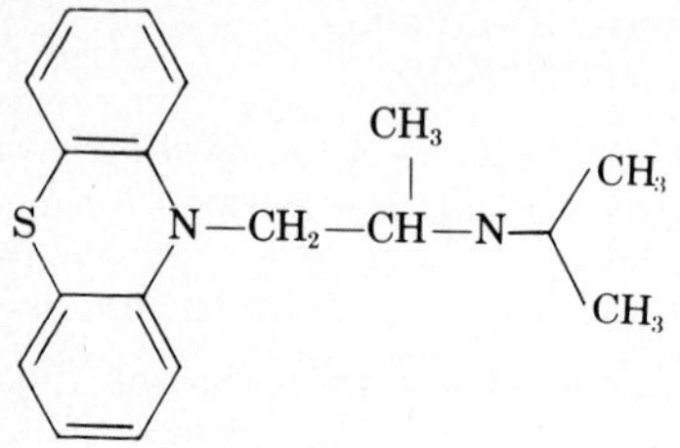

Promethazine

      b. Dosage: 12.5 mg PO 4id; 25 mg PO hs.

      c. Packaging and cost:
        25-mg tablets: as promethazine, 1000/$9.00
                        as Phenergan, 1000/$163.00

   2. Trimeprazine tartrate (Temaril)

      a. Structure

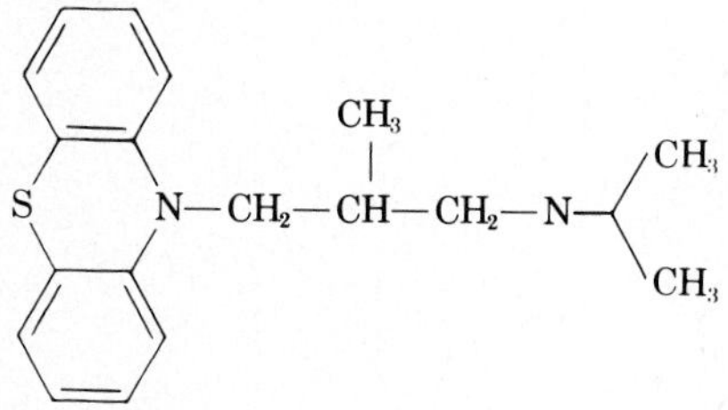

Trimeprazine

      b. Dosage: 2.5 mg PO q4h.

      c. Packaging and cost:
        2.5-mg tablets: as Temaril, 100/$15.00

   3. Methdilazine (Tacaryl) is another phenothiazine derivative antihistamine.

F. Piperidine derivatives

   1. Cyproheptadine hydrochloride (Periactin) is an antihistamine in which antiserotonin activity has been demonstrated both in vivo and in vitro. As yet, however, there is no evidence that this action contributes to clinical therapeutic effects.

a. Structure

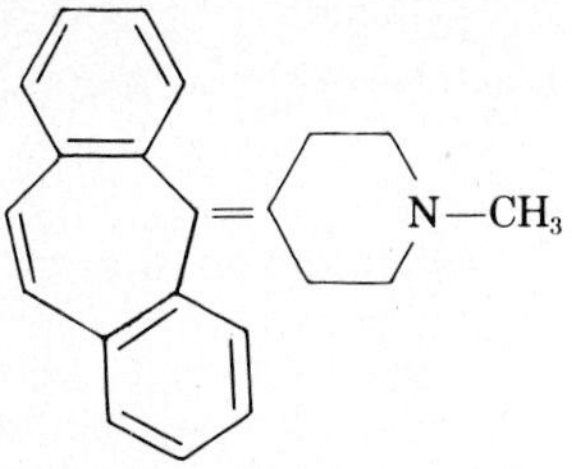

Cyproheptadine

b. Dosage: 4 mg PO q4h.

c. Packaging and cost:
4-mg tablets: as Periactin, 100/$18.25

2. Azatadine maleate (Optimine) is another piperidine antihistamine.

G. Piperazine antihistamines are H1 blocking agents that include chlorcyclizine hydrochloride (Fedrazil, Mantadil), cyclizine hydrochloride (Migral, Marezine), buclizine hydrochloride (Bucladin-S), and meclizine hydrochloride (Bonine, Antivert).

H. Thioguanidine derivatives block histamine H2 receptors.

1. Cimetidine (Tagamet) is used principally for the treatment of peptic ulcer through blocking gastric parietal cell receptors and gastric acid secretion.

a. Structure:

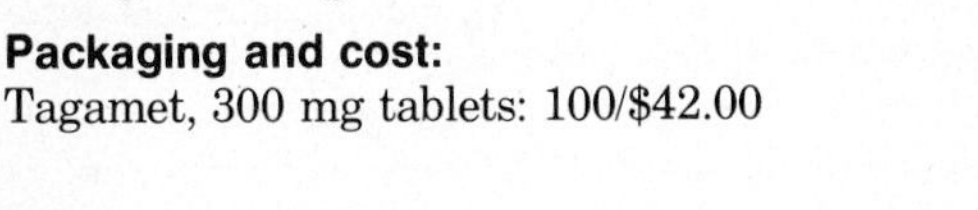

Cimetidine

b. Dosage: 300 mg PO 4id.

c. Packaging and cost:
Tagamet, 300 mg tablets: 100/$42.00

References

ANTIHISTAMINES

Beaven, M. A.   Histamine. *N. Engl. J. Med.* 294:30–35, 1976.

Davies, M. G., and Greaves, M. W.   The current status of histamine receptors in human skin: Therapeutic implications. *Br. J. Dermatol.* 104:601–606, 1981.

Fisher, A. A.   The antihistamines. *J. Am. Acad. Dermatol.* 3:303–306, 1980.

Hagermark, O.   Influence of antihistamines, sedatives and aspirin on experimental itch. *Arch. Derm. Venereol.* (Stockh.) 53:363–368, 1973.

Rhoades, R. B., Leifer, K. N., Cohan, R., and Wittig, H. J. Suppression of histamine-induced pruritus by three antihistamine drugs. *J. Allergy Clin. Immunol.* 55:180–185, 1975.

Savin, J. A. Do systemic antipruritic agents work? *Br. J. Dermatol.* 102:113–118, 1980.

Anti-infective agents

I. **Antibacterial and antiseptic agents, topical. Antiseptic agents** are applied to tissue to destroy microorganisms or inhibit their reproduction or metabolic activity. The major uses of antiseptics are as hand scrubs, cleansers, irrigants, and protective dressings. Commonly used antiseptics include ethyl and isopropyl alcohols, cationic surfactants (e.g., benzalkonium), chlorhexidine, iodine compounds, and hexachlorophene. **Disinfectants** are used on nonliving agents to destroy microorganisms and prevent infection. Some diluted disinfectants are used as antiseptics. The most commonly used disinfectants are the aldehydes (formaldehyde and gluteraldehyde), elemental chlorine, and cresol (a phenolic compound). Topical antibiotics have long been used to prevent or treat cutaneous bacterial infection yet it is only recently that the effectiveness of this therapy has been critically evaluated.

Numerous antibacterial agents are available for topical use. In general, those of most benefit are either combinations of the "nonabsorbable" antibiotics (bacitracin, gramicidin, neomycin) or the iodophors (e.g., povidone-iodine). Topical erythromycin is also effective and is the drug of choice when contact irritation or sensitivity occurs to the poorly absorbed agents. Use of broad-spectrum germicides or of topical antibiotics, singly or as mixtures, is justified for many reasons: (1) They can treat a wide range of potential pathogens in mixed infections—frequently more than one pathogen is present and quick identification of organisms is difficult. (2) They are used in small amounts and thus permit use of drugs that are relatively toxic when given systemically. Percutaneous absorption of antibiotics from normal skin or from psoriatic or eczematous areas cannot be detected in blood or urine— the possibility of producing nephrotoxicity or ototoxicity is extremely unlikely. Neomycin is the only potential allergen, and between 3.7 and 60% of individuals with chronic dermatoses have been shown to be allergic by patch testing. The incidence of sensitization of normal subjects in the general population is not known. (3) The concentration of the drugs is high, though the total amounts are small; this represents large multiples of the minimum effective concentration for potential pathogens. (4) Topically administered drugs are in more direct contact with organisms so that the problems of absorption, distribution, and availability to the infected site are not involved. (5) The combined effects of bactericidal agents such as bacitracin, neomycin, and polymyxin B are predominantly synergistic, thus increasing the rate of bactericidal action and killing large numbers of bacteria more rapidly, and probably increasing the spectrum of their action. *Staphylococcus aureus* is highly susceptible to the bactericidal action of neomycin and static action of tetracyclines, while *Streptococcus pyogenes* is particularly susceptible to bacitracin and neomycin. Neomycin is approximately 50 times more active against staphylococci than bacitracin (by weight), but bacitracin is 20 times more active against streptococci. Of gram-negative invaders, all but *Proteus* species are sensitive to polymyxin B and all but *Pseudomonas* are sensitive to neomycin—thus, to cover this spectrum, combinations of two or three antibiotics may be necessary. (6) Another combined effect is to delay and depress the development of resistance or emergence of resistant mutants. This is true particularly with regard to neomycin and to gentamicin. Although outbreaks of neomycin-resistant infections have been noted in closed communities, the incidence of resistance to this antibiotic has not materially changed during the last 20 years.

With regard to treatment of infected dermatoses, agents that modify the underlying inflammatory condition (e.g., corticosteroids) seem to be as effective as topical antibiotics or antibiotic-corticosteroid combinations. Local treatment does not diminish the reservoir of pathogens in the lesion or on the rest of the body, however; systemic antibiotics are best for that task. Similarly, impetigo should be treated with systemic antibiotics as discussed on p. 25. There is as yet no evidence to show whether topical antibiotics applied to the first wound in the skin would prevent it from becoming impetiginous, but once established, pyodermas are best treated with systemic agents.

Review of the data indicates that topical antibiotic preparations may effectively control the bacteria usually found in superficial wounds. They can reduce colony counts of bacteria and hence are effective for axillary deodorization or controlling nasal carriage of staphylococci. These antibiotics may also be useful in preventing infections in clean wounds, and when used early, might diminish the amount of infection, hasten healing, and reduce systemic effects of infection in infected wounds such as incisions, lacerations, or burns. Some topical antibiotics and antibiotic-corticosteroid creams have been classified by the FDA as lacking adequate evidence of effectiveness.

These preparations should be applied frequently (3–6 times a day) after the skin is cleansed of adherent crusts and debris and should not be applied under occlusive dressings.

A. **Aluminum** salts have strong antibacterial effects. 1% aluminum chlorohydrate, 10% aluminum acetate, and 30% aluminum chloride hexahydrate completely inhibit representative dermatophytes, yeasts, and gram-positive and gram-negative bacteria in vitro. In vivo, 20% aluminum chlorohydrate, 10–20% aluminum acetate, and 20–30% aluminum chloride hexahydrate have appreciable direct killing effects with the chlorohydrate salt being most potent. Recommended use concentrations (1:20 and 1:40) of 5% aluminum diacetate (Burow's solution) exert no in vivo bacteriostatic or bactericidal effects. Aluminum chloride hexahydrate 20–30% solution is effective in treating symptomatic interdigital tinea pedis because of bacterial killing effects as well as this salt's unique astringent (drying) properties, and 6% aluminum chloride hexahydrate has been found useful for treatment of folliculitis, notably of the buttocks. Aluminum salts are also effective as antiperspirants (see p. 286) and used as topical therapy for acne (see p. 7).

1. **Packaging and cost:**
   20% aluminum chloride hexahydrate (Drysol), 34.5 ml/$6.25
   6.25% aluminum chloride hexahydrate (Xerac-AC), 30 ml/$5.75
   Aluminum chloride hexahydrate crystals (AluWets), 6 packets/$3.25
   20–30% aluminum chloride hexahydrate solution may be compounded by dissolving AluWets crystals in absolute ethyl alcohol.

B. **Bacitracin.** This polypeptide antibiotic, which is produced from *Bacillus subtilis,* interferes with cell wall growth and is bactericidal against many gram-positive organisms such as streptococci, staphylococci, and pneu-mococci, but is inactive against most gram-negative organisms. All an-aerobic cocci, *Neisseria,* and the tetanus and diphtheria bacilli are also sensitive to bacitracin. Resistance is rare, but some staphylococcal strains are inherently resistant. Hypersensitivity reactions are uncommon. Bacitracin is stable in petrolatum (but not water-miscible preparations) and is available as an ointment or as a component of antibiotic mixtures.

1. Structure

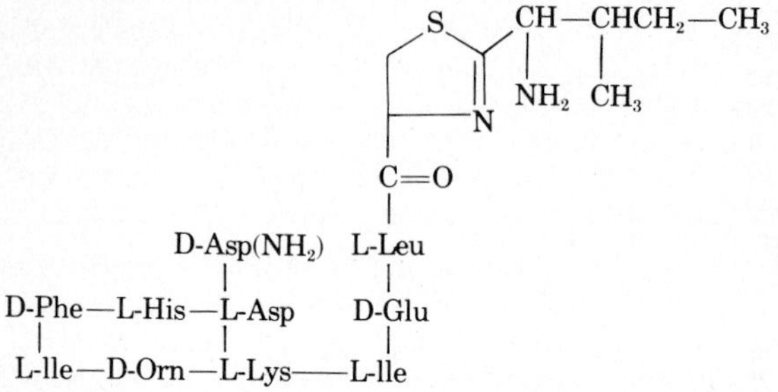

Bacitracin

2. Use: Clean wound and apply 4–6 times a day.

3. Packaging and cost:
500 units/gm: 15-gm tube/$1.25

C. Chlorhexidine. This topical antiseptic product acts rapidly but like hexachlorophene persists on the skin to give a cumulative, continuing antibacterial effect. Like iodophors and alcohol it is active against gram-positive and gram-negative bacteria as well as common yeasts and fungi. It does not lose effectiveness in the presence of whole blood. In many centers it is currently the antiseptic of choice for skin cleansing and sur-gical scrubs.

1. Structure:

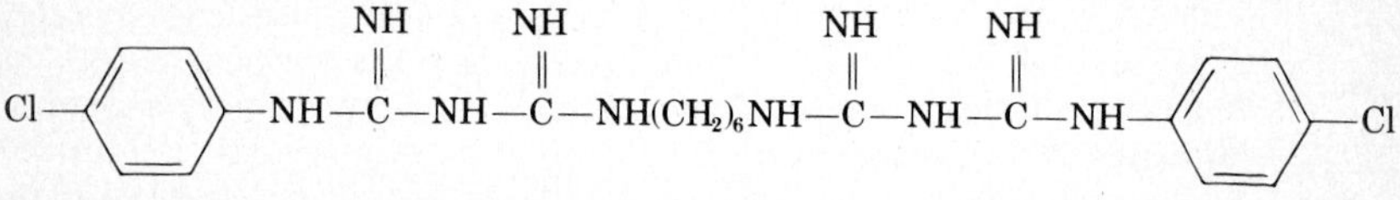

Chlorhexidine

2. Packaging and cost:
Hibiclens Skin Cleanser, 4% chlorhexidine gluconate in sudsing base, 120 ml/$4.25
Hibistat Germicidal Hand Rinse, 0.5% chlorhexidine in 70% isopropyl alcohol, 120 ml/$2.60

D. Gentamicin (Garamycin). This antibiotic is a combination of three re-lated aminoglycoside agents obtained from cultures of *Micromonospora purpurea* and acts by interfering with the bacterial synthesis of protein. Its antibiotic spectrum is similar to that of neomycin and cross resistance does occur. Gentamicin is active against gram-negative organisms in-cluding *Escherichia coli* and a high percentage of strains of species of

Pseudomonas and other gram-negative bacteria. *Proteus* organisms show a variable degree of sensitivity. Some gram-positive organisms, including *S. aureus* and group A beta-hemolytic streptococci, are also affected. In general, higher concentrations are needed to inhibit streptococci than are needed to inhibit staphylococci and many gram-negative bacteria. The most important use of gentamicin is in the treatment of systemic gram-negative infections, particularly those due to *Pseudomonas* organisms. Widespread topical use is unwarranted, since equally effective drugs are available, and widespread utilization will increase the background of gentamicin-resistant organisms as well as the incidence of allergic sensitization.

1. Structure

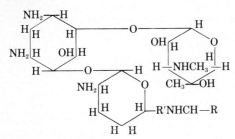

Gentamicin sulfate

Gentamicin	R	R′
C_1	CH_3	CH_3
C_2	CH_3	H
C_{1A}	H	H

2. Use: Clean lesion and apply 4–6 times a day.

3. Packaging and cost:
   15-gm cream or ointment: as Garamycin/$6.00

E. Iodophors. These consist of a water-soluble organic complex of iodine with a carrier that slowly liberates iodine on contact with reducing substances in body tissues. These broad-range germicidal antiseptics are effective against bacteria, fungi, viruses, protozoa, and yeasts. They are water-soluble, nonirritating, and nonstinging, but may lose effectiveness on contact with whole blood or serum. They are often used for preoperative skin cleansing and surgical scrubbing and as treatment for skin infections and burns. They are available in many vehicles. The solubilizing carrier substances include polyvinyl-pyrrolidone (povidone-iodine, as in Betadine products, or available as generics) and poloxamer-iodine complexes.

1. Structure

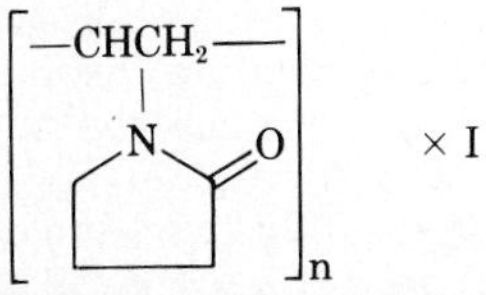

$$\left[\begin{array}{c} -CHCH_2- \\ | \\ N \diagdown \diagup O \end{array} \right]_n \times I$$

Povidone-iodine

2. **Packaging and cost** (as Betadine microbicidal antiseptics):
Solution: 15 ml/$1.25
Surgical scrub: 480 ml with pump/$10.50
Douche: 240 ml/$10.00
Ointment: 30 gm/$4.50
Shampoo: 120 ml/$5.75
Skin cleanser: 120 ml/$5.00
as generic: surgical scrub: 500 ml/$3.50
            solution: 500 ml/$4.25

F. **Neomycin sulfate.** This drug is obtained from species of the actinomycete *Streptomyces* and is an aminoglycoside antibiotic (as are streptomycin, gentamicin, and kanamycin) effective against most gram-negative organisms. Group A streptococci are relatively resistant. Neomycin acts by inhibiting protein synthesis, as do all aminoglycosides. It is responsible for a greater incidence of allergic contact sensitivity than any other topical antibiotic. This diagnosis often remains hidden, since morphologically the eruption is of a mild eczematous nature, and it frequently appears as if the original cutaneous disease were unaffected by treatment.

1. **Structure**

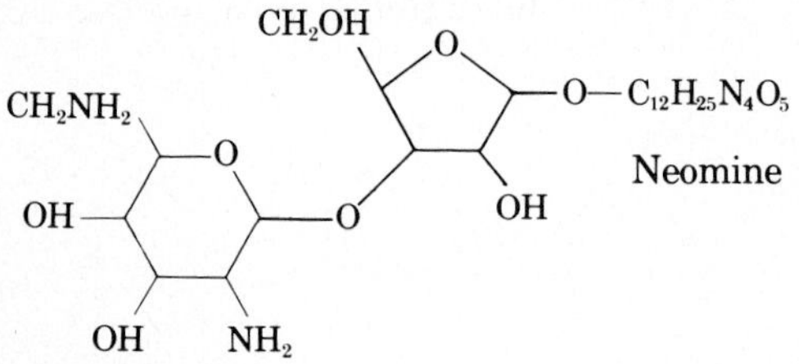

Neomycin B

2. **Use:** Apply 4–6 times a day.

3. **Packaging and cost:**
15-gm ointment/$1.25

G. **Polymyxin B.** Polymyxin B is one of a group of cyclic polypeptides, elaborated by *Bacillus polymyxa*. The drug is a surface-active agent and is thought to alter the lipoprotein membrane of bacteria so that it no longer functions as an effective barrier, and thereby allows the cell contents to escape. Polymyxin B is effective against *Pseudomonas* and other gram-negative bacteria except the *Proteus* and *Serratia* species and has little effect on gram-positive organisms.

H. **Tyrothricin.** Tyrothricin, containing **gramicidin** and **tyrocidine,** is a mixture of polypeptide antibiotics bactericidal for common gram-positive organisms but generally inactive against gram-negative organisms. Gramicidin uncouples oxidative phosphorylation, while tyrocidine decreases bacterial cell respiration, with concomitant leakage of amino acids into the surrounding medium. Tyrothricin has the advantage of a wide gram-positive spectrum, no sensitizing properties or tissue toxicity, and rarity of acquired resistance. It is frequently found as a component of antibacterial mixtures for topical use.

I. Combination topical preparations

1. Neo-Polycin ointment

a. **Contains:** per gm, 8000 units polymyxin B sulfate, 400 units zinc bacitracin, 3 mg neomycin sulfate (as base).

b. **Dosage:** Apply 4–6 times a day.

c. **Packaging and cost:**
as generic, 15-gm tube/$1.25
as Neo-Polycin, 15-gm tube/$4.00

2. Neosporin aerosol

a. **Contains:** per 90 gm, 100,000 units polymyxin B sulfate, 8000 units zinc bacitracin, 70 mg neomycin sulfate (as base).

b. **Dosage:** Apply 4–6 times a day.

c. **Packaging (R$_x$) and cost:**
90-gm can/$7.25

3. Neosporin ointment

a. **Contains:** per gm, 5000 units polymyxin B sulfate, 400 units zinc bacitracin, 3.5 mg neomycin sulfate (as base).

b. **Dosage:** Apply 4–6 times a day.

c. **Packaging and cost:**
as generic, 15-gm tube/$1.25
as Neosporin, 15-gm tube/$4.25

4. Neosporin powder

a. **Contains:** per gm, 5000 units polymyxin B sulfate, 400 units zinc bacitracin, 3.5 mg neomycin sulfate (as base).

b. **Dosage:** Apply 4–6 times a day. Neosporin powder is particularly useful in the therapy of erosions and ulcers.

c. **Packaging (R$_x$) and cost:**
10-gm shaker-top container/$5.25

5. Neosporin G cream

a. **Contains:** per gm, 10,000 units polymyxin B sulfate, 3.5 gm neomycin sulfate (as base), and 0.25 mg gramicidin.

b. **Dosage:** Apply 4–6 times a day.

c. **Packaging (R$_x$) and cost:**
15-gm tube/$3.00

6. Polysporin ointment

a. **Contains:** per gm, 10,000 units polymyxin B sulfate with 500 units zinc bacitracin.

b. **Packaging and cost:**
15 gm/$4.00

References

ANTI-INFECTIVE AGENTS

Anderson, V. (ed.).   Over-the-counter topical antibiotic products: Data on safety and efficacy. *Int. J. Dermatol.* (Suppl.) 15:2, 1976.

Fisher, A. A., and Adams, R. M.   Alternative for sensitizing neomycin topical medicaments. *Cutis* 28:491–503, 1981.

Leyden, J. J., and Kligman, A. M.   Aluminum chloride in the treatment of symptomatic athlete's foot. *Arch. Dermatol.* 111:1004–1010, 1975.

Leyden, J. J., and Kligman, A. M.   Criticism of "the case against topical antibiotics." *Prog. Dermatol.* 11:7–8, 1977.

Leyden, J. J., and Kligman, A. M.   Rationale for topical antibiotics. *Cutis* 22:515–527, 1978.

Leyden, J. J., Stewart, R., and Kligman, A. M.   Updated *in vivo* methods for evaluating topical antimicrobial agents on human skin. *J. Invest. Dermatol.* 72:165–170, 1979.

Peterson, A. F., Rosenberg, A., and Alatary, S. D.   Comparative evaluation of surgical scrub preparations. *Surg. Gyn. Obs.* 146:63–65, 1978.

Prystowsky, S. D., Allen, A. M., Smith, R. W., Nonomura, J. H., Odom, R. B., and Akers, W. A.   Allergic contact hypersensitivity to nickel, neomycin, ethylenediamine and benzocaine: Relationships between age, sex, history of exposure, and reactivity to standard patch tests and use tests in a general population. *Arch. Dermatol.* 115:959–962, 1979.

Rasmussen, J. E.   The case against topical antibiotics. *Prog. Dermatol.* 11:1–4, 1977.

Rasmussen, J. E.   Criticism of "the case for topical antibiotics." *Prog. Dermatol.* 11:5–7, 1977.

Shelley, W. B., and Hurley, H. J.   Anhydrous formulation of aluminum chloride for chronic folliculitis. *J. A. M. A.* 244:1956–1957, 1980.

II. Antifungal agents

A. Discussion. See Fungal Infections, p. 79.

B. Prescription drugs

    1. Acrisorcin (Akrinol) cream is effective in vitro against a variety of bacteria, fungi, and protozoa. Clinically, it is used solely for the topical therapy of tinea versicolor.

        a. Dosage: See p. 89.

        b. Packaging (R$_x$) and cost:
           50-gm tube/$7.25

    2. Amphotericin B (Fungizone) is one of the polyene group of antifungal antibiotics used topically in the treatment of superficial *Candida albicans* infection and is the therapy of choice for many systemic fungal infections. It is ineffective against dermatophytes. The drug is yellow orange, odorless, and may stain skin.

a. Structure

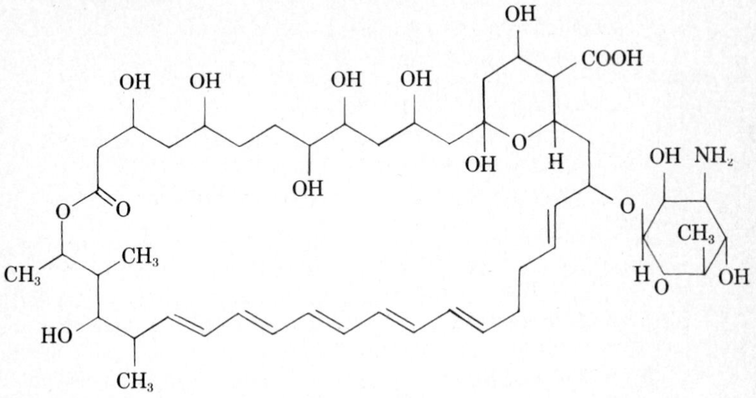

Amphotericin B

b. Dosage: Apply 4–6 times a day.

c. Packaging (Rₓ) and cost:
as Fungizone: 3% cream and ointment, 20 gm/$12.00
3% lotion, 30 ml/$16.00

3. **Candicidin (Candeptin, Vanobid)** is a polyene antifungal antibiotic similar chemically and in spectrum to amphotericin B. It is used topically only in the treatment of monilial vulvovaginitis.

a. Packaging (Rₓ) and cost:
Ointment: 75 gm × 2/$11.00
Vaginal tablets: package of 28/$8.50

4. **Clotrimazole (Lotrimin, Mycelex)** is a synthetic imidazole agent used for treatment of superficial fungal infections and *C. albicans* infections. It inhibits the growth of most dermatophyte species, is as active as nystatin against *C. albicans,* inhibits growth of some gram-positive bacteria, and in high concentrations is active against *Trichomonas* species. Its mechanism of action is not clear but probably involves damage to the cell wall in a fashion similar to that of the polyene antibiotics.

a. Structure

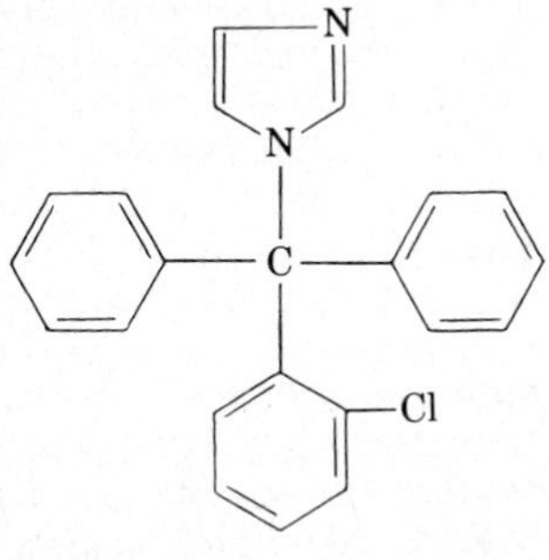

Clotrimazole

   b. **Dosage:** Apply 2–3 times a day until eruption clears (see p. 86).

   c. **Packaging (R$_x$) and cost:**
      Cream: 15-gm tube/$5.50
      45-gm tube/$11.00
      Solution: 10 ml/$4.75
      30 ml/$10.00
      Vaginal tablets (Gyne-Lotrimin): pkg of 7/$10.00
      Vaginal Cream (Gyne-Lotrimin): 45 gm/$9.75

5. **Griseofulvin** is an antifungal antibiotic effective against all dermatophyte fungi, but not against *C. albicans* or tinea versicolor. It causes stunting and curling of hyphae growing in vitro and was initially called the "curling factor." Griseofulvin resembles colchicine structurally and can cause metaphase arrest in rapidly dividing cells. It is absorbed by the gastrointestinal tract more rapidly after a fatty meal, but total absorption after 24 hr is constant and is not affected by taking griseofulvin with or between meals, or in single or divided doses. Absorption may possibly be greater if the drug is taken during the middle of the day. Microsize griseofulvin is produced by a special process that fractures the particles into minute crystals of irregular shape that offer a greater surface for increased gastrointestinal absorption. Further process to achieve ultramicrosize particles has been found to almost double the bioavailability; 125 mg were thought to be equivalent to 250 mg of microsize griseofulvin, but recent data indicate that it takes 150–200 mg to achieve bioequivalent plasma levels. Griseofulvin enters the epidermis by diffusion forces from extracellular fluid (through transepidermal water loss) and from sweat and reaches higher concentrations in the horny layer than in serum. With excessive sweating in hot, humid climates the amount of griseofulvin in skin is likely to be reduced, and more of the drug should be taken. The response to therapy depends on the rate of keratinization and the time necessary for desquamation of infected keratinized structures. Its use is contraindicated in patients with porphyria.

Griseofulvin may cause a reversal of the hypoprothrombinemic effect of anticoagulants, necessitating an increase in the dose of anticoagulant to maintain a therapeutic range of anticoagulation. This effect occurs through increased synthesis of drug-metabolizing liver enzymes, leading to more rapid inactivation of anticoagulants. Phenobarbital has been postulated to decrease the gut absorption of griseofulvin, thus decreasing blood levels and presumably decreasing antifungal action. Griseofulvin has the following cure rates (Anderson, 1965): tinea capitis, 93.1%; tinea of the glabrous skin, 64.8%; tinea of the palms and soles, 53.3%; tinea of the fingernails, 56.9%; and tinea of the toenails, 16.7%. Failure of fungal infection to respond to this therapy may occur because of inadequate dosage, poor compliance, inadequate absorption, microsomal enzyme inactivation and drug interaction, failure of griseofulvin to enter the site of infection or diminished activity within that site, or infection with an organism not sensitive to griseofulvin. The latter had been postulated but only recently was it shown that for *T. rubrum* infections of body, palms, and soles, a poor clinical response correlates with a diminished in-vitro sensitivity to this antimycotic. Minimal inhibitory concentration determinations for griseofulvin can be used to determine the appropriateness of this therapy.

a. Structure

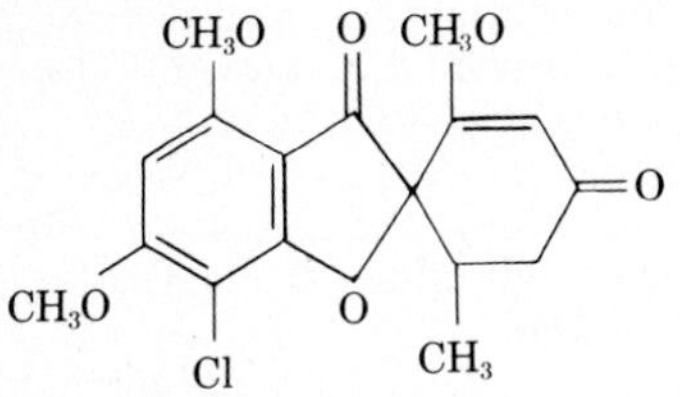

Griseofulvin

b. Dosage: See Fungal Infections, p. 87.

c. Packaging (R$_x$) and cost:
Microcrystalline (Fulvicin-U/F, Grifulvin V, Grisactin):
  100 250-mg caps/$30.00
  100 500-mg caps/$52.00
Ultramicrosize dispersion in polyethylene glycol (Grisactin Ultra, Gris-PEG):
100 125-mg tablets/$18.00 (Fulvisin P/G; Grisactin Ultra; Gris-PEG)
  100 250-mg capsules/$52.00
  100 165-mg tablets (Fulvicin P/G)/$20.00
  100 330-mg tablets (Fulvicin P/G)/$36.00
Generic, microcrystalline: 100 250-mg caps/$22.00
Grifulvin V microcrystalline suspension (125 mg/5 ml): 120 ml/$7.50.

6. **Haloprogin (Halotex)** is a synthetic chlorinated iodopropynyl trichlorophenyl ether antifungal agent used in the topical treatment of dermatophyte infections and tinea versicolor. It is also active in vitro against staphylococci, streptococci, and *C. albicans*.

a. Structure

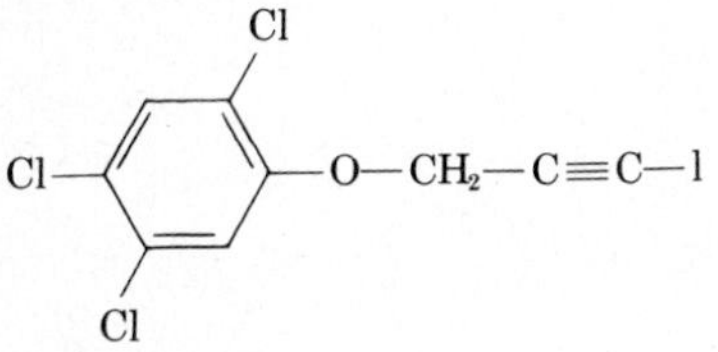

Haloprogin

b. Dosage: Apply 3id.

c. Packaging (R$_x$) and cost:
1% cream: 30 gm/$10.00
1% solution: 10 ml/$5.00
        30 ml/$10.00

7. **Ketoconazole (Nizoral)** is a water-soluble imidazole derivative with a wide spectrum of activity against pathogenic fungi at concen-

trations achievable with oral treatment. Unlike miconazole, it is well absorbed after oral administration, and unlike clotrimazole, it does not induce a liver enzyme that inactivates any absorbed drug. This drug, like other imidazoles, affects fungi by mechanisms involving increased membrane permeability, inhibition of uptake of precursors of RNA and DNA, and synthesis of oxidative and peroxidative enzymes. Ketoconazole's spectrum of activity includes *Candida* species, *Cryptococcus neoformans, Coccidioides immitis, Histoplasma capsulatum, Blastomyces dermatitidis,* and pathogenic dermatophytes. It is highly effective in chronic dermatophyte infections, including those resistant to griseofulvin and is effective for treatment of chronic mucocutaneous candidiasis.

Adverse effects appear to be few and only wider clinical experience will tell. Mild nausea and occasional vomiting may occur but can be controlled by taking the tablets with meals. There are rare reports of rash, hypoesthesias, gynecomastia. Abnormal liver function tests, hepatitis, and several cases of hepatic necrosis have been reported. Liver function tests should be monitored in patients on ketoconazole therapy. Ketoconazole is administered orally once daily with a meal. After gastric acidity solubilizes the tablet, maximum serum concentration is reached 2–4 hr later. This falls to 50% by 8 hr and to 20% of maximum at 24 hr. It penetrates poorly into the cerebrospinal fluid and is probably excreted in mother's milk. Ketoconazole is extensively degraded in the body and very little active drug is excreted either by renal or biliary pathways. The dose need not be modified for renal failure.

a. Structure:

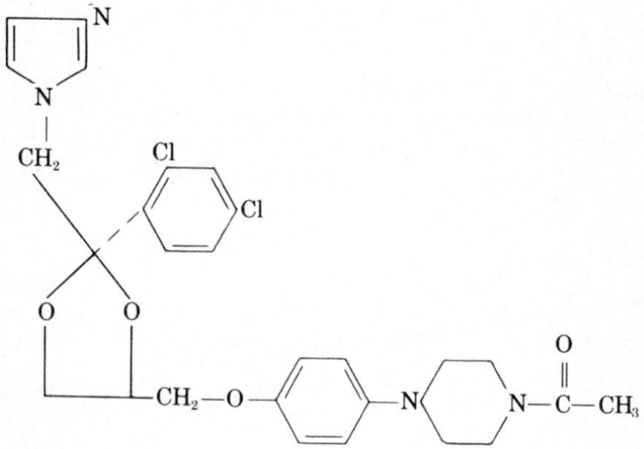

Ketoconazole

b. Dosage: See Fungal Infections, p. 88.

c. Packaging and cost:
100 200-mg tablets/$75–100.00.

8. **Nystatin,** a polyene antibiotic derived from a species of the actinomycete *Streptomyces noursei,* binds to sterols in fungal membranes, causing a change in the permeability of cell membranes and leakage

of cell components. It is nontoxic and available for oral, vaginal, and topical administration. Nystatin is poorly absorbed from the gastrointestinal tract and will thus rid the oral and gastrointestinal mucosa of *Candida* but have no effect on systemic or cutaneous lesions when given orally. Nystatin is unstable to heat, light, moisture, and air. Aqueous-alcohol suspensions are stable for 10 days under refrigeration.

a. Dosage: See Fungal Infections, p. 80.

b. Packaging (R_x) and cost:
Ointment and cream (100,000 units/gm) (Candex, Mycostatin, Nilstat): 15 gm/$6.75
Nystatin ointment and cream (100,000 units/gm) generic: 15 gm/$2.75
Powder (100,000 units) (Mycostatin): 15 mg/$10.00
Tablets (500,000 units) (Mycostatin): 100/$38.00
Tablets (500,000 units) generic: 100/$12.00
Oral suspension (100,000 units/ml) (Mycostatin): 60 ml/$15.00
Vaginal tablets (Mycostatin): 15/$8.50
Vaginal tablets, generic: 15/$8.50
Nystatin, neomycin sulfate, gramicidin, 0.1% triamcinolone acetonide (Mycolog) cream and ointment:
15 gm/$9.00
60 gm/$29.00

9. **Miconazole** (Monistat-Derm) is a synthetic imidazole antifungal compound effective against most dermatophyte species and against *C. albicans*. It is similar to clotrimazole (p. 259) in structure and efficacy, and can be used intravenously for systemic fungal infections. It destroys fungi presumably by inhibiting cell wall synthesis.

a. Structure

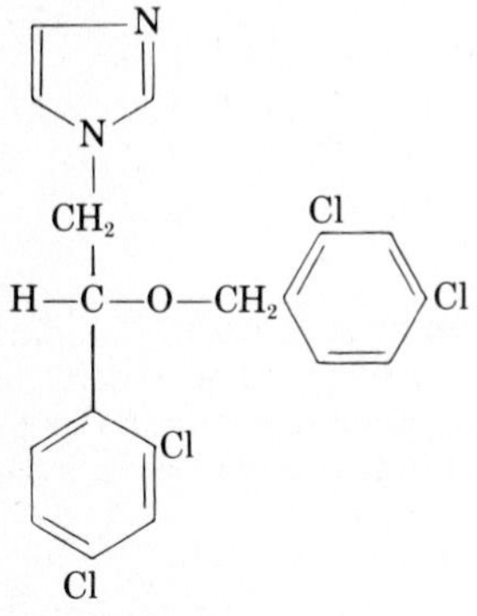

Miconazole

b. Dosage: Apply 2–3 times a day until eruption clears (see p. 80).

c. Packaging (R_x) and cost:
Monistat-Derm, 2% cream: 15 gm/$4.75
Monistat-Derm, 2% cream: 85 gm/$17.00
Monistat-Derm, 2% lotion: 30 ml/$10.00
Monistat-7, 2% vaginal cream: 47-gm tube with applicator/$10.00

10. **Tinver** contains 25% sodium thiosulfate ($Na_2S_2O_3$), 1% salicylic acid, and 10% alcohol and is used in treatment of tinea versicolor.

    a. **Dosage:** See p. 89.

    b. **Packaging (R_x) and cost:**
       180-ml lotion/$9.00

11. **Thymol** is an alkyl derivative of phenol with bactericidal and fungicidal properties. It is chiefly of value as a fungicide.

    a. **Structure**

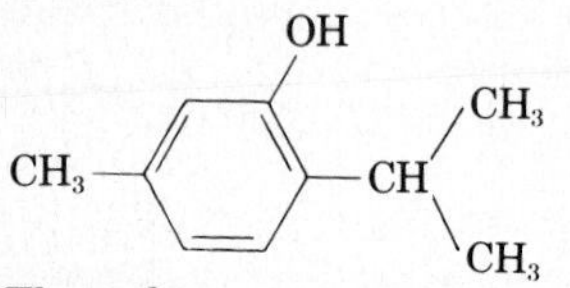

    Thymol

    b. **Dosage:** See p. 81.

C. OTC preparations

1. **Benzoic (12%) acid and salicylic (6%) acid (Whitfield's) ointment** is a potent keratolytic agent and is used in the treatment of dermatophyte infections (see also p. 86). It has, however, a strong potential for causing irritant reactions. It is also available in half-strength (6%/3%) concentration.

    a. **Structure**

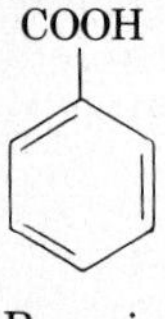

    Benzoic acid

    b. **Dosage:** Apply 2–4 times a day.

    c. **Packaging and cost:**
       30 gm/$1.00

2. **Carbol-fuchsin solution (Castellani's paint)** is a dark purple liquid that appears red on the skin. It has local anesthetic, bactericidal, and fungicidal properties and is applied topically in the treatment of subacute and chronic superficial fungal infection. It is particularly effective in intertriginous inflammation.

    a. **Structure**

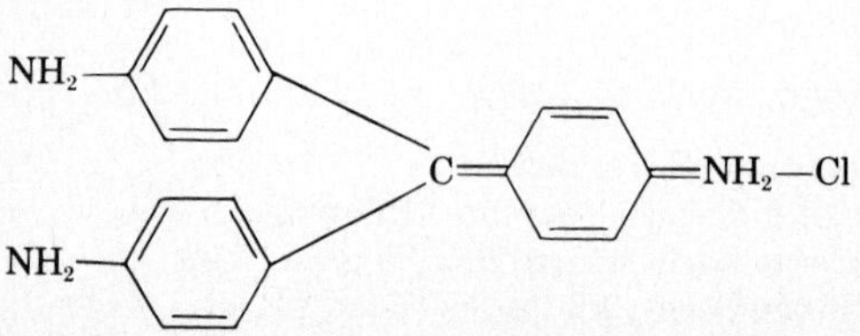

    Fuchsin (pararosaniline hydrochloride)

b. **Contains:**

Boric acid	1.0%
Phenol	4.5%
Resorcinol	10.0%
Fuchsin	0.3%
Acetone	5.0%
in water	

c. **Dosage:** Apply 1–3 times a day with swab. Clean skin with soap and water prior to application.

d. **Packaging and cost:** May be compounded by a pharmacist and is available generically or as Castaderm, 120 ml/$4.00.

3. **Gentian (crystal, methyl) violet (methylrosaniline chloride),** 0.5–3.0%, is used in the treatment of infections due to yeasts and molds. This triphenylmethane dye has also been effective in therapy of Vincent's angina and secondarily infected dermatoses and dermatophytoses.

a. **Structure**

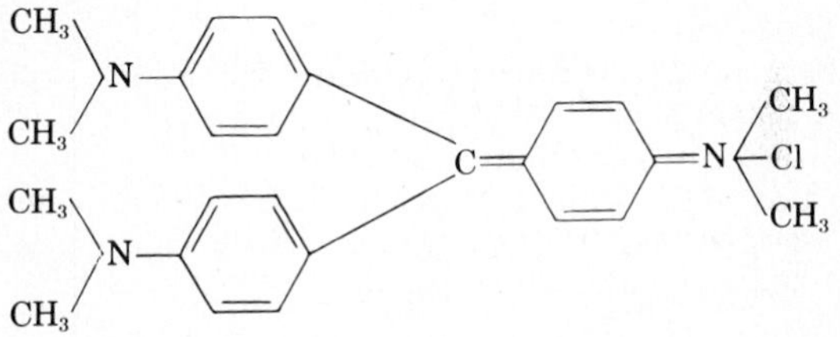

Gentian violet (methylrosaniline chloride)

b. **Dosage:** Apply with cotton 2id.

c. **Packaging and cost:**
1% solution: 30 ml/$1.25

4. **Sodium thiosulfate ($Na_2S_2O_3 \cdot 5\ H_2O$), 25%,** is an effective and inexpensive medication used in the treatment of tinea versicolor. The odor of sulfur sometimes offends patients.

a. **Packaging and cost:**
Compounded by the pharmacist to order, a typical cost would be 480 ml/$5.00.

5. **Tolnaftate (Tinactin and others)** is an odorless and nonstaining synthetic antifungal agent effective against all dermatophyte fungi and tinea versicolor. However, it is ineffective against *C. albicans* and bacteria.

a. **Structure**

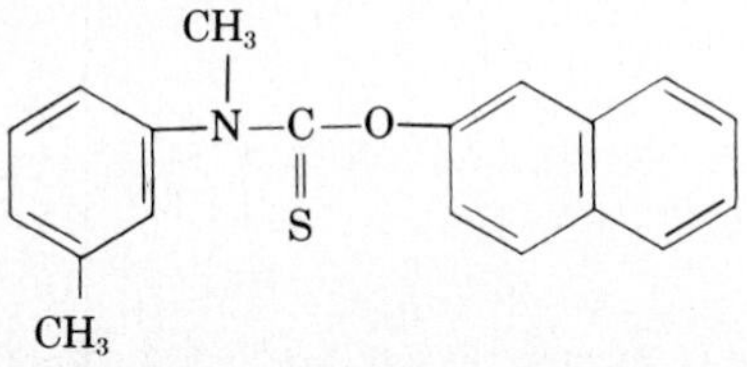

Tolnaftate

b. **Dosage:** Apply 2–3 times a day until the eruption has cleared (2–6 weeks) (see pp. 86, 89).

c. **Packaging and cost:**
Cream: 15 gm/$4.50
1% powder: 45 gm/$3.25
1% solution: 10 ml/$4.00

6. There are numerous **OTC antifungal remedies** that contain fatty acids and fatty acid salts (undecylenic acid $CH_2 = CH \ (CH_2)_8COOH$, proprionic acid), organic acids and their salts (benzoic acid, salicylic acid), and miscellaneous other compounds. They are all reasonably effective (see p. 86). Some common preparations and costs follow.

a. **Packaging and cost:**
Desenex
Ointment (5% undecylenic acid, 20% zinc undecylenate): 54 gm/ $4.50
Powder (2% undecylenic acid, 20% zinc undecylenate): 90 gm/$4.00

b. **Verdefam**
Solution (2% sodium proprionate, 2% sodium caprylate, 3% proprionic acid, 5% undecylenic acid, 5% salicylic acid, 0.5% copper undecylenate): 60 ml/$3.75
Cream (1% sodium proprionate, 1% sodium caprylate, 3% proprionic acid, 2% undecylenic acid, 3% salicylic acid, 0.5% copper undecylenate): 30 gm/$3.75

References

ANTIFUNGAL AGENTS

Cox, F. W., Stiller, R. L., South, D. A., and Stevens, D. A.   Oral ketoconazole for dermatophyte infections. *J. Am. Acad. Derm.* 6:455–462, 1982.

Graybill, J. R., and Drutz, D. J.   Ketoconazole: A major innovation for treatment of fungal disease. *Ann. Intern. Med.* 93:921–923, 1980.

III. Antiviral agents

A. **Acyclovir** is a drug that inhibits replication of herpesvirus in vitro and is being used and further evaluated for the prevention or treatment of infections with herpes simplex virus and varicella-zoster virus (see pp. 96, 97, 103). To inhibit the growth of herpes simplex virus and presumably that of varicella-zoster virus, acyclovir must first be phosphorylated to the respective monophosphates by virus-specific thymidine kinase and must then be converted by cellular enzymes to the respective triphosphates, which are the active and selective inhibitors of herpesvirus-specific DNA polymerase.

B. **Adenine arabinoside (vidarabine) (VIRA-A)** is a purine nucleoside which interferes with the early steps of viral DNA synthesis of herpes simplex, zoster-varicella, and vaccinia viruses.

1. **Dosage:** Apply 3id into conjunctival sac for herpes simplex keratitis.

2. **Packaging and cost:**
   3.5 gm/$12.00

C. **Idoxuridine (2′-Deoxy-5-iodouridine) (Dendrid, Herplex, Stoxil).** This is an antiviral agent that interferes with viral DNA synthesis. It is of proven value in the treatment of dendritic keratitis.

1. **Structure**

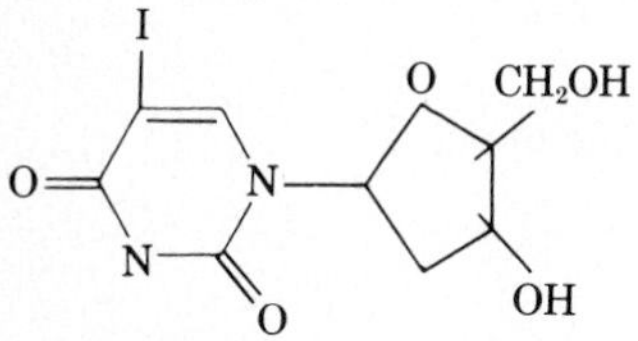

Idoxuridine

2. **Dosage:** See Herpes Simplex, p. 96.

3. **Packaging (R_x) and cost:**
   0.5% ointment (Stoxil): 4 gm/$8.50
   0.1% solution (Stoxil): 15 gm/$8.50

IV. **Scabicides and pediculicides.** (For discussion, see Infestations, p. 118.)

A. **Benzyl benzoate, 20–25%,** is effective in scabies and has been used to treat pediculosis capitis and pubis.

1. **Structure**

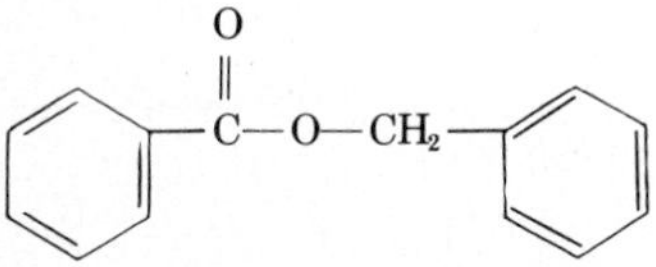

Benzyl benzoate

2. **Packaging and cost**
   as 50% emulsion: 500 ml/$5.25

B. **Chlorophenothane, USP (DDT)** (10% powder, 10% solution [R_x]) eradicates body lice and bedbugs and is an excellent insecticide for flies, mosquitoes, ants, cockroaches, and spiders.

1. **Structure**

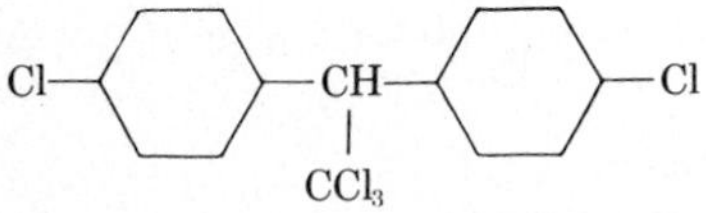

DDT

C. **Crotamiton (N-ethyl-o-crotonotoluide) (Eurax)** is used for the prevention and treatment of scabies.

1. **Structure**

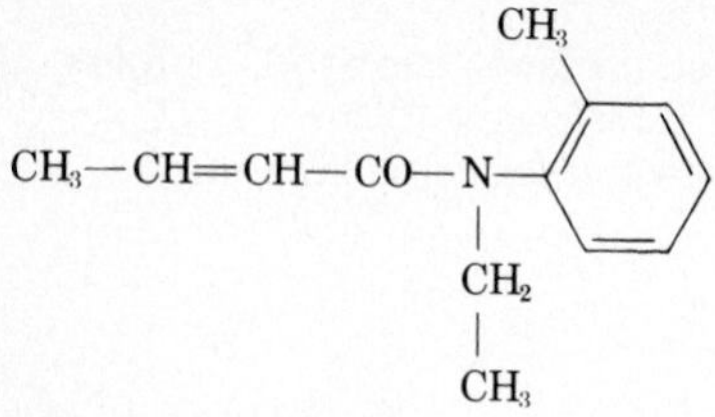

$$CH_3-CH=CH-CO-N \begin{array}{c} CH_3 \\ \hline \\ CH_2 \\ | \\ CH_3 \end{array}$$

Crotamiton (N-ethyl-o-crotonotoluide)

2. **Packaging (R_x) and cost:**
   10% cream: 60 gm/$4.00
   10% lotion: 60 ml/$4.50

D. **Gamma benzene hexachloride (Gamene, Kwell).** This a highly effective scabicide and pediculicide (see p. 118).

1. **Structure**

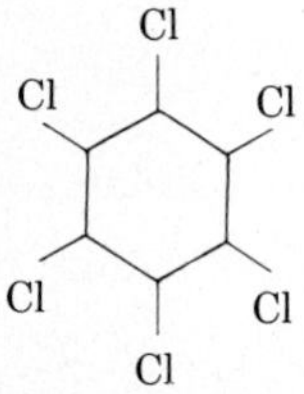

Gamma benzene hexachloride

2. **Packaging (R_x) and cost** (as Kwell):
   Cream: 60 ml/$4.75
   Lotion: 60 ml/$4.00; 500 ml/$28.00
   Shampoo: 60 ml/$4.00

E. **Malathion** (0.5% lotion, 1% powder) is effective in the prevention and treatment of pediculosis.

1. **Structure**

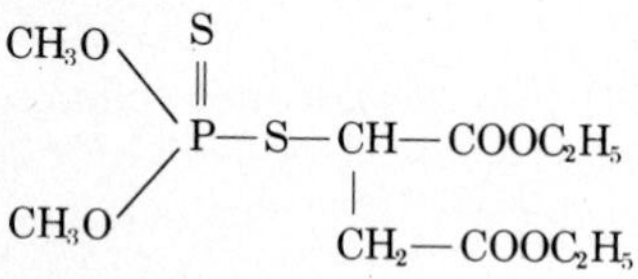

$$\begin{array}{c} CH_3O \\ \\ CH_3O \end{array} P-S-CH-COOC_2H_5 \\ | \\ CH_2-COOC_2H_5$$

Malathion

F. **Pyrethrin** compounds are used for the treatment of pediculosis (see p. 120).

1. **Packaging (R_x) and cost:**
   Gel (A-200 Pyrinate): 30 gm/$4.00
   Liquid (A-200 Pyrinate, RID): 60 ml/$4.00

V. **Miscellaneous Agents**

A. **Iodochlorhydroxyquin (Vioform),** containing 40% iodine, was originally developed as a substitute for iodoform as an antiseptic dusting powder.

While its most effective use is in the treatment of amebiasis, it also has mild antibacterial and antifungal effects and may be used alone or with steroids in the treatment of eczematous and impetiginized processes and some dermatophyte, yeast, and *Trichomonas* infections. However, more specific agents are available. The medication may stain the skin, hair, and clothing yellow and may induce contact allergy.

1. Structure

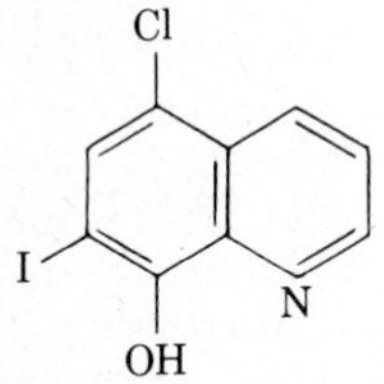

Iodochlorhydroxyquin

2. Dosage: Apply 1–3 times a day.

3. Packaging (R$_x$) and cost:
3% cream or ointment:
  as Vioform, 30 gm/$3.50
  as iodochlorhydroxyquin, 30 gm/$1.50
3% cream with 1% hydrocortisone:
  as Vioform hydrocortisone, 20 gm/$9.00
  as iodochlorhydroxyquin hydrocortisone, 20 gm/$2.50

B. Mafenide (α-amino-p-toluenesulfonamide, Sulfamylon) is a synthetic antibacterial agent related chemically, but not pharmacologically, to the sulfonamides. The drug appears to interfere with bacterial cellular metabolism and is not antagonized by para-aminobenzoic acid, pus, or serum. It is bacteriostatic against many gram-positive and gram-negative organisms, including staphylococci, streptococci, and *Pseudomonas* species. After percutaneous absorption the drug is metabolized; it acts as a weak carbonic anhydrase inhibitor and may therefore cause systemic acidosis.

Mafenide is used primarily in the treatment of burn wounds. It may be painful on application, and active allergic contact sensitivity may develop.

1. Structure

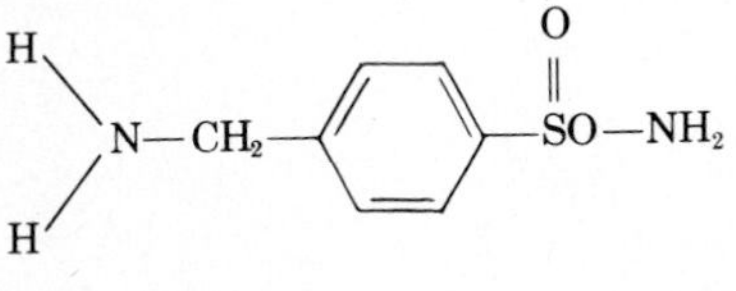

Mafenide

2. Dosage: Apply 2id with hand in a sterile glove.

3. Packaging (R$_x$) and cost:
Cream (as acetate):   60 gm/$5.00
                      120 gm/$9.00

C. **Mercurial compounds** have bacteriostatic effects, most likely mediated through inhibiting sulfhydryl enzymes, but fall far short of being ideal antibacterial compounds. Mercurial compounds may be absorbed and can sensitize; more effective and less hazardous antiseptic agents are available.

1. **Insoluble mercury compounds** are used as antibacterial and antiparasitic agents. **Yellow mercury oxide ointment** has been used for pediculosis involving the eyelashes; **ammoniated mercury,** containing 78% mercury, has been utilized in pyoderma and scaling processes.

2. The **organic mercurial antiseptics** are more bacteriostatic and less irritating and toxic than inorganic salts. Merbromin (Mercurochrome), containing 25% mercury, is not particularly strongly active and further suffers from having its activity decreased in the presence of organic material. Thimerosal (Merthiolate), containing 49% mercury, has the same drawbacks but is more effective.

D. **Nitrofurazone (Furacin),** a synthetic nitrofuran derivative with a broad antibacterial spectrum, can be used for prophylaxis and treatment of infections of the skin. It is rarely used by dermatologists, however, as it carries a high risk of acquired contact sensitivity.

1. **Structure**

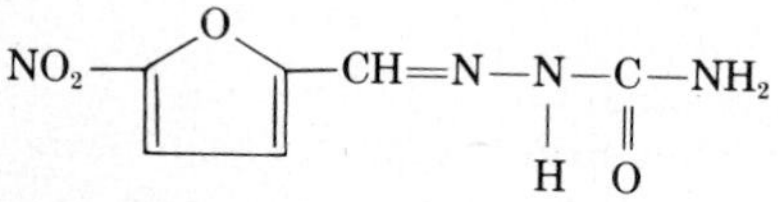

Nitrofurazone

E. **Silver sulfadiazine (Silvadene)** represents an effort to combine the beneficial properties of silver nitrate and sulfonamides such as mafenide. It is used primarily in the prevention and treatment of wound sepsis in patients with second- and third-degree burns. It is bactericidal against many gram-positive and gram-negative bacteria as well as *C. albicans* and is reasonably effective against *Pseudomonas aeruginosa* and *S. aureus.* Bacteria susceptible to sulfadiazine but resistant to silver nitrate, as well as those sensitive to silver nitrate but resistant to sulfadiazine, have shown good response to silver sulfadiazine. It does not stain, is unlikely to produce electrolyte imbalance, and does not cause systemic acidosis. Some patients note a stinging sensation on application, and because this compound can be absorbed, systemic sulfonamide reactions may occur that are similar to those caused by sulfonamides.

1. **Structure**

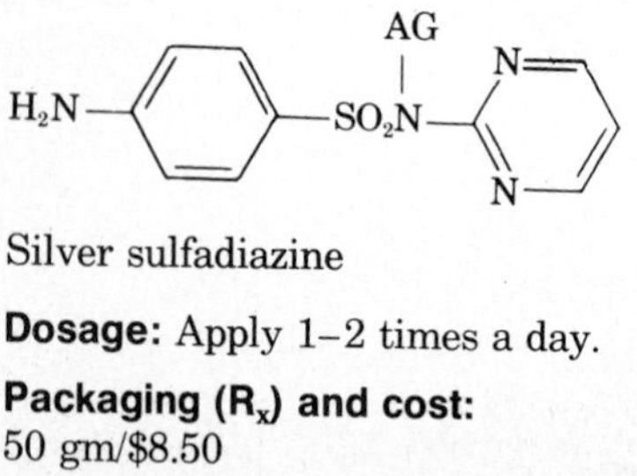

Silver sulfadiazine

2. **Dosage:** Apply 1–2 times a day.

3. **Packaging (R$_x$) and cost:**
   50 gm/$8.50

Reference

MISCELLANEOUS AGENTS

Maibach, H. I. Iodochlorhydroxyquin-hydrocortisone treatment of fungal infection: A double-blind trial. *Arch. Dermatol.* 114:1774–1775, 1978.

Anti-inflammatory agents

Topical Corticosteroids

I. Corticosteroids are the most potent and effective local anti-inflammatory medications available and also have a striking ability to inhibit cell division. They are the therapy of choice in all inflammatory, pruritic eruptions (e.g., dermatitis and eczema) and are also effective in hyperplastic disorders (e.g., psoriasis) and infiltrative disorders (e.g., sarcoid, granuloma annulare). Since 1952, when these preparations first became commercially available, hundreds have been marketed. Their continuous wide usage has been assured by their numerous desirable qualities: broad applicability in treating a wide variety of common eruptions, rapidity of action in small amounts, ease of use, absence of pain or odor, lack of sensitization, prolonged stability, compatibility with almost all commonly used topical medications, and rarity of untoward clinical systemic effects from percutaneous absorption.

The effectiveness of a topical corticosteroid is related to the potency of the drug and its percutaneous penetration. Approximately 1% of a hydrocortisone solution will penetrate normal skin on the forearm. There is a marked regional variation in corticosteroid penetration; compared to the forearm data, hydrocortisone is absorbed 0.14 times as well through the plantar foot arch, 0.83 times through the palm, 1.7 times through the back, 3.5 times through the scalp, 6.0 times through the forehead, 13 times through the cheeks at the jaw angle, and 42 times through scrotal skin. If the skin is completely hydrated, absorption will be increased four- or fivefold. Inflamed skin, such as is found with atopic dermatitis, allows increased percutaneous penetration; with conditions such as exfoliative psoriasis there seems to be little barrier to absorption at all. Small changes in molecular structure related to enhancing the intrinsic activity of the corticosteroid moiety, increasing lipophilicity to facilitate better skin penetration, and retarding the metabolic inactivation of the molecule, result in enormous alterations in clinical effectiveness. To be active, cortisone must be reduced to cortisol (hydrocortisone), just as prednisone must be converted to prednisolone before it can be utilized. Addition of halogen atoms to the steroid nucleus may dramatically increase activity. The potency of topical corticosteroids is most often assessed in vivo by their ability to produce vasoconstriction on human skin, and results of this bioassay correlate well with clinical trials. Other potency assays include suppression of experimentally induced allergic contact dermatitis (e.g., to Rhus antigen) or irritant dermatitis (produced by kerosene or croton oil), or reduction in size of histamine-induced wheals. Antimitotic activity may be assessed by in vitro fibroblast inhibition and/or in vivo epidermal mitotic assay.

In 1960 it was discovered that placing corticosteroids under occlusion with thin, pliable plastic wraps dramatically increased their efficacy (up to 100-fold); occlusion causes hydration of the stratum corneum, increases the surface area of skin almost 40%, and appears to induce a reservoir of cortico-steroid in the horny layer that persists for several days after application. Percutaneous absorption of steroids under wrap, particularly through al-tered skin, always occurs. It should be assumed that all patients under sub-stantial occlusive therapy have temporary suppression of the hypothal-mic-pituitary-adrenal (HPA) axis. Adults applying a potent steroid in excess of 50–100 gm weekly (10–20 gm in small children) for 2 or more weeks face the probability of having HPA-axis suppression. Normal function returns within days to weeks after dressings are discontinued, depending on the duration, extent, and intensity of prior therapy. Undesirable effects from occlusive therapy include infection, miliaria, folliculitis, a disagreeable odor, interfer-ence with heat exchange, increased ease of sunburn, and atrophy and striae.

There are multiple adverse effects from use of topical corticosteroids. Burn-ing, itching, irritation, and dryness are the most common problems and are usually related to the vehicle of the steroid preparation and to the pretreat-ment state of the skin. Ointments are better tolerated on inflamed skin than are creams or gels. Miliaria, folliculitis, and maceration may occur from ex-cessive occlusion and plastic films. Atrophy and telangiectasia are frequent findings if potent corticosteroids have been used over prolonged periods, par-ticularly with use of occlusive techniques. Purpura may be found in atrophic areas. Thinning with or without atrophic striae can be seen within 1 month of use on more susceptible sites such as face, intertriginous, and anogenital areas. The more potent the corticosteroid, the more rapidly and more severe the adverse effects will be. Complications are related to potency but not to halogenation of the corticosteroid molecule; any effective agent including 1% hydrocortisone can have these side effects. Most adverse effects such as at-rophy and telangiectasia will slowly disappear within 6 months of discon-tinuing the drug. Striae are irreversible. Less common side effects include perioral dermatitis or a rosacealike dermatitis, acneform lesions, hyper-trichosis, hypopigmentation, contact dermatitis to the vehicle or to the actual corticosteroid, and ocular hypertension from application in or around the eyes.

Injection of small amounts of corticosteroids (betamethasone sodium phos-phate and betamethasone acetate suspension, triamcinolone acetonide, triamcinolone diacetate, triamcinolone hexacetonide, and methylpred-nisolone) into cutaneous lesions has the advantage of achieving high local concentration with prolonged depot effects and no systemic side effects. In-tralesional use is of particular value in the treatment of acne cysts, psoriatic plaques, circumscribed neurodermatitis, keloids, and, occasionally, chronic plaques of nummular eczema, insect bite reactions, alopecia areata, discoid lupus erythematosus, sarcoidosis, myxoid cysts, and nail disorders. Local ad-verse reactions include atrophy (especially when the concentration is too high or the steroid is injected too high in the dermis), hypopigmentation of deeply pigmented skin, growth of occasional tufts of hair in susceptible indi-viduals, infection, and ulceration. Injection with a 1-ml tuberculin syringe using a 30-gauge needle is best. Air-powered guns can be used but are less precise, disrupt the dermis, and are associated with increased risk of infec-tion. Usually a 1:4 dilution of the medication (i.e., to 2.5 mg/ml triam-cinolone acetonide) will provide enough steroid to reduce inflammation while avoiding these problems. (See discussion of individual diseases for proper dilution.)

II. Dosage considerations

A. **Dose-response relationship.** It is usually possible to observe a clear dose-response relationship in the use of topical corticosteroids. Compounds vary markedly in their potency and efficacy, and most products are available in standard concentrations and diluted 1:2 or 1:4 concentrations; some may also be obtained in high-potency concentrations. Efficacy may also be strikingly altered by method of use (e.g., prior hydration, occlusion).

Ointment vehicles generally give better biologic activity to the incorporated steroids than do cream or lotion vehicles. Preparations containing urea may also enhance penetration of accompanying corticosteroids. In most instances, initial therapy should be with one of the most potent compounds, and maintenance therapy with either a less concentrated fluorinated compound or with 1% hydrocortisone. At least 33–50% of patients can be managed with medium- to low-strength topical corticosteroids and this should always be tried. The less potent corticosteroid formulations (e.g., 1% hydrocortisone) should be used for the scrotum, groin, axillae, eyelids, and face. When possible, apply medications to moist skin after bathing or soaking the area in water.

B. **Frequency of application.** There is a paucity of pharmacokinetic data dealing with the optimal dose-response characteristics of topical corticosteroid use. One study of 12 patients with corticosteroid-responsive dermatoses found that six treatments per day were no more effective than three applications per day. In animals with skin absorption similar to that of humans, the percutaneous penetration of hydrocortisone has been shown to be substantially increased when a large amount is applied as a single daily dose as compared to one-third that dose applied either 1 or 3 times daily. Yet another study demonstrated that a once-daily application was as effective as applying 3 times a day in 95 patients with psoriasis and atopic dermatitis. Overnight application of corticosteroids to hydrated skin, used with or without occlusion, may be as effective and far less costly than multiple daily applications. During the day simple lubricants can be used. If desired, topical corticosteroids may be used 3 times a day but there is no data supporting the notion that more frequent use leads to better or faster resolution of hyperplasia or inflammatory processes.

C. **Tachyphylaxis.** Repeated application of a potent topical steroid may result in a diminished effect of that preparation. This may occur within 1 week of initial use, but the ability to respond fully returns within a week of stopping drug application. It is therefore best to treat effectively for short periods of time (days to 2 weeks) and then leave corticosteroid-treatment-free intervals of a week or more during which time lubricants alone are applied. This regimen also avoids the possible increased percutaneous absorption of topical corticosteroids that may occur after long-term administration.

D. **Relative potency.** It is possible to list the potency of topical corticosteroid preparations based on bioassay tests and literature reviews. Table 4 is modified from Stoughton (1977). There are no significant differences within each group.

Table 4. Topical corticosteroid potency

1 (most potent)	Amcinonide ointment 0.1% (Cyclocort) Betamethasone dipropionate ointment 0.05% (Diprosone) Desoximetasone cream 0.25% (Topicort) Diflorasone diacetate ointment 0.05% (Florone, Maxiflor) Fluocinonide cream, ointment, gel 0.05% (Lidex and Lidex-E cream, Lidex ointment, Topsyn gel) Halcinonide cream 0.1% (Halog)
2	Betamethasone benzoate gel 0.025% (Benisone, Uticort) Betamethasone dipropionate cream 0.05% (Diprosone) Betamethasone valerate ointment 0.1% (Valisone) Diflorasone diacetate cream 0.05% (Florone, Maxiflor) Triamcinolone acetonide cream 0.5% (Aristocort)
3	Amcinonide cream 0.1% (Cyclocort) Betamethasone valerate lotion 0.1% (Valisone) Fluocinolone acetonide cream 0.2%, ointment 0.025% (Fluonid, Synalar) Flurandrenolide ointment 0.05% (Cordran) Hydrocortisone valerate ointment 0.2% (Westcort) Triamcinolone acetonide ointment 0.1% (Aristocort, Kenalog)
4	Betamethasone valerate cream 0.1% (Valisone) Clocortolone pivalate cream 0.1% (Cloderm) Fluocinolone acetonide cream 0.025% (Fluonid, Synalar) Flurandrenolide cream 0.05% (Cordran) Hydrocortisone valerate cream 0.2% (Westcort) Triamcinolone acetonide cream 0.01%, lotion 0.025% (Kenalog, Aristocort)
5	Desonide cream 0.05% (Tridesilon) Flumethasone pivalate 0.03% (Locorten)
6 (least potent)	Dexamethasone 0.1% (Decadron Phosphate) Fluorometholone 0.025% (Oxylone) Hydrocortisone 0.25, 0.5, 1.0, 2.5% (generic, Hytone, Nutraderm, Synacort, others) Methylprednisolone 1% (Medrol) Prednisolone 0.5% (Meti-Derm)

Source: Modified from Stoughton (1976, 1980).

E. **Occlusive therapy.** Some conditions, such as psoriasis, lichen simplex chronicus, and hand eczema, respond poorly, if at all, to creams alone. The use of **occlusive (airtight) dressings** will increase the efficacy of these preparations. Patients should be instructed to:

1. **Soak the area in water, or wash it well.**

2. **While the skin is still moist,** rub medication into lesions.

3. **Cover the area with a plastic wrap** (Saran Wrap, Handi Wrap), plastic gloves for hands, plastic bags for feet, bathing cap for scalp, vinyl exercise suit for large areas of the legs or torso. Tubular plastic dressings (see Fig. 6) are also useful.

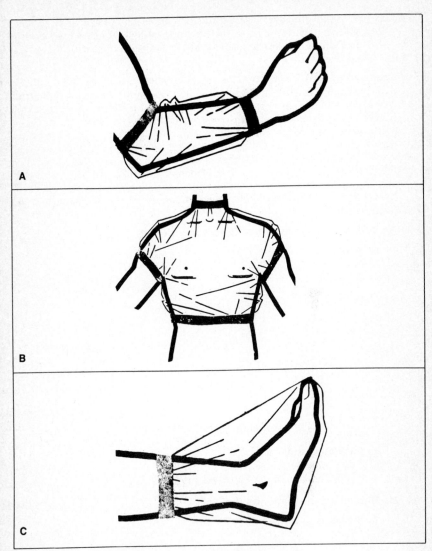

Figure 6. Plastic dressings applied to (A) arm, (B) body, (C) foot.

4. **Seal edges with tape** or cover plastic with an ace bandage, a long stocking, panty hose, or any dressing that will ensure close adherence to skin. Blenderm tape will stick particularly well to skin. Paper tape may be less irritating.

5. **Use for at least 6 hr.** Overnight application is usually sufficient to induce clinical remission, but such a technique may also be used during the day. Occlusion for even a few hours, however, may be very beneficial.

As noted previously, significant percutaneous absorption of steroids will occur with occlusive therapy, and patients undergoing stressful procedures (i.e., operations) should be supplemented with IV corticosteroids.

III. Packaging (all R$_x$) and cost. As topical corticosteroids are stable preparations, buying in bulk is feasible and will frequently result in significant cost savings to the patient. Some pharmacies and institutions will buy 5-lb containers and repackage, with resultant enormous decreases in unit cost. With corticosteroids the cost of purchasing multiple small tubes is particularly high in contrast to buying one larger size. For example, the price of four 15-gm tubes of Lidex is 170% that of one 60-gm tube, and the cost of nine 5-gm Valisone tubes is 215% that of one 45-gm tube. All topical corticosteroids are available by prescription only with the exception of 0.25 and 0.5% hydrocortisone, which are OTC. Selected agents will be discussed in more detail below.

A. Betamethasone benzoate (Benisone; Uticort)

  1. Structure

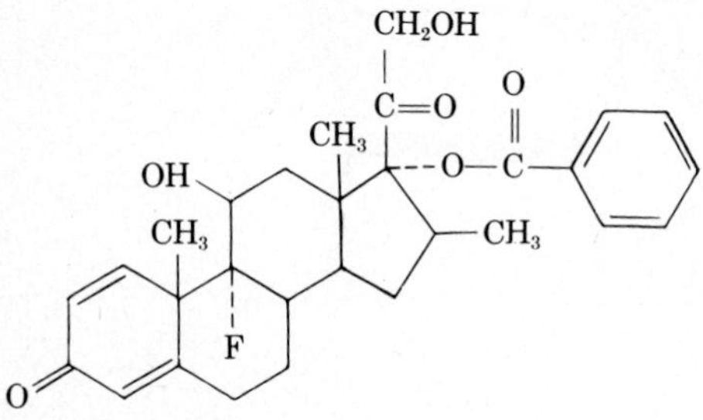

Betamethasone benzoate

  2. Packaging and cost:
    0.025% gel: 15 gm/$5.25, 60 gm/$14.50
    0.025% cream: 15 gm/$5.25, 60 gm/$14.50

B. Betamethasone valerate (Valisone)

  1. Structure

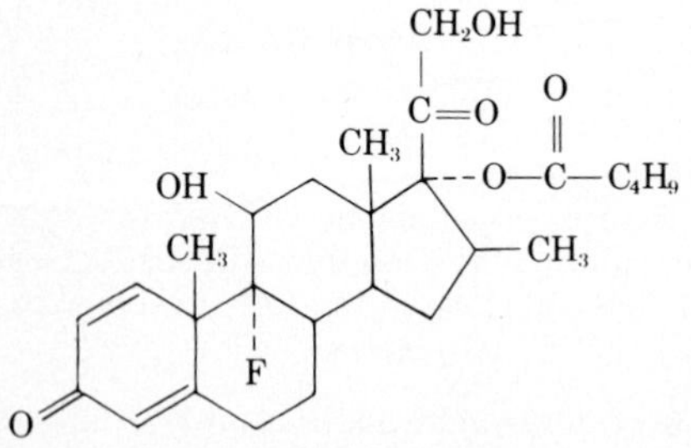

Betamethasone valerate

2. **Packaging and cost:**
   0.01% cream: 15 gm/$4.25, 60 gm/$9.75
   0.1% cream or ointment: 5 gm/$3.50, 15 gm/$7.00, 45 gm/$13.75
   0.1% lotion: 20 ml/$8.75, 60 ml/$17.50
   0.15% aerosol: 85 gm/$7.00

C. Desonide (Tridesilon)

1. Structure

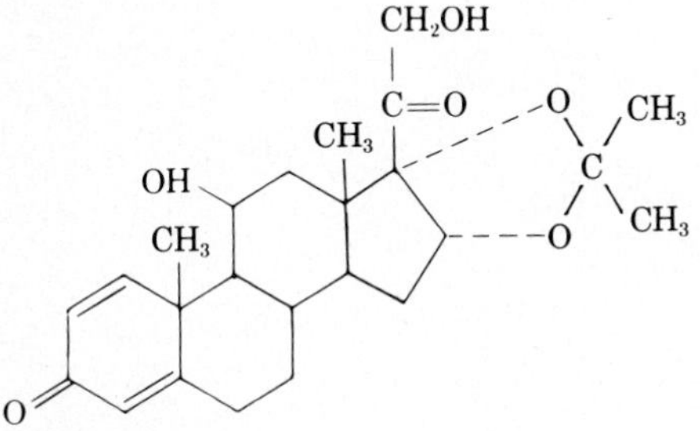

Desonide

2. Packaging and cost:
0.05% cream and ointment: 15 gm/$5.50, 60 gm/$14.50

D. Fluocinolone acetonide (Fluonid, Synalar)

1. Structure

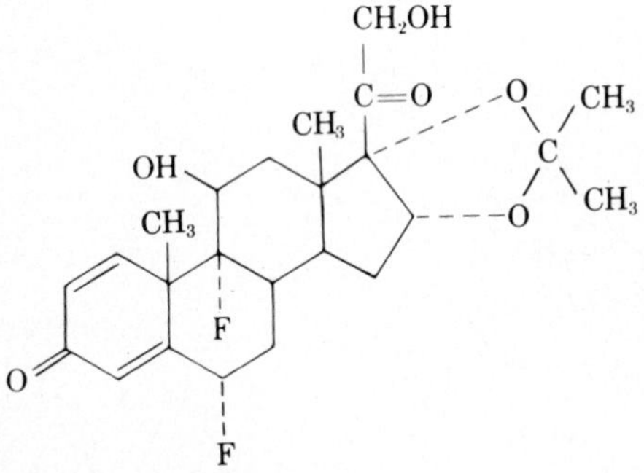

Fluocinolone acetonide

2. Packaging and cost:
0.025% cream, ointment, and emollient cream (Synemol): 15 gm/
$6.00, 60 gm/$13.50, 120 gm/$24.50, 425 gm/$77.00
0.01% cream: 15 gm/$5.25, 60 gm/$9.75, 120 gm/$13.50
0.2% (HP) cream: 12 gm/$14.00
0.01% solution: 20 ml/$6.75, 60 ml/$13.50
(Institutions may purchase five 425-gm jars of full-strength [0.025%]
or ten 425-gm jars of 0.01% cream or ointment at reduced costs.)

E. Fluocinonide (Fluocinolone acetonide acetate; Lidex cream and ointment, Lidex E cream, Topsyn gel)

1. **Structure**

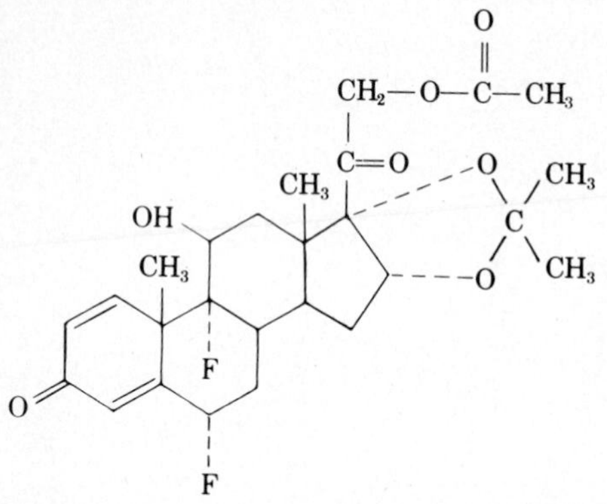

Fluocinonide fluocinolone acetonide acetate

2. **Packaging and cost:**
   0.05% cream, ointment, or gel: 15 gm/$6.50, 60 gm/$15.00

F. Flurandrenolide (Cordran; flurandrenolone) is available as 0.05% and 0.025% cream, ointment, and lotion, and 0.05% tape.

1. **Structure**

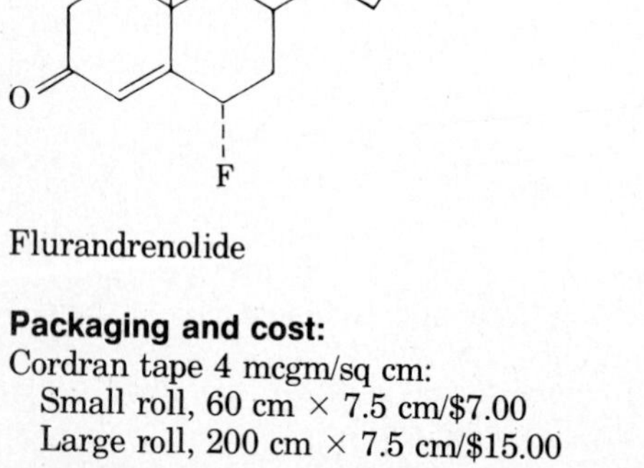

Flurandrenolide

2. **Packaging and cost:**
   Cordran tape 4 mcgm/sq cm:
     Small roll, 60 cm × 7.5 cm/$7.00
     Large roll, 200 cm × 7.5 cm/$15.00

G. Halcinonide (Halog) is available as 0.1% and 0.025% cream, ointment, and solution, and as Halciderm cream or ointment.

1. **Structure**

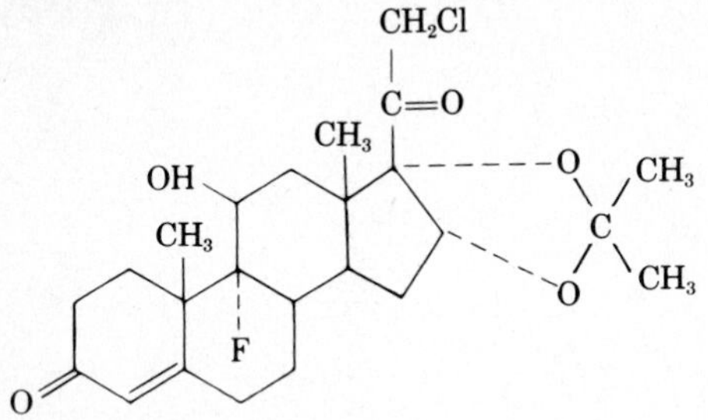

$$CH_2Cl$$
$$C{=}O$$

Halcinonide

2. **Packaging and cost:**
   0.1% cream: 15 gm/$5.50, 60 gm/$15.00, 240 gm/$40.00
      as Halciderm cream or ointment: 0.1%: 15 gm/$6.50, 60 gm/$17.00

H. Hydrocortisone may be purchased as a generic drug.

1. **Structure**

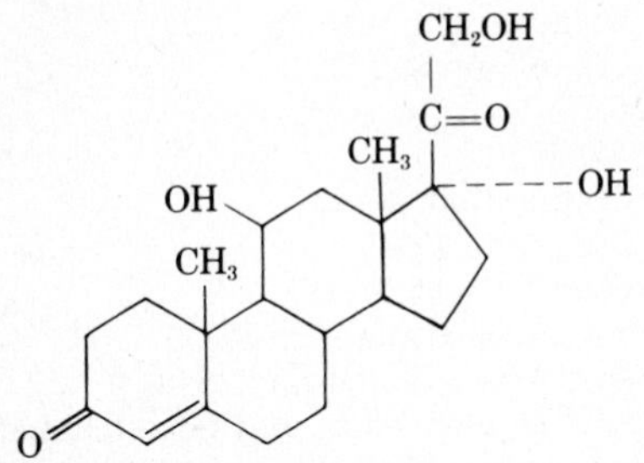

$$CH_2OH$$
$$C{=}O$$

Hydrocortisone

2. **Packaging and cost:**
   0.5% cream or ointment (OTC): 30 gm (as Cortaid)/$7.00
                                         30 gm (as generic)/$2.00
   0.5% lotion (OTC):   60 ml (as Cortaid)/$9.75
                       120 ml (as generic)/$4.25
   1% cream or ointment: 30 gm (as Hytone)/$4.65
                           30 gm (as generic)/$2.50
                       120 gm (as Nutracort)/$12.90
   1% lotion: 120 ml (as generic)/$8.50
             120 ml (as Nutracort)/$13.50
   1% gel: 60 ml (as Nutracort)/$9.25
   2.5% cream: 20 gm (as generic)/$3.50
               30 gm (as Hytone)/$7.30

I. Triamcinolone acetonide (Kenalog) or triamcinolone diacetate (Aristocort)

1. **Structure**

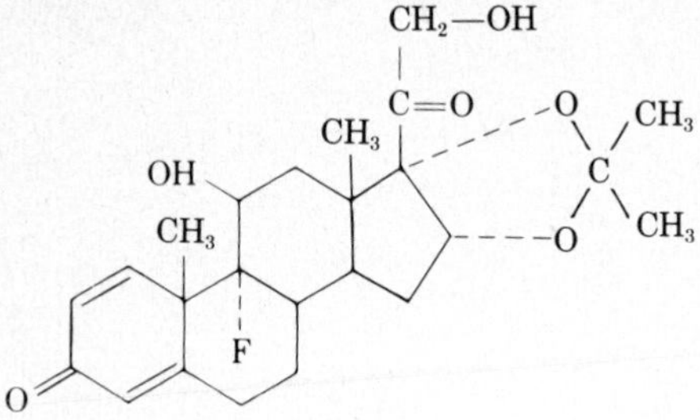

Triamcinolone acetonide

2. **Packaging and cost:**
   0.025% cream or ointment: 15 gm/$2.25
      80 gm (as Kenalog)/$12.00
      75 gm (as Aristocort A)/$15.00
   0.1% cream or ointment: 15 gm/$6.75
      60 gm (as Kenalog-H)/$18.50
      50 gm (as Aristocort-A)/$18.00
   0.5% cream or ointment (as Aristocort-A): 15 gm/$21.00
   0.1% in Orabase (as Kenalog): 5 gm/$5.75
   0.1% spray: 23 gm/$7.25, 63 gm/$12.75
   0.1% lotion: 60 ml/$16.75
   0.025% lotion: 60 ml/$18.00
   Aqueous suspension for injection:
      10 mg/ml (as Kenalog): 5 ml/$7.25
      25 mg/ml (as Aristocort): 5 ml/$20.00
      40 mg/ml (as Kenalog, Aristocort): 1 ml/$6.00
      40 mg/ml (as Kenalog, Aristocort): 5 ml/$25.00
   (2400 gm [5.25 lb] of 0.1% triamcinolone may be purchased directly by institutions or pharmacies for $110.00, or 2400 gm of 0.025% for $49.00.)

J. **Steroid combinations.** There are hundreds of topical corticosteroid preparations available in different vehicles and in combination with antibiotics (most frequently, neomycin), other antiseptics (iodochlorhydroxyquin), and other agents (tars, keratolytic agents). Some combinations are useful, but there is more flexibility and control over therapy, often at a lower cost to the patient, if separate identifiable agents are used.

Systemic corticosteroids

I. **Discussion.** Systemic corticosteroids are used in the treatment of a number of skin diseases, ranging from pemphigus vulgaris to severe cases of allergic contact dermatitis. Because of their well-known and serious side effects, the decision to use them must be based on careful consideration of the indications, alternatives, contraindications, and risks in each clinical situation. Fortunately, many of the instances for which they are utilized in dermatology are either short-lived or rapidly responsive, so that "short courses" of treatment, for which the risks are significantly diminished, may be used.

Virtually every aspect of inflammation and immunologic reactivity is altered—usually diminished—by corticosteroids. For example, neutrophil migration and adherence to endothelium are reduced, capillary permeability and blood flow are diminished, the passage of immune complexes across basement membranes is decreased, and it is thought that lysosomal membranes are stabilized by corticosteroids, among many other effects.

Systemic corticosteroids are either proved or generally acknowledged to be of benefit in the treatment of pemphigus vulgaris, bullous pemphigoid, id (autosensitization) reactions, and severe allergic contact dermatitis (such as poison ivy). They are also often prescribed for severe erythema multiforme, severe cutaneous drug reactions, toxic epidermal necrolysis, and severe sunburn, though their efficacy in these conditions is based largely on anecdotal clinical experience and has not been unequivocally proved. Experimentally, for example, prednisone was unable to alter the development or course of sunburn erythema induced artificially on small areas of the skin. On the other hand, it is probably true that patients with severe sunburn and toxic symptoms (e.g., fever and chills) may feel better when treated with systemic steroids. Corticosteroids have also been recommended for the prevention of postherpetic neuralgia, particularly when they can be given early enough in the course of herpes zoster in elderly patients (see p. 104).

II. General principles of corticosteroid use in cutaneous disorders

A. Overall assessment of indications, risks, benefits, and alternatives.

B. Evaluation for contraindications and consideration of side effects. See Tables I and II.

C. Corticosteroids are generally considered to be contraindicated in psoriasis, in which their withdrawal may incite a generalized pustular flare, and in atopic dermatitis, in which withdrawal may be extremely difficult and may be accompanied by exacerbation.

D. Diagnose and treat any secondary infection (such as impetigo, cellulitis, or erysipelas) before starting steroids.

Table I. Contraindications to corticosteroid treatment

Absolute
  Ocular herpes simplex
  Untreated tuberculosis
Relative
  Acute or chronic infections
  Pregnancy
  Diabetes mellitus
  Hypertension
  Peptic ulcer
  Osteoporosis
  Psychotic tendencies
  Renal insufficiency
  Congestive heart failure (excluding CHF secondary to active rheumatic carditis)
  Diverticulitis
  Recent intestinal anastomoses

Source: Modified from Storrs (1979).

Table II. Common corticosteroid complications

Obesity
Striae
Bruisability
Growth disturbances
Hypertension
"Moon face"
Excessive appetite
Decreased cell-mediated immunity
Neutrophilia
Lymphocytopenia
Monocytopenia
Increased infections
Delayed wound healing
Increased excretion of sodium and potassium
Carbohydrate intolerance
Personality disturbances
Posterior subcapsular cataracts*

*This is the only side effect of those listed that is not decreased with alternate-day rather than daily therapy.
Source: Storrs (1979).

E. If acute infection, trauma, or surgery occurs during treatment, the steroid dose must be increased appropriately.

F. Hypothalamic-pituitary-adrenal (HPA) axis suppression must be considered even after short courses. Although short courses are not as likely to cause problems as longer ones, recent work indicates that pituitary-adrenal reserve in response to stress may be diminished for as long as 5 days after a 5-day course of 25 mg PO twice daily. A single injection of triamcinolone acetonide may suppress adrenal responsiveness for 2 to 3 weeks or more. Patients should be informed of this potential risk.

G. In most instances, the route of administration of choice is oral and the drug of choice is prednisone, which is short-acting and inexpensive. In order to be active, prednisone must be converted to prednisolone in the liver (Table III). Potency and duration of action vary among the multiple drugs available (Table III; sec. **IV** following). Intramuscular injections are preferred by some dermatologists under some circumstances (sec. **V** following). (For detailed information on HPA axis suppression, steroid withdrawal, alternate versus daily and divided versus single daily dose schedules, as well as arguments favoring one route of administration over another, the reader is referred to the references at the end of this chapter.)

H. The association of corticosteroids with peptic ulceration remains controversial. In the absence of a clear past history or symptoms of peptic ulcer disease, the routine use of either antacids or cimetidine is probably *not* warranted. In the presence of such a history or if symptoms develop, cimetidine and/or antacids as well as medical evaluation, may be indicated.

Table III. Relative potencies of some systemic glucocorticoids

Drug	Equivalent dose (mg)
Cortisone	25
Cortisol (hydrocortisone)	20
Prednisone, prednisolone	5
Methylprednisolone, triamcinolone	4
Betamethasone	0.60
Dexamethasone	0.75

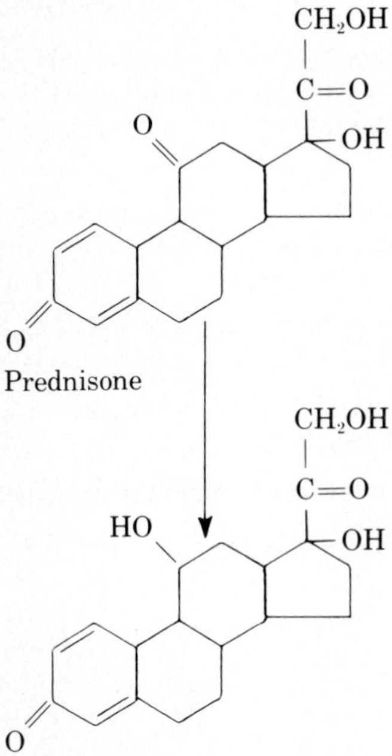

Prednisone

Prednisolone

1. Cimetidine (Tagamet)
   When indicated: 300 mg PO qid with meals and at bedtime.

2. Antacids
   An antacid of choice may be taken prn for symptoms or on a regular basis (e.g., q2–4h).

III. **Dosage considerations in acute dermatoses.** In order to achieve maximal therapeutic benefit, systemic corticosteroids must be given in adequate dosage for a sufficient length of time. It is also desirable to commence treatment as early as possible in the course of the illness. Alternate-day therapy must be considered when use for more than 1 month is necessary. The initial dose of prednisone for an adult with conditions such as allergic contact dermatitis should be at least 60 mg every day. The course should be no less than 2–3 weeks. If the dose is too small or duration of treatment too short, a rebound phenomenon with generalized exacerbation of the rash and symptoms can occur.

The prednisone should be given as a single daily dose (before 8:00 A.M.) in order to minimize suppression of the normal diurnal cortisol secretions. Used in this fashion for 2 or 4 weeks, there is no strong evidence that cortico-steroids need be slowly tapered. Suggested regimens for acute dermatoses are given below.

A. Preferred methods

1. Prednisone 60 mg PO each morning for 5 days, 40 mg each morning for 5 days, 20 mg each morning for 5 days; then discontinue. This is the easiest and least expensive regimen and uses thirty 20-mg tablets over 15 days.

2. Prednisone 60 mg PO each morning for 7 days, followed by prednisone 30 mg PO each morning for 7 days, then discontinue (126 5-mg tablets, or 63 10-mg tablets over 14 days).

B. Other schedules

1. Prednisone 60 mg PO each morning for 3 days, 50 mg each morning for 3 days, 40 mg each morning for 3 days, and then taper by 5 mg per day to 0 (120 5-mg tablets over 16 days).

2. Prednisone starting with 60 mg PO the first day and decreasing by 5 mg per day (i.e., 60, 55, 50, 45 . . . 0; 78 5-mg tablets over 12 days).

The total amount and duration of treatment may be varied; a certain amount of empiricism and art is often in order.

IV. Glucocorticoid adrenocorticotropic hormone (ACTH) suppression of oral corticosteroids; representative costs[*]

A. Short-acting (24–36 hr)
Cortisone
Cortisol (hydrocortisone)
Prednisone
Prednisolone
Methylprednisolone

1. Packaging and cost:
Prednisone:
1 mg, 100 tablets/$3.50
5 mg, 100 tablets/$2.25
10 mg, 100 tablets/$4.50
20 mg, 100 tablets/$7.50

B. Intermediate-acting (48 hr)
Triamcinolone

1. Packaging and cost:
as Aristocort, 4 mg, 100 tablets/$68.00
as generic, 4 mg, 100 tablets/$6.75

C. Long-acting (over 48 hr)
Betamethasone
Dexamethasone

[*] Modified from Storrs (1979).

1. **Packaging and cost:**
   Dexamethasone:
   Decadron, 0.75 mg, 100 tablets/$26.50
   generic, 0.75 mg, 100 tablets/$7.50

V. Injectable glucocorticoids.* Time noted is the duration of their ability to suppress an inflammatory reaction (see pp. 272, 276).

A. Short-acting (hours–days)
Dexamethasone sodium phosphate (Decadron)

B. Intermediate-acting (1–2 weeks)
Betamethasone acetate
Betamethasone sodium phosphate (Celestone, Soluspan)
Dexamethasone acetate (Decadron-LA)
Triamcinolone diacetate (Aristocort)

C. Long-acting (3–4 weeks)
Triamcinolone acetonide (Kenalog)
Triamcinolone hexacetonide (Aristospan)

References

TOPICAL CORTICOSTEROIDS

Allenby, C. F., and Sparkes, C. G.   Halogenation and topical corticosteroids: A comparison between the 17-butyrate esters of hydrocortisone and clobetasone in ointment bases. *Br. J. Dermatol.* 104:179–183, 1981.

Callen, J. P.   Intralesional corticosteroids. *J. Am. Acad. Dermatol.* 4:149–151, 1981.

Chernosky, M. E., and Schmidt, J. D.   Atrophy, telangiectasia, and purpura after topical fluorinated corticosteroid therapy. *Cutis* 13:383–386, 1974.

de Vivier, A.   Tachyphylaxis to topically applied steroids. *Arch. Dermatol.* 112:1245–1248, 1976.

Eaglstein, W. H., Farzad, A., and Capland, L.   Topical corticosteroid therapy: Efficacy of frequent application. *Arch. Dermatol.* 110:955, 1974.

Fredriksson, T., Lassus, A., and Bleeker, J.   Treatment of psoriasis and atopic dermatitis with halcinonide cream applied once and three times daily. *Br. J. Dermatol.* 102:575–577, 1980.

Goette, D. K., and Odom, R. B.   Adverse effects of corticosteroids. *Cutis* 23:477–487, 1979.

Guin, J. D.   Complications of topical hydrocortisone. *J. Am. Acad. Dermatol.* 4:417–422, 1981.

Jarratt, M. T., Spark, R. F., and Arndt, K. A.   The effects of intradermal steroids on the pituitary-adrenal axis and the skin. *J. Invest. Dermatol.* 62:463–466, 1974.

Kligman, A. M., and Kaidby, K. H.   Hydrocortisone revisited. An historical and experimental evaluation. *Cutis* 22:232–244, 1978.

Munro, D. D., and Wilson, L. (eds.).   Steroids and the Skin. Proceedings of a Conference held in Edinburgh, Oct., 1975. *Br. J. Dermatol.* (Suppl. 12) 94:1976.

Robertson, D. B., and Maibach, H. I.   Topical corticosteroids. *Intern. J. Med.* 21:59–67, 1982.

* Modified from Storrs (1979).

Scoggins, R. B., and Kliman, R.   Percutaneous absorption of corticosteroids: Systemic effects. *N. Engl. J. Med.* 273:831–840, 1965.

Stoughton, R. B.   A Perspective of Topical Corticosteroid Therapy. In Farber, E. M., and Cox, A. J. (eds.), *Psoriasis: Proceedings of the Second International Symposium.* New York: York Medical Books, 1976.

Stoughton, R. B.   Principles of Topical Steroid Treatment in Skin Diseases. In *Topics in Internal Medicine.* Baltimore: Williams & Wilkins, 1980.

Stoughton, R. B., and August, P. J.   Cushing's syndrome and pituitary-adrenal suppression due to clobetesol proprionate. *Br. Med. J.* 2:419–421, 1975.

Wester, R. C., Noonan, P. K., and Maibach, H. I.   Effect of frequency of application on percutaneous absorption of hydrocortisone. *Arch. Dermatol.* 113:620–622, 1977.

Wester, R., Noonan, P., and Maibach, H.   Percutaneous absorption of hydrocortisone increases with long-term administration in the rhesus monkey. *Arch. Dermatol.* 116:186–188, 1980.

SYSTEMIC CORTICOSTEROIDS

Axelrod, L.   Glucocorticoid therapy. *Medicine* 55:39–65, 1976.

Byyny, R. L.   Withdrawal from glucocorticoid therapy. *N. Engl. J. Med.* 295:30–32, 1976.

Conn, H. O., and Blitzer, B. L.   Nonassociation of adrenocorticosteroid therapy and peptic ulcer. *N. Engl. J. Med.* 294:473–479, 1976.

Fauci, A. S.   Alternate-day corticosteroid therapy. *Am. J. Med.* 64:729–731, 1978.

Garber, E. K., Fan, P. T., and Bluestone, R.   Realistic guidelines of corticosteroid therapy in rheumatic disease. *Sem. Arth. Rheum.* 11:231–256, 1981.

Greenwald, J., Parrish, J. A., Jaenicke, K. F., and Anderson, R. R.   Failure of systemic administered corticosteroids to suppress UVB-induced delayed erythema. *J. Am. Acad. Dermatol.* 5:197–202, 1981.

Keczkes, K., and Basheer, A. M.   Do corticosteroids prevent post-herpetic neuralgia? *Br. J. Dermatol.* 102:551–555, 1980.

Storrs, F. J.   Use and abuse of systemic corticosteroid therapy. *J. Am. Acad. Dermatol.* 1:95–105, 1979.

Streck, W. F., and Lockwood, D. H.   Pituitary adrenal recovery following short-term suppression with corticosteroids. *Am. J. Med.* 66:910, 1979.

Antiperspirants and medications used in the treatment of hyperhidrosis

I. **For hyperhidrosis of palms and soles**

    A. **Aldehydes.** Aldehydes induce anhidrosis probably by producing a blockage within the stratum corneum. Either formalin (5–10%) or nonalkalinized glutaraldehyde applied with a cotton swab is effective. Unbuffered generic glutaraldehyde is available as a 50% solution through drug supply houses; 2% glutaraldehyde is most easily used as Cidex solution or Cidex Formula 7 Long-Life solution.

        1. **Glutaraldehyde** solution is applied 3 times a week for 2 weeks, and then once weekly or as needed. A 10% solution is used for the feet. It will cause a temporary brown discoloration to appear, but this will diminish as frequency of application decreases. A 2% solution, which

will not stain, may be used on the palms; however, this concentration produces only slight diminution in sweating.

2. **Methenamine** is a structure that, when applied to the skin, hydrolyzes to ammonia and formaldehyde. A 5% methenamine stick or 10% solution is effective in mild to moderate hyperhidrosis.

   a. **Structure**

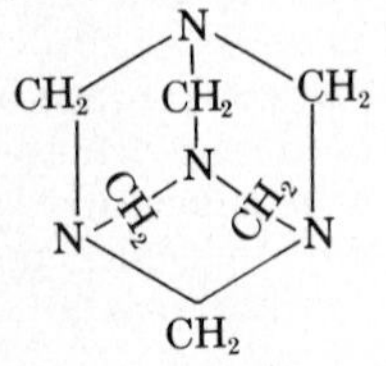

   Methenamine

B. **Aluminum** compounds may be used as noted below.

C. **Iontophoresis with tap water or anticholinergic drugs** such as glycopyrrolate will induce hypohidrosis of palms or soles for several weeks. The drugs are safe, and sensitization does not occur.

   1. **Structure**

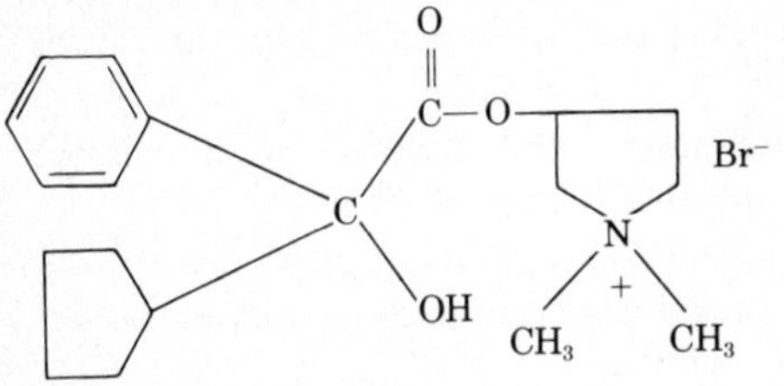

   Glycopyrrolate

D. **Systemic anticholinergic drugs** are usually not tolerated in the required doses but may be tried (glycopyrrolate [Robinul PH 2 ml] 3–5 times a day initially, then decrease). Sedatives or tranquilizing drugs are sometimes helpful.

E. **Relaxation techniques** including biofeedback training may decrease excessive palmoplantar and axillary sweating and the symptoms of chronic hyperhidrosis.

II. For axillary hyperhidrosis

A. **Glutaraldehyde** is generally not effective in the axillae.

B. **Aluminum compounds** (see p. 253).

   1. For initial treatment of axillary hyperhidrosis apply 20–25% aluminum chloride hexahydrate in absolute alcohol (Drysol) to dry axillae at bedtime. Use for 2–7 consecutive nights and then as needed. Discomfort or irritation can be kept to a minimum by avoiding use on

moist skin and by using 1% hydrocortisone cream in the morning if necessary. Sweating should decrease to less than 50% of pretreatment levels within 4 weeks. If this treatment process is unsatisfactory, use with occlusion as follows:

Apply 20% solution of aluminum chloride hexahydrate in 80% absolute anhydrous ethyl alcohol (Drysol: liquid, 37.5 ml/$6.25; "Dab-o-matic," 30 ml/$6.75) to absolutely dry axillae at bedtime and cover with plastic wrap. Do not wash the area closer than 2 hr before applying. Use a shirt (not tape) to keep wrap in place 6–8 hr (overnight) and wash medication off in the morning. Use for two consecutive nights or more the first week until the desired anhidrosis is achieved, then 1–3 times weekly thereafter. For treatment of palms and soles, initial treatment may have to be for 3–5 nights and follow-up treatment more often (every 4–5 days). For regular use, plastic wrap can be sewn into the foot of a sock or used inside a glove.

2. The antiperspirant action of aluminum salts appears to involve physical blockage of sweat ducts by an aluminum-containing cast. Within the distal intraepidermal portion of the eccrine duct aluminum hydroxide is deposited and forms a plug. Some plugs may extend to the mid-dermis. Within the axillae less than half of the eccrine glands are susceptible to aluminum antiperspirants, whereas all seem to be inhibited in other regions of the body. A single adequate exposure every 1–2 weeks may keep sweat ducts in a permanent state of blockage.

C. **Scopolamine hydrobromide** 0.025% applied topically can be an effective antiperspirant. Higher concentrations produce side effects such as diplopia.

D. **Systemic anticholinergic and sedative (tranquilizing) drugs, iontophoresis, and relaxation techniques** may be of value.

E. **Excision** of the sweat-gland-containing axillary vault is a simple surgical procedure and is the management of choice in some patients with severe hyperhidrosis.

References

ANTIPERSPIRANTS AND MEDICATIONS USED
IN THE TREATMENT OF HYPERHIDROSIS

Abell, E., and Morgan, K. The treatment of idiopathic hyperhidrosis by glycopyrronium bromide and tap water iontophoresis. *Br. J. Dermatol.* 91:87–91, 1974.

Brandrup, F., and Larsen, P. O. Axillary hyperhidrosis: Local treatment with aluminum chloride hexahydrate 25% in absolute alcohol. *Acta Dermatol. Venerol.* 58:401–405, 1978.

Cullen, S. I. Topical methenamine therapy for hyperhidrosis. *Arch. Dermatol.* 111:1158–1160, 1975.

Duller, P., and Gentry, W. D. Use of biofeedback in treating chronic hyperhidrosis: A preliminary report. *Br. J. Dermatol.* 103:143–146, 1980.

Eiseman, G. Surgical treatment of axillary hyperhidrosis as an out-patient procedure. *Cutis* 16:69–72, 1975.

Gordon, B. I. "No sweat." *Cutis* 15:401–404, 1975.

Gordon, H. H. Hyperhidrosis: Treatment with glutaraldehyde. *Cutis* 9:375–378, 1972.

Harahap, M. Management of hyperhidrosis axillaris. *J. Derm. Surg. Oncol.* 5:223–225, 1979.

Holzle, E., and Kligman, A. M. Mechanism of antiperspirant action of aluminum salts. *J. Soc. Cosmet. Chem.* 30:279–295, 1979.

Kinmont, P. P. C. Deodorants. *Practitioner* 202:88–94, 1969.

Levit, F. Treatment of hyperhidrosis by tap water iontophoresis. *Cutis* 26:192–194, 1980.

Munro, D. D., Verbov, J. L., O'Gorman, D. J., and du Vivier, A. Axillary hyperhidrosis: Its quantification and surgical treatment. *Br. J. Dermatol.* 90:325–329, 1974.

Sato, K., and Dobson, R. L. Mechanism of the antiperspirant effect of topical glutaraldehyde. *Arch. Dermatol.* 100:564–569, 1969.

Sato, K., and Dobson, R. L. Mechanism of the antiperspirant effect of topical glutaraldehyde. *Arch. Dermatol.* 100:564–569, 1969.

Scholes, K. T., Crow, K. D., Ellis, J. P., Harman, R. R., and Saihan, E. M. Axillary hyperhidrosis treated with alcoholic solution of aluminum chloride hexahydrate. *Br. Med. J.* 2:84–85, 1978.

Shelley, W. B., and Hurley, H. J. Studies on topical antiperspirant control of axillary hyperhidrosis. *Acta Dermatol. Venerol.* (Stockh.) 55:241–260, 1975.

Shrivastava, S. N., and Singh, G. Tap water iontophoresis in palmoplantar hyperhidrosis. *Br. J. Dermatol.* 96:189–195, 1977.

Antipruritic and external analgesic agents

I. **Discussion.** Pruritus is a symptom, not a disease, but the intense discomfort it can produce should not be underestimated. Complete investigation into the systemic or cutaneous cause of the itching is of primary importance, but whatever the cause, the complaint requires prompt and effective therapy. Topical corticosteroids and emollients are often useful. This section will discuss some of the more traditional dermatologic antipruritic agents and formulations. Pruritus is a complicated sensation involving neurophysiologic and psychologic considerations not yet fully understood; this naturally increases the difficulty of treatment. See also Antihistamines, p. 246.

A. **Camphor** is a ketone that, when applied in 1–3% concentration, has mild antipruritic effects through its anesthetic properties. It is used in various OTC topical analgesic products in concentrations as high as 9%.

1. **Structure**

Camphor

B. **Menthol,** a cyclic alcohol (derived from peppermint, other mint oils, or prepared synthetically), relieves itching by substituting a cool sensation. It is usually used in 0.25–2.0% concentration but is present in concentrations as high as 16% in some OTC products.

   1. Structure

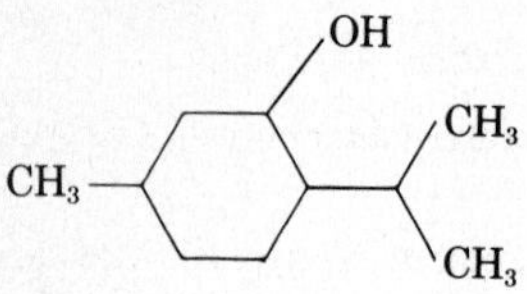

   Menthol

C. **Phenol** in dilute solution (0.5–2.0%) decreases itch by anesthetizing the cutaneous nerve endings.

   1. Structure

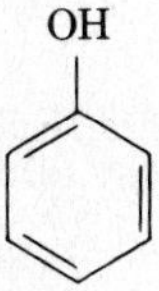

   Phenol

D. **Salicylic acid** (1–2%) and **tars** (coal tar solution, 3–10%) are also occasionally useful, although their mode of action is not known.

   1. Structure

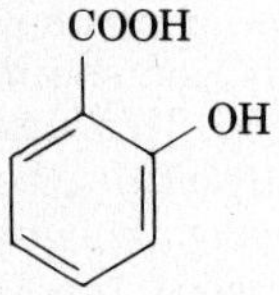

   Salicylic acid

E. Local **anesthetics** are often used to allay pruritus by blocking nerve impulses at sensory nerve endings. See also section on Anesthetics, p. 243.

F. Other ingredients in OTC analgesics include:

   1. Methyl salicylate, occurring naturally as wintergreen or sweet-birch oil, which when rubbed on the skin produces mild irritation and is absorbed to an appreciable extent. **Triethanolamine salicylate** 10% acts as an analgesic without irritant properties and is readily absorbed.

   2. Thymol (see p. 264).

   3. Turpentine oil is used for its "counterirritant" properties. Counterirritants induce other sensations such as warmth and "crowd out" the perception of pain.

4. **Allyl isothiocyanate,** volatile oil of mustard, acts as a powerful local irritant.

5. **Clove oil,** which contains **eugenol** as its main constituent, is used in ointments and widely used in toothache preparations.

6. **Capsicum oleoresin,** an irritant product of cayenne pepper, produces a feeling of warmth when applied to intact skin.

7. **Methacholine chloride, histamine dihydrochloride,** and **methyl nicotinate** are used for their local vasodilating properties.

8. Other volatile oils in OTC preparations include **wormwood** and **eucalyptus oils.**

G. **Dermatologic antipruritic formulations**

1. **Lotions, liniments, emulsions**

   *a. Calamine lotion, USP (drying):

Calamine (zinc oxide with 0.5% ferric oxide for coloring)	8 gm
Zinc oxide	8 gm
Glycerin	2 ml
Bentonite magma (suspending agent)	25 ml
Calcium hydroxide solution, to make	100 ml

   (1) Packaging and cost:
   120 ml/$1.00
   500 ml/$2.50

   *b. Phenolated calamine, USP:
   1% phenol added to calamine formulations. Cost is the same as for plain calamine lotion.

   *c. Alcoholic calamine lotion (more drying):

Calamine	10 gm
Zinc oxide	10 gm
Bentonite	2 gm
Talc	10 gm
Glycerin	10 gm
Alcohol	40 ml
Water, to make	100 ml

   *d. Calamine liniment (less drying):

Calamine	15 gm
Peanut oil	50 ml
Calcium hydroxide, to make	100 ml

   e. Menthol lotion with phenol (Schamberg's):

Menthol	0.5 gm
Phenol	1 gm
Zinc oxide	20 gm
Calcium hydroxide solution	40 ml
Peanut oil, to make	100 ml

*Menthol, phenol, or camphor may be added to any of the calamine lotions.

(1) Packaging and cost:
500 ml/$7.00

f. Menthol   0.25 gm
Phenol   1 gm
In O/W or W/O base such as Eucerin, to make   100 gm

(1) Packaging and cost:
Menthol 0.5%, phenol 0.1% in W/O emulsion base
(Ambix Labs), 454 gm/$7.75

g. Menthol   0.5–1.0 gm
Phenol   0.5–1.0 gm
Benzyl alcohol   5–10 gm
Olive oil   5 ml
Propylene glycol   5 ml
Camphor water, to make   100 ml

h. Menthol   0.25 gm
Phenol   0.50 gm
Coal tar solution   5.0 gm
Zinc oxide   15.0 gm
Talc   15.0 gm
Glycerin   10.0 ml
Isopropanol 25% (less drying)–70% (more   qs 100 ml
drying)

2. Gels, ointments, and oils

a. Camphor
Menthol
Benzyl alcohol, 9%
Isopropyl alcohol, 30%
In mildly drying, greaseless gel base

(1) Packaging and cost:
60-gm tube (as Topic)/$3.00

b. Phenol   1 gm
Menthol   0.25 gm
Salicylic acid   1 gm
Coal tar   2 gm
Hydrophilic ointment, to make   100 gm

c. Phenol   0.5 gm
Menthol   0.5 gm
Camphor   0.5 gm
Liquid petrolatum, to make   100 ml

d. Salicylic acid   3%
Phenol   1%

(1) Packaging and cost (as Panscol):
Ointment, 90 gm/$4.25
Lotion, 120 ml/$4.75

3. Impregnated pads

a. Glycerin   10%
Witch hazel (contains gallic acid, tannin,
and volatile oils)   50%
Water   40%

        (1) Dosage: Apply prn as replacement for toilet tissue or as cleansing and antipruritic wipe in prevention and therapy of pruritus ani and other perineal pruritic processes.

        (2) Packaging and cost:
           as Tucks: box of 40/$3.50
                     box of 100/$5.25

  4. Miscellaneous antipruritic preparations (some contain potential allergic sensitizers such as benzocaine and diphenhydramine).

    a. Calamatum contains benzocaine (1.05% in spray, 3% in ointment), calamine, zinc oxide, menthol (in aerosol), camphor, phenol (in ointment), isopropanol (in spray).

        (1) Packaging and cost:
           aerosol, 85 gm/$4.00
           ointment, 45 gm/$4.00
           lotion, 113 ml/$4.75

    b. Caladryl contains 1% diphenhydramine, 1% camphor, calamine, 2% alcohol.

        (1) Packaging and cost:
           lotion, 180 ml/$4.00

  5. Miscellaneous external analgesic products. These multi-ingredient preparations are used by many patients for aches and pains.

    a. Ben-Gay lotion contains 15% methyl salicylate, 7% menthol; Extra-Strength Balm contains 30% methyl salicylate, 8% menthol.

    b. Mentholatum ointment contains 9% camphor, 1.35% menthol and aromatic oils. Mentholatum Deep Heating ointment contains 12.7% methyl salicylate, 6% menthol, eucalyptus oil and turpentine oil.

    c. Sloan's liniment contains 46.7% turpentine oil, 6.7% pine oil, 3.3% camphor, 2.6% methyl salicylate, 0.6% capsicum, and 40% kerosene.

    d. Absorbent Rub lotion contains 1.6% camphor, 1.6% menthol, 0.7% methyl salicylate, 0.6% wormwood oil, 0.5% sassafras oil, and 0.03% capsicum. The other ingredients are 69% isopropyl alcohol, 1.16% green soap, 0.9% pine tar soap, 0.5% o-phenylphenol, and 0.5% benzocaine.

References

ANTIPRURITIC AND EXTERNAL ANALGESIC AGENTS

Ayres, S.   The fine art of scratching. *J. A. M. A.* 189:1003–1007, 1964.

Epstein, E., and Pinsky, J. B.   A blind study. *Arch. Dermatol.* 89:548–549, 1964.

Fischer, R. W.   Comparison of antipruritic agents administered orally: A double blind study. *J. A. M. A.* 203:418–419, 1968.

Herndon, J. H.   Itching: The pathophysiology of pruritus. *Int. J. Dermatol.* 14:465–484, 1975.

Lyell, A.   The itching patient: A review of the causes of pruritus. *Scott. Med. J.* 17:334–347, 1972.

Cleansing agents

I. **Discussion.** Soaps are alkaline (pH 9–10) sodium or potassium salts of fatty acids. Anionic surfactants and cationic detergent cleansers emulsify fats with water and help remove foreign particles from the skin. Their surfactant and alkaline properties may, however, lead to primary irritation of intact or already damaged skin.

   A. Soaps or cleansing bars are manufactured in many ways, all of which are said to make them "milder" on the skin.

      1. **Neutral soaps** or soaplike preparations contain synthetic surfactants and have a pH of 7.5 or less. Preparations include: Alpha Keri, Aveenobar (contains 50% oatmeal), Dove, Lowila Cake, Neutrogena, pHisoDerm, Purpose.

      2. **Superfatted soaps** contain increased fat or oil on the assumption that they leave a film of protective oil on the skin. Preparations include Basis, Emulave, Oilatum Soap.

      3. **Antimicrobial bar soaps** contain topical antiseptics such as carbanilide, triclocarban, or the substituted phenol, triclosan. They have some deodorant action by inhibiting bacterial growth. Representative soaps include Coast, Dial, Lifebuoy, Safeguard, and Zest.

   B. A new chamber test for assessing the **irritant qualities of soaps** has been utilized to test 18 commonly used brands. Great differences were noted, but most soaps had appreciable potential for irritating the skin.

      1. The only soap which could be classified as "mild" was Dove.

      2. The mid-range group included Aveenobar, Purpose, Dial, Alpha Keri, Fels Naphtha, Neutrogena, Ivory, Oilatum, and Lowila.

      3. Zest, Camay, and Lava were classified as "harsh."

   C. **Shampoos** are liquid soaps or detergents used for cleansing and/or therapeutic measures. Individual preparations are discussed elsewhere (see p. 156).

      1. **Selenium sulfide suspension** (SeS_2, Exsel, Iosel, Selsun) is a mixture of selenium monosulfide and a suspension of solid selenium and amorphous sulfur. Selenium acts by inhibiting cellular proliferation and has high substantivity. Little or no toxicity has been observed when applied directly to normal skin or hair, but these products should not be used on inflamed or exudative skin where absorption may be increased. They are used in the control of seborrheic dermatitis, dandruff, and tinea versicolor.

         a. **Packaging and cost:**
            Exsel (R_x), Selsun (R_x), 2.5% suspension, 120 ml/$5.50
            Iosel (R_x), 2.5% suspension, 240 ml/$7.50
            Generic (R_x), 2.5% suspension, 240 ml/$2.75
            Selsun Blue, 1% cream, 105 gm/$3.25
                          1% lotion, 120 ml/$2.75
            Generic, 1% liquid, 120 ml/$1.50

2. **Zinc pyrithrione** is the active ingredient in several shampoos used to control dandruff and seborrheic dermatitis (see p. 156) and is also effective in the therapy of tinea versicolor (see p. 89). It was originally added to dandruff shampoos for its antimicrobial properties, but those characteristics seem unrelated to its unquestionable effectiveness. When added to cultures of skin epithelial fibroblast cultures, zinc pyrithrione has a rapid cytotoxic effect and no apparent inhibition of mitosis. It is substantive to the skin allowing continuing therapeutic effect after washing.

a. **Structure**

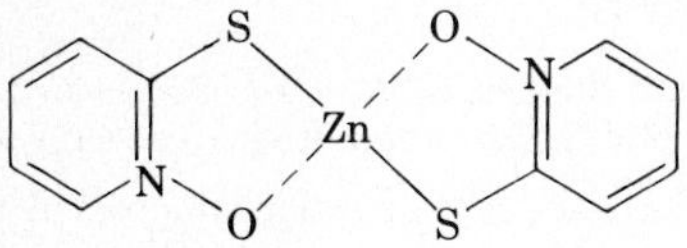

Zinc pyrithrione

b. **Packaging:** Shampoos including Breck (1%), Danex (1%), DHS-Zinc (1%), Head and Shoulders (2%), Zincon (1%).

References

CLEANSING AGENTS

Blank, I. H.   Action of soaps and detergents on the skin. *Practitioner* 202:147–151, 1969.

Frosch, P. J., and Kligman, A. M.   The soap chamber test: A new method for assessing the irritancy of soaps. *J. Am. Acad. Derm.* 1:35–41, 1979.

Frost, P., and Horwitz, S. N.   *Principles of Cosmetics for the Dermatologist.* St. Louis: Mosby, 1982.

Priestly, G. C., and Brown, J. C.   Acute toxicity of zinc pyrithione to human skin cells in vitro. *Acta Derm. Venerol.* (Stockh.) 60:145–148, 1980.

Spoor, H. J.   Shampoos and hair dyes. *Cutis* 201:189–190, 1977.

Cosmetics and covering agents
(See also p. 230)

I. **Hypoallergenic cosmetics**

A. So-called hypoallergenic cosmetics abound, but only a few manufacturers will supply the physician with a list of the nonallergenic ingredients of their products. The term *hypoallergenic* means only that all product ingredients are chemically pure, but **not** that they are less likely to cause allergic reactions. Pharmaceutical companies specifically involved in the manufacture of less allergenic compounds include Almay and Ar-Ex.

II. **Covering agents**

A. **Covermark** (Lydia O'Leary) is a tinted, inert, opaque makeup that is highly effective in covering pigmentary, vascular, and scarring lesions. It is, in addition, an effective sunscreen. A waterproof form is available.

1. Packaging and cost:
Cream: 22.5 gm/$6.50
　　　 85.5 gm/$15.00
Stick form, as Spotstick/$4.00

B. Erace (Max Factor) is an effective covering agent available in lipstick form.

C. Covering agents and stains for vitiligo are discussed on p. 112.

References

COSMETICS AND COVERING AGENTS

Estrin, N. F., Crosley, P. A., and Haynes, C. R.　*CFTA Cosmetic Ingredient Dictionary.* Washington, D.C.: Cosmetic, Toiletry and Fragrance Association, Inc., 1982.

Maltz, B.　Cosmetics: Reactions of the skin to various components. *Weekly Update: Dermatology* 1(24):2–5, 1979.

Spoor, H. J.　Cosmetic review. *Cutis* 18:30–39, 1976.

Depilatories and removal of excessive hair

I. Hypertrichosis

A. Mild hypertrichosis, most often familial in nature, is a cause for cosmetic concern for many women. It is mandatory that endocrine or local factors be ruled out before dismissing excessive hair as a simple cosmetic difficulty.

II. Hair removal

A. There are several ways by which to decrease the amount or appearance of excessive hair.

1. Bleaching fine hair will make it less obvious. A 6% solution of hydrogen peroxide, commonly known as 20-volume peroxide, is most often used. It may be used alone, but the addition of an alkali, usually 10 drops of ammonia per 30 ml of peroxide, immediately before use will activate the hydrogen peroxide and permit more intense bleaching.

2. Plucking hair is painful but effective. Each pluck will start another growing cycle in the hair root.

3. Wax epilation is essentially just widespread plucking. A warm wax is placed on the skin, allowed to dry, and then, as it is peeled off, the hairs are pulled out.

4. Shaving is quick and effective and does *not* cause the hair to regrow more rapidly or more abundantly.

5. Rubbing with a pumice stone will remove fine hair.

6. Depilatories disintegrate and destroy hair on topical application by degrading disulfide bonds. The hair is left as a gelatinous mass, which is easily wiped off the skin. Two active ingredients are currently used:

a. Sulfides of alkali metals and alkaline earths are the most effective, but they also develop a disagreeable hydrogen sulfide odor and are more irritating than thioglycollate products. Preparations available include Magic Shaving Powder and Royal Crown Shaving Powder. Both contain barium sulfide and calcium hydroxide.

   b. Thioglycollate-containing agents require increased contact time, but are more easily perfumed and are less irritating than other preparations. Preparations available include Better Off, Nair, Neet, Nudit, Shimmy Shins, Sleek, Surgi Cream.

7. Electrolysis is the only permanent method of hair removal. In this procedure the hair bulb is destroyed by a high-frequency electric current, and the hair will not grow back later. When performed in a skillful fashion, this is a useful technique. Pitlike perifollicular scarring and regrowth of incompletely destroyed hairs may follow electrolysis. Self-use, home electrolysis units are instruments that some patients may easily learn to use to yield effective results.

References

DEPILATORIES AND REMOVAL OF EXCESSIVE HAIR

Spoor, H. J.   Depilation and epilation. *Cutis* 21:283–287, 1978.

Sternberg, T. H.   Clinical study of self-use electrolysis. *Derm. Digest* 7:20–27, 1976.

Dermatologic topical preparations and vehicles

(See also p. 228)

Lotions, creams, ointments, and powders can be used alone or may act as vehicles for pharmacologically active substances. Ideally, they are nontoxic, stable, and do not sensitize with repeated use. It should not be assumed that "inert" vehicles or bases have no effect on the skin or epithelial metabolism. Petrolatum, for example, has been shown to interfere with the oxidation of arachidonic acid and inhibit synthesis of prostaglandins in animal skin. It also appears to retard the rate of epidermal healing, whereas O/W creams and lotions increase this rate.

I. Constituents of dermatologic products. Dermatologic vehicles are often complex substances that contain many additives.

   A. Emulsifying or dispensing agents provide stability and homogeneity. Glyceryl monostearate, polyethylene glycol derivatives (polyoxyl 40 stearate, polysorbate 80), and sodium lauryl sulfate are such agents used in preparations containing oily components and water. Sodium lauryl sulfate may act as an irritant.

   B. The consistency and appearance of creams are improved by the addition of additives such as ethylenediamines (frequent allergic sensitizers in products such as Mycolog cream), and cetyl palmitate and related esters.

   C. Lubricants, emollients, and/or antifoaming agents include stearic acid and stearyl alcohol.

   D. Methylcellulose and gum tragacanth are used as suspending agents in pastes and ointments.

E. Preservatives include the parabens (short alkyl esters of parahydroxybenzoic acid), oxyquinoline sulfate, organic quaternary ammonium compounds, hexachlorophene, parachlorometaxylenol, and chlorobutenol. Methyl and propylparaben may act as allergic sensitizers.

II. Lotions, creams, ointments, and powders

A. Lotions are suspensions of a powder in water that require shaking before application. Many are now held in more or less permanent suspension by suspending or surface-active agents. They provide a protective, drying, and cooling effect and may act as a vehicle for other agents. The addition of alcohol increases the cooling effect. If an astringent, such as aluminum, is present, it will precipitate protein and dry and seal exudating surfaces.

1. Calamine lotion (see Antipruritic Agents, p. 289).

2. Alcohol, zinc oxide, and talc lotion (more drying):

Zinc oxide	15 gm
Talc	15 gm
Glycerin	10 gm
Alcohol	30 ml
Water, to make	100 ml

3. Burow's emulsion, modified (less drying):

Zinc oxide	10 gm
Talc	10 gm
Olive oil	45 ml
Anhydrous lanolin	10 gm
Aluminum acetate solution	2.5 ml
Water, to make	100 ml

4. Neutrogena Vehicle/N is a topical vehicle system for extemporaneous compounding. Multiple drugs are soluble in Vehicle/N and stable for at least 3 months. These include clindamycin HCl, erythromycin base and stearate, camphor, menthol, hydrocortisone (alcohol), liquid carbonis detergens, and some corticosteroids.

a. Vehicle/N contains: ethyl alcohol 47.5%, isopropyl alcohol 4.0%, propylene glycol, laureth-4.
Vehicle/N mild contains: alcohol 41.5%, isopropyl alcohol 6%, laureth-4.

b. Packaging and cost:
50 ml/$4.50

B. Oil-in-water and water-washable creams are easily washable and will take up water but are not in themselves soluble.

1. Hydrophilic ointment, USP contains polyoxyl 40 stearate as an emulsifying and wetting agent, stearyl alcohol as a stabilizer, and parabens (parahydroxybenzoic acid) as preservatives. It is a good vehicle for water-soluble medications. If hydrophilic ointment is used under occlusion, an irritant contact dermatitis may result. Sodium lauryl sulfate is the provocative agent.

a. **Contains:**

Methylparaben	0.025 gm
Propylparaben	0.015 gm
Sodium lauryl sulfate	1.0 gm
Stearyl alcohol	25 gm
White petrolatum	25 gm
Propylene glycol	12 gm
Polyoxyl 40 stearate	5 gm
Water, to make	100 ml

b. **Packaging and cost:**
   480 gm/$5.00

2. **Glycerin** is frequently found in moisturizing creams (such as Acid Mantle, Aquacare, Emulave, Lubriderm, Jergens). This agent has been termed a humectant, which is a substance that is purportedly absorbed into the skin to help replace missing hygroscopic substances, or if absorption does not occur, to attract water from the atmosphere and serve as a reservoir for the stratum corneum. In fact, glycerin does appear to be effective in treating dry skin but its mechanism of action is not known.

3. Commercially available oil-in-water emulsion bases include Acid Mantle cream, Nivea cream, Purpose Dry Skin cream, Lubriderm.

C. **Ointments.** These bland bases may have an antimitotic effect on stripped epidermis, perhaps related to the effects of physical occlusion. The "stickiest" preparations are the most inhibitory.

1. **Water-soluble ointments (Polyethylene glycols) (Carbowax)** are completely water soluble and may also act as lubricants or as water-soluble bases.

2. **Emulsifiable ointments**

   a. **Water-in-oil absorbent ointments** are difficult to wash off and are insoluble in water, but will take up water in significant amounts.

   (1) **Hydrous wool fat, USP (lanolin),** although insoluble in water, is capable of absorbing twice its weight in water. It is a yellow white preparation containing 28% water and is the purified, fatlike substance from the wool of sheep, *Ovis aries* Linné.

   Anhydrous lanolin, a brown yellow absorbent ointment that contains less than 0.25% water, is more greasy and occlusive.

   (a) **Packaging and cost:**
       480 gm/$6.00

   (2) **Cold cream, USP (rose water ointment)** is a pleasant-smelling, soft base used chiefly because of its cosmetic appearance and for its lubricating, emollient, and cooling effects (hence its name, cold cream). These preparations are good vehicles for the incorporation of many substances. The official cold cream is a water-in-oil (W/O) emulsion, but there are many variations that approach oil-in-water (O/W) emulsions. These

creams are the basis of many cosmetic products such as cleansing, night, moisturizing, and eye creams.

(a) Contains:

Spermaceti	12.5 gm
White wax	12.0 gm
Mineral oil	56.0 gm
Sodium borate	0.5 gm
Water	19.0 ml
	100.0 gm

(b) Packaging and cost:
454 gm/$5.50

b. Similar bases consisting of oils and emulsifying agents but no water are termed **absorbent ointments.** They are difficult to wash off and are insoluble in water, but they will soak up water to become water-in-oil emulsions.

(1) Hydrophilic petrolatum, USP is characterized by its ability to take up large amounts of water. It is less greasy than petrolatum but more greasy than hydrophilic ointment.

(a) Contains:

Cholesterol	3 gm
Stearyl alcohol	3 gm
White wax	8 gm
White petrolatum, to make	100 gm

(b) Packaging and cost:
454 gm/$10.75

(2) Commercially available hydrophilic (W/O) bases include Eucerin (which is equal parts Aquaphor and water), Keri Cream, Nivea oil and cream, Polysorb, and Aquaphor, the latter two when hydrated.

3. Water-repellent ointments consist of inert oils, are insoluble in water, are difficult to wash off, will not dry out, and change little with time.

a. Petrolatum, USP is a semisolid mixture of hydrocarbons obtained from petrolatum and is the most commonly used base for ointments. **White petrolatum (decolorized petrolatum)** is more esthetically appealing and is most often used.

(1) Packaging and cost:
454 gm/$2.25

b. Liquid petrolatum, USP (mineral oil, liquid paraffin) is a mixture of purified hydrocarbons obtained from petrolatum.

(1) Packaging and cost:
500 ml/$2.25

4. Silicone (dimethicone) ointments are excellent water-protective agents because they have an extremely low surface tension and penetrate crevices in the skin to form a plasticlike barrier. Further, they are nontoxic, inert, stable, and water-repellent. As such, they are useful as barrier creams in industry or wherever constant or frequent exposure to aqueous compounds is a problem. They will not, however, protect well against solvents, oils, or dusts. Silicone preparations are available as sprays, liquids, ointments, and creams.

a. Structure

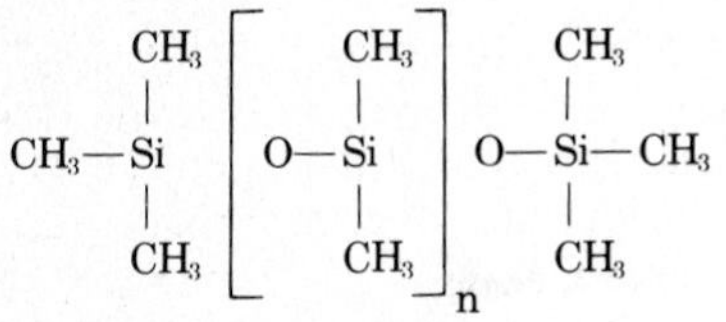

$$CH_3 - \underset{\underset{CH_3}{|}}{\overset{\overset{CH_3}{|}}{Si}} \left[O - \underset{\underset{CH_3}{|}}{\overset{\overset{CH_3}{|}}{Si}} \right]_n O - \underset{\underset{CH_3}{|}}{\overset{\overset{CH_3}{|}}{Si}} - CH_3$$

Dimethicone

b. Packaging and cost:
10% silicone ointment, 60 gm/$3.25
30% silicone ointment, 60 gm/$4.25

As there are no all-purpose effective protective agents, it is essential to choose a particular cream for protection against a specific hazard, i.e., against dusts and particulate matter, aqueous compounds, or solvents (see p. 52).

D. Pastes are made by incorporating a fine powder into an ointment. The base is usually petrolatum, and the powders, which constitute 20–50% of the paste, are usually zinc oxide, talc, starch, bentonite, aluminum oxide, or titanium dioxide. Pastes are more absorptive, less greasy, and less effective vehicles than ointments and are less efficient at preventing water evaporation. However, they are excellent protective compounds and may be used in subacute and chronic dermatoses. Pastes should be applied evenly with a tongue blade or finger and may be removed most easily with a cloth soaked in mineral or vegetable oil.

Zinc oxide paste, USP (Lassar's):

Zinc oxide	25 gm
Starch	25 gm
White petrolatum, to make	100 gm

Packaging and cost:
30 gm/$1.25
454 gm/$3.25

E. Powders increase evaporation, reduce friction, and provide antipruritic and cooling sensations. Zinc oxide or stearate, magnesium stearate, talc, cornstarch, bentonite, and titanium dioxide may either be used as dusting powders or incorporated into pastes or shake lotions. Talc is the most lubricating, but it does not absorb water; starch is less lubricating and absorbs water; zinc oxide has absorptive properties intermediate between the two. Zeasorb powder, which contains 45% microporous cellulose, has a relative absorbency of water almost twice that of talc-based powders. Talc can cause a granulomatous reaction in wounds, and starch may be metabolized by organisms and cause an increase in *Candida* overgrowth.

Talc, USP (talcum) is hydrous magnesium silicate that sometimes contains a small amount of aluminum silicate.

Packaging and cost:
454 gm/$3.00

F. Miscellaneous

1. **Collodion** is a mixture of pyroxylin (a nitrocellulose derivative), ether, and alcohol that forms an adherent film on the skin after drying. **Flexible collodion** contains collodion, camphor 0.2%, and castor oil 0.3%. It is used as a vehicle for salicylic and lactic acids in the treatment of warts (see p. 306), as a protective film over herpes zoster lesions (see p. 104), and over fissures as present in chronic hand dermatitis.

   a. **Packaging and cost:**
   Flexible collodion, 120 ml/$1.75.

References

DERMATOLOGIC TOPICAL PREPARATIONS AND VEHICLES

Bergstresser, P. R., and Eaglstein, W. H.   Irritation by hydrophilic ointment under occlusion. *Arch. Dermatol.* 108:218–219, 1973.

Eaglstein, W. H., and Mertz, P. M.   "Inert" vehicles do affect wound healing. *J. Invest. Dermatol.* 74:90–91, 1980.

Pennys, N. S.   Inhibition of arachidonic acid oxidation *in vitro* by vehicle components. *Acta Derm. Venerol.* (Stockh.) 62:59–61, 1982.

Pennys, N. S., Eaglstein, W. H., and Ziboh, V.   Petrolatum: Interference with the oxidation of arachidonic acid. *Br. J. Dermatol.* 103:257–262, 1980.

Tree, S., and Marks, R.   An explanation for the "placebo" effect of bland ointment bases. *Br. J. Dermatol.* 92:195–198, 1975.

Insect repellents

I. **Discussion.** See Bites and Stings, p. 29.

II. Effective preparations contain either **diethyltoluamide (deet), ethyl hexanediol (E-H),** or multiple ingredients. The amount of active ingredients varies greatly and generally is highest in the liquid products. Efficacy is related to the amount of active ingredients present.

A. **Diethyltoluamide** (see p. 34) is an organic liquid that is an excellent mosquito repellent and is in commercial preparations such as sprays, creams, and lotions that vary in concentrations from 6% to more than 50%. The U.S. Army standard insect spray contains 75% deet.

B. **Ethyl hexanediol** will not irritate human skin but can cause a chemical conjunctivitis. It is a standard repellent for chiggers, mosquitoes, black flies, and other biting flies, and is more useful when combined with dimethyl phthalate and indalone. The mixture of these three chemicals will repel ticks and flies when it is applied to clothing.

C. **Dimethyl carbate** can be applied to clothing in order to repel ticks.

D. **Butopyronoxyl** is not water soluble and can be applied to skin and clothing to repel biting stable flies, Lone Star ticks, dog and cat fleas, and chiggers.

E. **Butylethylpropandiol** is used together with benzyl benzoate as the U.S. Army Standard for clothing impregnation to repel ticks and chiggers.

F. **Benzyl benzoate** (see p. 267) can be used in a 5% emulsion to repel many anthropods and can be used as a lotion to treat sarcoptic mange and canine pediculosis.

Keratolytic, cytotoxic, and destructive agents

I. **Anthralin,** a synthetic substance prepared from anthracene, is used in the therapy of psoriasis. It is most effective when incorporated into a thick paste containing salicylic acid. Anthralin reduces epidermal mitotic activity and in cultured human cells anthralin inhibits both replication and repair synthesis of DNA. It may act as an irritant and will stain skin and clothing (see p. 145).

A. **Structure**

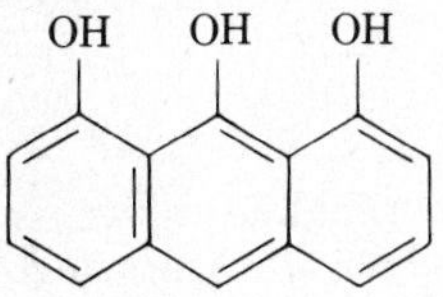

Anthralin

B. **Packaging and cost:**
   Anthra-Derm Ointment contains anthralin (0.10%, 0.25%, 0.50%, 1%), petrolatum, and a fatty acid ester: 45 gm/$6.50
   Lasan Unguent contains 0.4% anthralin with salicylic acid in a water-washable base: 120-gm jar/$10.75
   Drithocreme contains 0.1, 0.25, or 0.5% anthralin in a vanishing cream base: 50-gm tube/$13.50

II. **Cantharidin** (Spanish fly, Russian fly) causes intraepidermal vesiculation and is used in the treatment of warts and other benign cutaneous lesions (see p. 194).

A. **Structure**

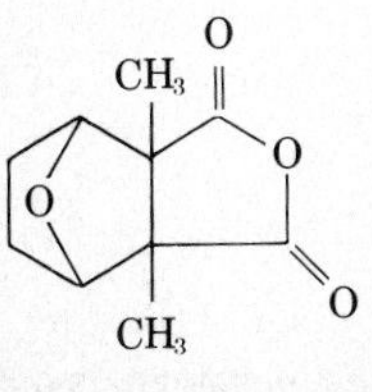

Cantharidin

B. **Packaging and cost:**
Cantharone (0.7% cantharidin, in equal amounts of flexible collodion and acetone): 7.5 ml/$20.00
Verrusol (1% cantharidin, 5% podophyllin, 30% salicylic acid): 7.5 ml/$4.20 (sold to physicians only)

III. **Caustics** are used alone in some circumstances, and are often used to obtain hemostasis. They are also used in combination with electrosurgery for the superficial treatment of hyperplastic cutaneous lesions (warts, keratoses, xanthelasmas, basal cell carcinoma) and are also utilized in cosmetic therapy for aging, wrinkled facial skin.

A. **Mono-, di-, and trichloroacetic acids** (CCl_3COOH [trichloroacetic acid]) are rapid and effective local cauterizing agents. They are strongly corrosive and act by precipitation and coagulation of skin proteins. Saturated solutions are often used. The monochloroacetic derivative is more deeply destructive than the trichloroacetic preparation; 35–50% trichloroacetic acid is the most useful preparation for general use.

B. **Silver nitrate** ($AgNO_3$) in solid form or in solutions stronger than 5%, is used for its caustic action; 5–10% solutions may be applied to fissures or excessive granulation tissue. **Silver nitrate sticks** consist of a head of toughened silver nitrate (>94.5%) prepared by fusing the silver salt with sodium chloride. They are dipped in water and applied as needed.

Packaging and cost:
100 sticks/$4.00

IV. **Fluorouracil (Efudex, Fluoroplex, 5-FU)** is a pyrimidine antagonist that interferes with DNA synthesis by inhibiting thymidylate synthetase activity. It is used topically, for the treatment of multiple actinic keratoses (see p. 131), superficial basal cell carcinomas, and Bowen's disease; it has also been found useful in therapy of some types of warts (see pp. 194, 197).

A. **Structure**

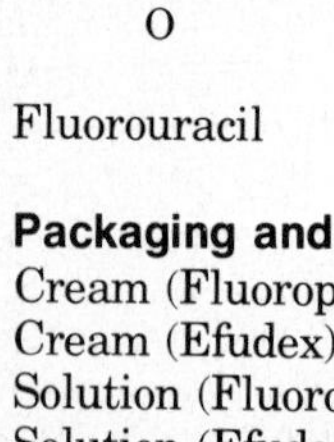

Fluorouracil

B. **Packaging and cost:**
Cream (Fluoroplex), 1%: 30 gm/$9.75
Cream (Efudex), 5%: 25 gm/$11.75
Solution (Fluoroplex), 1%: 30 ml/$9.75
Solution (Efudex), 2%: 10 ml/$7.25
Solution (Efudex), 5%: 10 ml/$10.50

V. **Podophyllum resin (Podophyllin)** is a resinic extract obtained from the roots of either of two plant species: *Podophyllum peltatum* or *P. emodi* (called also mandrake or May-apple) and is used in the treatment of condyloma acuminatum and other warts. Lesional necrosis and involution are caused by the lignans present in concentrations of 15–20% in *P. peltatum* and 30–40% in *P. emodi* resins—podophyllin is chemically highly variable. In vitro, podophyllin inhibits RNA synthesis. Podophyllotoxin, an active component of podophyllum resin, binds to intracellular microtubular proteins, prevents the development of the mitotic spindle and thereby exerts its effects on the G_2 phase of the cell cycle. Podophyllin can induce severe erosive changes in adjacent tissue, which thus must be protected from its action. Patients have developed serious systemic intoxication after application of abundant amounts of podophyllin to large lesions or onto mucous membranes. It is applied as a 25% suspension in compound tincture of benzoin or in alcohol (see p. 196). Recent studies demonstrate efficacy of a standardized method based on the repeated application of 0.5% podophyllotoxin in ethanol 2id for 3 days.

A. Structure

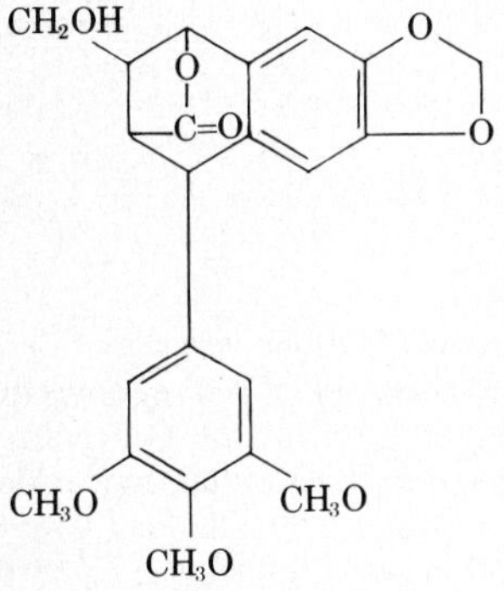

Podophyllotoxin

B. Packaging and cost:

Podoben (25% podophyllin in compound benzoin tincture 10% and isopropyl alcohol 70%): 5 ml/$5.50

Podophyllin resin, 30 ml/$25.00

Verrex (podophyllin 10%, salicylic acid 7%): 7.5 ml, sold to physicians only.

Verrusol (podophyllin 5%, salicylic acid 30%, cantharidin 1%): 7.5 ml, sold to physicians only.

VI. Propylene glycol solution (40–60%, v/v, $CH_2CH[OH]CH_2OH$, propylene glycol) applied to the skin under plastic occlusion hydrates the skin and causes desquamation of scales. Propylene glycol, isotonic in 2% concentration, is a widely used vehicle in dermatologic preparations. Hydroalcoholic gels containing propylene glycol or other substances augment the keratolytic action of salicylic acid. Keralyt gel consists of 6% salicylic acid, 19.4% alcohol, hydroxypropylcellulose, propylene glycol and water and is an extremely effective keratolytic agent. Overnight occlusion is used nightly until improvement is evident, at which time the frequency of therapy can be decreased to every third night or once weekly. This therapy is well tolerated, is usually nonirritating, and has been most successful in patients with X-linked ichthyosis and ichthyosis vulgaris (see p. 69). Burning and stinging may occur when applied to damaged skin. Patients with other abnormalities of keratinization with hyperkeratosis, scaling, and dryness may also benefit. Used concomitantly with Topsyn gel under occlusion, this combination is very useful in thickly-scaling psoriasis.

Packaging and cost:
30 mg (Keralyt gel)/$6.75

VII. Resorcinol (resorcin), a phenol derivative, is less keratolytic than salicylic acid. This drug is an irritant and sensitizer and is said to be both bactericidal and fungicidal. Solutions containing 1–2% have been used in preparations for seborrhea, acne, and psoriasis.

A. Structure

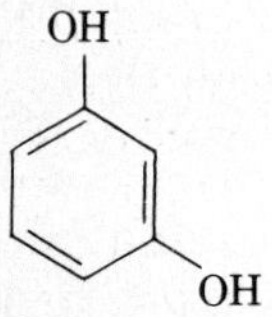

OH

OH

Resorcinol

VIII. Retinoids (see pp. 11, 69, 147, 237)

IX. Salicylic acid is keratolytic and at concentrations between 3% and 6% causes softening of the horny layers and shedding of scales. It produces this desquamation by solubilizing the intercellular cement and enhances the shedding of corneocytes by decreasing cell-to-cell cohesion. In concentrations greater than 6% it can be destructive to tissue. Salicylic acid is used in the treatment of superficial fungal infections, acne, psoriasis, seborrheic dermatitis, warts, and other scaling dermatoses. When combined with sulfur, some believe a synergistic keratolytic effect is produced. Common preparations include a 3% and 6% ointment with equal concentration of sulfur; 6% propylene glycol solution (Keralyt); 5–20% with equal parts lactic acid in flexible collodion for warts (Duofilm, Tiflex); in a cream base at any concentration for keratolytic effects; as a 60% ointment for plantar warts; and in a 40% plaster on velvet cloth for the treatment of calluses and warts (40% salicylic acid plaster).

A. Structure

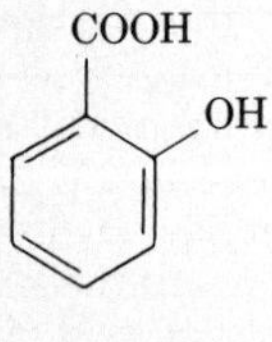

COOH

OH

Salicylic acid

B. Packaging and cost:
Duofilm, 16.7% salicylic acid, 16.7% lactic acid in flexible collodion: 15 ml/$5.25

Keralyt gel, 6% salicylic acid in hydroalcoholic propylene glycol gel: 30 gm/$6.75

Whitfield's ointment, 12% benzoic acid, 6% salicylic acid: 30 gm/$1.00

Saligel, 5% salicylic acid in hydroalcoholic gel: 60 gm/$3.50

X. Selenium sulfide (see p. 294).

XI. Sulfur is incorporated into many preparations used in the treatment of acne, rosacea, ringworm, psoriasis, scabies, seborrheic dermatitis, and infestations. Sulfur inhibits the growth of microorganisms, particularly fungi and parasites. More effective keratolytic, antifungal, and antibacterial agents are available.

XII. Tar compounds. A tar is a product of destructive distillation of organic substances. Tar is obtained from various sources and thus there are different types. Wood tars include oil of cade, beech, birch, and pine. They do not photosensitize. Bituminous tars include ichthyol and ammonium ichthyosulphonate, a distillation of shale deposits containing fossilized fish. Coal tars are by-products of the destructive distillation of bituminous coals and are ill-defined, aromatic, complex substances. They contain 2–8% light oils (benzene, toluene, xylene), 2–10% middle oils (phenols, cresols, naphthaline), 8–10% heavy oils (naphthaline and derivatives), 16–20% anthracene oils, and about 50% pitch. Coal tars are brown black, slightly soluble in water, and partially soluble in many solvents. Only coal tar and coal tar pitch have photosensitizing properties.

In hairless mice coal tars have been shown to inhibit DNA synthesis. Five percent crude coal tar ointment applied to normal human skin causes an initial transient hyperplasia followed by a 20% reduction in viable epidermal thickness after 40 days' treatment. These findings indicate that tar by itself can act as a cytostatic agent. Although coal tars are carcinogenic for the skin of experimental animals and are often used along with another oncogenic agent, ultraviolet light, the risk of developing cancer from therapeutic coal tar products remains unclear. The presence of unidentified mutagenic material(s) in the urine of patients treated with coal tar has been recently reported.

Tars have long been found to be useful in patients with eczematous, pruritic, and hyperplastic disease. They are often used in combination with sulfur, salicylic acid, and topical steroids and are used with UVB ultraviolet light in the therapy of psoriasis (see p. 145).

A. Coal tar products are available over the counter or may be compounded to USP, NF, or other formulas.

1. **Pragmatar:**
Coal tar distillate	4%
Precipitated sulfur	3%
Salicylic acid in O/W base	3%

   a. **Packaging and cost:**
   30 gm/$2.75

2. **Estar gel:**
Tar (equivalent to crude coal tar) in hydroalcoholic base	5%

   a. **Packaging and cost:**
   90 gm/$5.75

3. **Tar ointment, USP:**

Coal tar	1 gm
Polysorbate 80	0.5 gm
Zinc oxide paste, to make	100 gm

a. **Packaging and cost:**
454 gm/$16.00

4. **James C. White's tar ointment:**

Coal tar	5 gm
Polysorbate 80	2.5 gm
Starch	45 gm
Zinc oxide	5 gm
Petrolatum, to make	100 gm

5. **Coal tar creams** include Tarbonis (5%) and Tegrin (5%).

6. **Tar gels** include Estar (5%), psoriGel (7.5%), and T-Gel (5.0%).

7. **Liquid tar preparations** are T/Derm (5%), Tar-Doak lotion (5%), Tegrin (5%), and Zetar emulsion (30%).

8. **Tar ointments** include Supertah (1.25%) and Unguentum Bossi (5%).

9. **Bath preparations** include Balnetar (2.5%), Lavatar (33.5%), Polytar (25%), and Zetar emulsion (30%).

10. **Shampoos** include DHS-T, Ionil T, Pentrax, Paytar, Sebutone, T/Gel, Tegrin, TiSeb-T, Vanseb-T, Zetar. T/Gel is the most pleasant to use and may be the most effective. **Tar soaps** are Packer's Pine Tar and Polytar.

B. **Coal tar solution (liquor carbonis detergens; LCD)** is prepared by extracting coal tar with alcohol and polysorbate (Tween) 80, an emulsifying agent. Each 100 ml of the solution represents 20 gm of coal tar. When mixed with water, a fine dispersion of coal tar results. LCD may be incorporated (at 2–5%) in creams or ointments, in tincture of green soap for a shampoo (10%), or added (60 ml) to the bath for antipruritic and other effects.

C. **Ichthammol (ichthyol)** is obtained by the destructive distillation of certain bituminous schists (shale rock). It is less irritating than coal or wood tars, is water soluble, stains linens, and is used at 2–5% in the treatment of some subacute and chronic dermatoses.

D. **Juniper tar, USP (cade oil)** is obtained by destructive distillation of the heartwood of *Juniperus oxycedrus*. It contains hydrocarbons, including phenolic compounds and aromatic compounds, and is used in the management of chronic eczema and psoriasis. It is available in an ointment, shampoo, bath solution, and soap.

XIII. **Urea-containing preparations** have a softening and moisturizing effect on the stratum corneum and at times may provide good therapy for dry skin and the pruritus associated with it. They appear to have an antipruritic effect separate from their hydrating qualities. Urea compounds disrupt the normal hydrogen bonds of epidermal proteins; thus their effect in dry hyperkeratotic diseases such as ichthyosis vulgaris and psoriasis is not only to make the skin more pliable but also to help remove adherent scales. Lactic acid is also thought to have a softening and moisturizing effect on the stratum corneum (see p. 69).

A. Packaging and cost:
Aquacare (2% urea)
    cream: 75 gm/$3.50
    lotion: 240 ml/$4.50
Aquacare HP (10% urea) cream: 75 gm/$3.75
Carmol-10 (10% urea) lotion: 180 ml/$3.50
Carmol-20 (20% urea) cream: 90 gm/$4.00
U-Lactin (urea and lactic acid) lotion: 240 ml/$4.75

XIV. Zinc pyrithrione (see p. 295).

References

KERATOLYTIC, CYTOTOXIC, AND DESTRUCTIVE AGENTS

Baden, H. P., and Alper, J. C.   A keratolytic gel containing salicylic acid in propylene glycol. *J. Invest. Dermatol.* 61:330–333, 1973.

Bickers, D. R.   The carcinogenicity and mutogenicity of coal tar—a perspective. *J. Invest. Dermatol.* 77:173–175, 1981.

Edinbinden, J. M., Parshly, M. S., Walzer, R. A., and Sanders, S. L.   The effect of cantharidin on epithelial cells in tissue culture. *J. Invest. Dermatol.* 52:291–303, 1969.

Farber, E. M.   Editorial. Tar. *Int. Psoriasis Bull.* 4(4):1–3, 1977.

Fine, J. D., and Arndt, K. A.   *Propylene Glycol: A review.* Princeton: Excerpta Medica, 1980.

Freedberg, I. M.   Effects of podophyllin upon macromolecular metabolism. *J. Invest. Dermatol.* 45:539–546, 1965.

Goldsmith, L. A., and Baden, H. P.   Propylene glycol with occlusion for treatment of ichthyosis. *J. A. M. A.* 220:579–580, 1972.

Lavker, R. M., Grove, G. L., and Kligman, A. M.   The atrophogenic effect of crude coal tar on human epidermis. *Br. J. Dermatol.* 105:77–82, 1981.

Lorenc, E., and Winkelmann, R. K.   Evaluation of dermatologic therapy: I. Sulfur and petrolatum. *Arch. Dermatol.* 83:761–767, 1961.

Lowe, N. L., Breeding, J. H., and Wortzman, M. S.   New coal tar extract and coal tar shampoos: Evaluation by epidermal cell DNA synthesis suppression assay. *Arch. Dermatol.* 118:487–489, 1982.

Roberts, D. L., Marshall, R., and Marks, R.   Detection of the action of salicylic acid on the normal stratum corneum. *Br. J. Dermatol.* 103:191–196, 1980.

Runne, U., and Kunze, J.   Short-duration ("minutes") therapy with dithranol for psoriasis: A new out-patient regimen. *Br. J. Dermatol.* 106:135–139, 1982.

Stoughton, R. B., DeQuoy, P., and Walter, J. F.   Crude coal tar plus near ultraviolet light suppresses DNA synthesis in epidermis. *Arch. Dermatol.* 114:43–48, 1978.

von Krogh, G.   Topical treatment of penile condyloma acuminatum with podophyllin, podophyllotoxin and colchicine: A comparative study. *Acta Dermatol. Venerol.* (Stockh.) 58:163–168, 1978.

von Krogh, G.   Podophyllotoxin in serum: Absorption subsequent to three-day repeated application of a 0.5% ethanolic preparation on condyloma acuminata. *Sex. Trans. Dis.* 9:26–33, 1982.

Wheeler, L. A., Saperstein, M. D., and Lowe, N. J.   Mutagenicity of urine from psoriatic patients undergoing treatment with coal tar and ultraviolet light. *J. Invest. Dermatol.* 77:181–185, 1981.

Wortzman, M., Breeding, J., and Lowe, N. Efficacy of a new coal tar extract and four coal tar shampoos by DNA synthesis suppression assay. *J. Invest. Dermatol.* 76:315, 1981.

Pigmenting and depigmenting agents, sunscreens

I. **Discussion.** See Hyperpigmentation and Hypopigmentation, p. 107.

II. **Agents that cause hypopigmentation**

A. **Hydroquinone products**

1. **Structure**

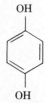

Hydroquinone

2. **Packaging and cost:**

Artra cream, 2%: 30 gm/$2.25
Eldopaque ointment with opaque base, 2%:
15 gm/$7.25
30 gm/$11.00
Eldopaque Forte ointment with opaque base, 4%:
15 gm/$8.50
30 gm/$15.00
Eldoquin
lotion, 2%: 15 ml/$7.50
cream, 2%: 30 gm/$11.00
Eldoquin Forte ointment, 4%: 30 gm/$15.50
Esoterica cream, 2%: 90 gm/$5.25
Melanex solution, 3%: 30 ml/$5.75
Solaquin, 2%, and Solaquin Forte, 4%, cream in PABA ester and benzophenone sunscreen:
30 ml (2%)/$10.00
30 ml (4%)/$14.00

B. **Monobenzone** products should be used only when permanent depigmentation is desired, only after careful consideration by the patient and
physician, and under close supervision.

1. **Structure**

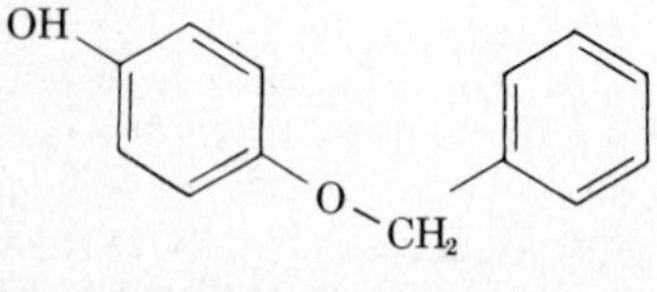

OH ... O–CH₂

Monobenzone

2. Packaging and cost:
Benoquin (R$_x$) 20% ointment: 37.5 gm/$11.50

III. Agents that induce hyperpigmentation and repigmentation

A. Trioxsalen (Trisoralen, trimethylpsoralen) followed by UVA exposure is used to repigment vitiliginous areas (see p. 110) and in photo-chemotherapy (see pp. 146, 220).

1. Structure

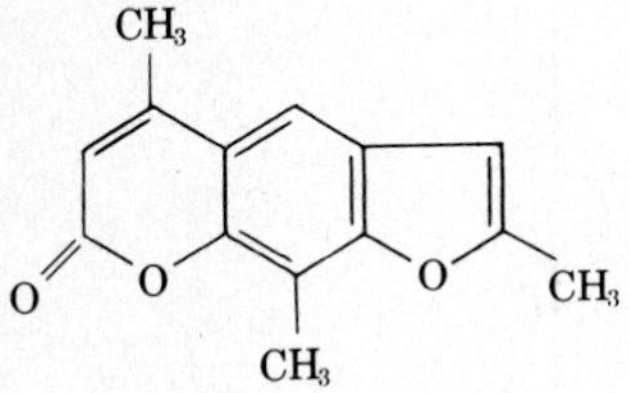

Trioxsalen

2. Packaging and cost:
Trisoralen, 5-mg tablets: 100/$50.00

B. Methoxsalen (methoxypsoralen, Oxsoralen) has effects similar to those of trioxsalen. Methoxsalen is superior to trioxsalen in producing erythema and tanning and is the drug used in PUVA therapy. Methoxsalen is also available as a 1% lotion.

1. Structure

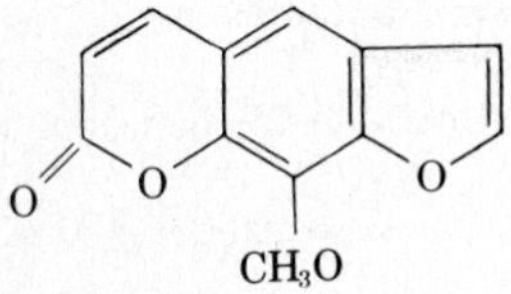

Methoxsalen

2. Packaging and cost:
Oxsoralen 10-mg capsules: 100/$55.00
Oxsoralen 1% lotion: 30 ml/$36.50

IV. Sunscreens (see p. 175).

A. Para-aminobenzoic acid (PABA) preparations absorb UVL between 280–320 nm. This acid will stain white fabrics, especially cotton. The esters of PABA are slightly less effective and do not stain as much.

1. Structure

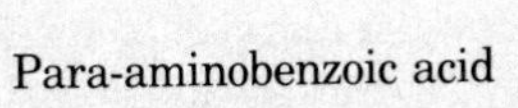

Para-aminobenzoic acid

2. **Packaging and cost:**
   Blockout (5% PABA esters in 70% alcohol): 120 ml/$5.25
   PreSun #4 (4% padimate-O, 10% alcohol): 120 ml/$4.25
   Pabanol (5% PABA in 70% alcohol): 120 ml/$4.75
   PreSun #8 (5% PABA in 55% alcohol): 120 ml/$4.25
   PreSun #8 cream (5% PABA, 15% alcohol): 120 ml/$5.00

B. **Benzophenone compounds** absorb UVL well from 250–365 nm and somewhat from 365–400 nm. They are less effective than PABA compounds in the UVB sunburn spectrum.

   1. **Structure**

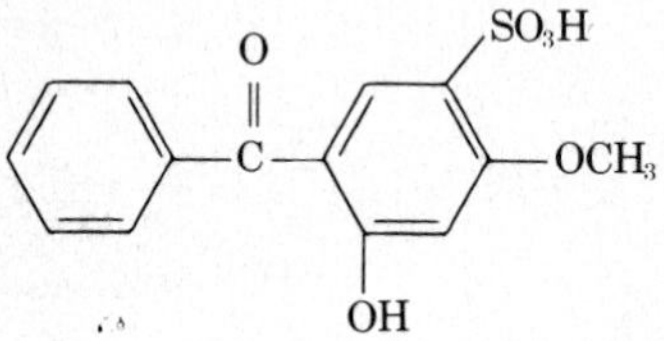

   Sulisobenzone

   2. **Packaging and cost:**
      Solbar (3% oxybenzone and 3% dioxybenzone): 75 gm/$6.50
      Uval (6% oxybenzone, 5% 2-ethylhexyl p-methoxycinna-mate): 75 gm/$5.50

C. **Multiple ingredient sunscreens:**

   1. **Packaging and cost:**
      PreSun #15 (5% PABA, 5% padimate-O, 3% oxybenzone, 50% alcohol): 120 ml/$4.75
      PreSun #15 Lip Protector (8% padimate-O, 3% benzophenone-3): 3.75 gm/$1.50
      Supershade 15 (7% PABA esters, 3% oxybenzone): 120 ml/$7.50

D. **Others**

   1. **RVP (red veterinary petrolatum)** has UVL-absorbing qualities to 340 nm and is also a water-protective agent because of its greasy base. It is available as a sunshade with zinc oxide added (RVPaque) and for lip protection with 5% PABA.

      Packaging and cost:
      RVP (95% RVP): 60 gm/$4.75
      RVPaba lipstick (20% RVP, 5% PABA): 3.75 gm/$2.00

   2. **Sunshades** physically block light and usually contain titanium dioxide or zinc oxide powders. They are not very effective unless a thick coat is applied.

      a. **Packaging and cost:**
         A-Fil (5% menthyl anthranilate, 5% titanium dioxide, in two shades): 45 gm/$3.25
         RVPaque (20% zinc oxide, 3% RVP, 1.5% cinoxinate): 15 gm/$4.25
         RVPlus (10% titanium-mica platelets, 30% RVP): 60 gm/$5.75
         Solar cream (4% PABA, 5% titanium dioxide): 30 gm/$5.50

Wet dressings, baths, astringents

I. Wet dressings

A. The effects of wet dressings have been previously discussed (see p. 228).

1. Open wet dressings are indicated in acute inflammatory states with exudation, oozing, and crusting. They are applied as follows:

a. The patient should be in a comfortable position, usually in bed, with an impermeable material under the area to be compressed to prevent wetting the mattress.

b. The dressings, which need not be sterile, should consist of 2- –4-inch-wide Kerlix, soft gauze (not 4 × 4), or soft linen such as old sheeting or pillowcases, handkerchiefs, or shirts.

c. Moisten dressings by immersing them in the solution and then gently wringing them out. They should be sopping wet, but not dripping. Solutions should be warm or tepid. Cover with a soft towel or cloth that will allow evaporation.

d. Apply or wrap around the skin loosely. Multiple layers, at least 6–8, should be applied to prevent rapid drying and cooling.

e. Dressings should be removed, remoistened, and reapplied every 10–15 min, for between 30 min and 2 hr 3id. It is difficult to completely moisten dressings in place, and resoaking is often needed to remove accumulated and adherent exudate and crusts. If frequent changes are impracticable, an IV bottle with the wet dressing solution may be suspended over the bed and the material slowly fed into the dressing through IV tubing. Alternatively, the dressing should simply be removed every 2–3 hr and reapplied. It is usually difficult for patients to care for their own dressings.

f. After dressings are removed, a lotion, powder, liniment, or paste may be applied to the skin. Occlusion of exudative skin with ointments should be avoided.

g. Dressing material should be discarded daily, but some, such as Kerlix, may be laundered and reused.

h. If large areas of skin are compressed at once, chilling and hypothermia may result. In general, no more than one-third of the body should be treated at any time.

2. Closed wet dressings will cause maceration and retain heat and are used in the treatment of conditions such as cellulitis and abscesses. The foregoing instructions should be followed, but warm dressings should be covered with plastic, oilcloth, or other impermeable material.

B. Solutions for wet dressings are either astringents or antiseptic agents. Astringents precipitate protein and thereby decrease oozing. The principal astringents are salts of aluminum, zinc, lead, iron, bismuth, tannins, or other polyphenolic compounds.

1. Aluminum acetate (Al [OCOCH$_3$]$_3$, Burow's solution), containing approximately 5% aluminum acetate, is diluted 1:10 to 1:40 for use.

Probably the most widely used astringent for wet dressings, it is easy to use, does not stain, and is drying and soothing (see p. 253). **Aluminum chloride hexahydrate,** potentially a better antibacterial and astringent, may be preferable for compresses.

Domeboro or Bluboro powder packets or tablets quickly dissolve in water to make fresh aluminum diacetate available. One packet or tablet in 1 pint of water yields a 1:40 dilution (two packets at 1:20 dilution); 30 min evaporation, however, will concentrate a 1:40 solution to 1:10, at which point the aluminum salts may become too irritating and drying. One package of **AluWets** dissolved in 12 oz (1½ cups) of water produces a 2% aluminum chloride hexahydrate solution for wet dressings.

a. **Packaging and cost:**
   Domeboro (aluminum sulfate and calcium acetate):
      12 packets/$4.00
      12 tablets/$4.00
   Bluboro (aluminum sulfate, calcium acetate,
      FD&C blue dye):
      1.9 gm packets/$4.00
   AluWets (aluminum chloride hexahydrate):
      6 packets/$3.25

2. **Potassium permanganate (KM_nO_4)** is an oxidizing agent that is rapidly rendered inactive in the presence of organic material. The oxidizing action of the chemical is purportedly responsible for its germicidal activity. It is also an astringent and a fungicide. This preparation stains the skin and clothing, and undissolved crystals will cause a chemical burn. It is used less commonly now than formerly (primarily as an antifungal agent) and may be little better than water as a wet dressing. A 1:4000 to 1:16,000 dilution is used on weeping or denuded surfaces (one crushed 65-mg tablet to 250 ml → 1000 ml; one 330-mg tablet to 1500 ml → 5.0 liter). For use as a medicated bath, 8 gm (about 2 tsp) should be dissolved in 200 liter (a full bathtub) of water to produce about a 1:25,000 dilution. Skin stains may be removed with a weak solution of oxalic acid or sodium thiosulfate.

3. **Normal saline (0.9% sodium chloride)** may be approximated by adding 1 level tsp of salt to 480 ml water.

4. **Copper and zinc sulfates and camphor solution (Dalibour solution, Dalidome)** is an effective, nonstaining, blue astringent.

5. **Boric acid** is not of any use as a topical agent; it is toxic when absorbed and has caused poisoning in children through percutaneous absorption.

6. **Silver nitrate, 0.1–0.5%,** is an excellent germicide and astringent. Its germicidal action is due to precipitation of bacterial protein by liberated silver ions. It may cause pain if applied in concentrations greater than 0.5%. A 0.25% solution may be prepared by adding 1 tsp of the stock 50% aqueous solution to 1000 ml of cool water. Silver nitrate stains skin dark brown after exposure to air and will stain black any metal container (including the teaspoon) and everything else that it touches.

7. **Compresses with 5% acetic acid** reduce the microbial count in infected wounds and are used primarily for infections involving *Pseudomonas aeruginosa*.

II. Baths

A. **Baths and soaks** are useful in treating widespread eruptions. Evaporation is impeded, and thus there is less drying and cooling. Nevertheless, baths and soaks may be very soothing, antipruritic, and somewhat anti-inflammatory. The tub should be half full (about 100 liter, or 25 gallons of water) and the duration of exposure limited to 30 min. Many of the bath oils make the tub very slippery.

1. **Soothing and antipruritic colloid additives**

   a. **Oatmeal** contains 50% starch with about 25% protein and 9% oil. Mix 1 cup Aveeno oatmeal and 2 cups of cold tap water, shake, and pour into tub of lukewarm water. Oilated Aveeno contains an additional 35% mineral oil and lanolin derivative for emollient action.

   Packaging and cost:
   Aveeno, 454 gm/$5.50
   Oilated Aveeno, 240 gm/$5.00

   b. **Starch baths** are best prepared by mixing 2 cups of a hydrolyzed starch, such as Linit, with 4 cups of cold tap water to form a paste, then adding this to a tub of lukewarm water. A mixture of equal parts of sodium bicarbonate (baking soda) and starch is often used as a soothing colloidal bath powder.

2. **Bath oils** are added to tub water to help prevent drying of the skin. Most contain a mineral or a vegetable oil and also a surfactant. Theoretically, the patient absorbs a portion of the oil around him. There are two types of bath oils: those that are dispersed throughout the bath, and those that lie on the surface of the water and coat the surface of the body as the patient leaves the tub. If nothing else, bath oils are pleasant, but patients occasionally note mild pruritus immediately after their use. All of the following are pleasing preparations; some patients will prefer one to another: Alpha Keri, Ar-Ex, Domol, Lubrex, Surfol. Some such as Alpha Keri may be applied after bathing by aerosol (spray).

References

WET DRESSINGS, BATHS, ASTRINGENTS

Hedberg, M., and Miller, J. K. Effectiveness of acetic acid, betadine, amphyll, polymyxin B, colistin and gentamicin against *Pseudomonas aeruginosa*. *Appl. Microbiol.* 18:854–855, 1969.

Quinones, C. A., and Winkelmann, R. K. Changes in skin temperature with wet dressing therapy. *Arch. Dermatol.* 96:708–711, 1967.

Wilkinson, D. S. Dermatological dressings. *Practitioner* 202:27–36, 1969.

General references

American Hospital Formulary Service. Washington: American Society of Hospital Pharmacists, 1981.

American Medical Association. *AMA Drug Evaluations* (4th ed.). Chicago: American Medical Association, 1980.

Drug Topics Red Book. Oradell, N. J.: Medical Economics, 1981.

Frazier, C. N., and Blank, I. H. *A Formulary for External Therapy of the Skin*. Springfield, Ill.: Thomas, 1954.

Gilman, A. G., Goodman, L. S., and Gilman, A. (eds.). *The Pharmacological Basis of Therapeutics* (6th ed.). New York: Macmillan, 1980.

Handbook of Nonprescription Drugs (6th ed.). Washington, D.C.: American Pharmaceutical Association, 1979.

Lerner, M. R., and Lerner, A. B. *Dermatologic Medications* (2nd ed.). Chicago: Year Book, 1960.

Lewis, A. J. (ed.). *Modern Drug Encyclopedia and Therapeutic Index: A Compendium* (15th ed.). New York: Yorke Medical Group, 1979.

Maddin, S. W. (ed.). *Current Dermatologic Therapy* (3rd ed.). Philadelphia: Saunders, 1982.

The United States Pharmacopoeia (20th ed.). Easton, Pa.: Mack, 1980.

Index

Index

Table 5. Amount of topical medication needed for single or multiple application(s)

Area Treated	One application (gm)	2id for 1 week (gm)	3id for 2 weeks (gm)	2id for 1 month (gm)	3id for 6 weeks (gm)
Hands, head, face, anogenital area	2	28	90 (3 oz)	120 (4 oz)	270 (9 oz)
One arm, anterior or posterior trunk	3	42	120 (4 oz)	180 (6 oz)	360 (12 oz)
One leg	4	56	180 (6 oz)	240 (8 oz)	540 (18 oz)
Entire body	30–60	420–840 (14–28 oz)	1.26–2.52 kg (42–84 oz; 2.5–5 lb)	1.8–3.6 kg (60–120 oz; 3.75–7.5 lb)	3.8–7.5 kg (126–252 oz; 7.5–15 lb)

Table 6. Metric measures with approximate equivalents

Liquid measure

4000.0 ml = 1 gallon (4 qt)
1000.0 ml
  (1 liter) = 1 quart (32 oz)
500.0 ml = 1 pint (16 oz)
250.0 ml = 8 fluid ounces
30.0 ml = 1 fluid ounce
15.0 ml = 1 tablespoon
5.0 ml = 1 teaspoon
4.0 ml = 1 dram
0.06 ml = 1 minim, the rough equivalent of 1 drop

Weight

1 kg = 2.20 pound (Av.)
.454 kg = 1 pound
454 gm = 16 oz (pound, Av.)
30 gm = 1 oz
4 gm = 60 grains (gr) (1 dram)
1 gm = 15 gr
60 mg = 1 gr

Length (exact equivalents)

1 meter = 39.37 in.
30.48 cm = 1 ft
2.54 cm = 1 in.
1 cm = 0.39 in.
1 mm = 0.04 in.

Note: A. 1 milliliter (ml) ≃ 1 cubic centimeter (cc); B. Most of these approximate dose equivalents have been approved by the Food and Drug Administration. They may be used as a convenience in prescribing, but must not be used for compounding specific pharmaceutical formulas.

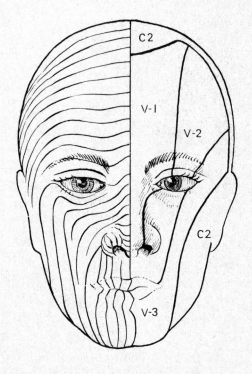

Left side: relaxed skin tension lines. Right side: dermatone chart—sensory root fields.

Note: The illustrations on the inside covers and facing back cover, dermatome charts and relaxed skin tension lines, represent approximations, since there is much overlap and individual variation. Denervation of one posterior root will *not* produce complete anesthesia within the corresponding dermatome. The direction of the relaxed skin tension lines (RSTL) should always be assessed before making an ellipsoidal incision parallel to, or a punch biopsy with skin stretched perpendicular to, these lines (see Fig. 1, p. 202). In areas of flexion creases, flex and note the direction of the majority of "wrinkle" lines, that is, the direction of the RSTL. In nonflexion areas, the RSTL is determined by picking up skin folds between thumb and index finger and pinching, proceeding in a clockwise direction, until it is clear in which direction wrinkle lines are most numerous, straight, and parallel to one another. In certain areas it is difficult or impossible to find the RSTL. In that situation, make a small circular incision or "punch" to see in which direction the ellipse forms.